Atlas of **Nuclear Cardiology**

Imaging Companion to Braunwald's Heart Disease

Atlas of Nuclear Cardiology

Imaging Companion to Braunwald's Heart Disease

Ami E. Iskandrian, MD, MACC, FASNC, FAHA

Distinguished Professor of Medicine and Radiology
Section Chief, Non-Invasive Cardiac Imaging
and Nuclear Cardiology
University of Alabama at Birmingham
Birmingham, Alabama

Ernest V. Garcia, PhD, FASNC, FAHA

Endowed Professor in Cardiac Imaging
Director, Nuclear Cardiology R&D Laboratory
Department of Radiology and Imaging Sciences
Emory University Hospital
Atlanta, Georgia

ELSEVIER
SAUNDERS

ELSEVIER
SAUNDERS

1600 John F. Kennedy Blvd.
Ste. 1800
Philadelphia, Pennsylvania 19103-2899

ATLAS OF NUCLEAR CARDIOLOGY:
IMAGING COMPANION TO BRAUNWALD'S
HEART DISEASE   978-1-4160-6134-2

Notices
Knowledge and best practice in this field are constantly changing. As new research and experience broaden our understanding, changes in research methods, professional practices, or medical treatment may become necessary.

Practitioners and researchers must always rely on their own experience and knowledge in evaluating and using any information, methods, compounds, or experiments described herein. In using such information or methods they should be mindful of their own safety and the safety of others, including parties for whom they have a professional responsibility.

With respect to any drug or pharmaceutical products identified, readers are advised to check the most current information provided (i) on procedures featured or (ii) by the manufacturer of each product to be administered, to verify the recommended dose or formula, the method and duration of administration, and contraindications. It is the responsibility of practitioners, relying on their own experience and knowledge of their patients, to make diagnoses, to determine dosages and the best treatment for each individual patient, and to take all appropriate safety precautions.

To the fullest extent of the law, neither the Publisher nor the authors, contributors, or editors, assume any liability for any injury and/or damage to persons or property as a matter of products liability, negligence or otherwise, or from any use or operation of any methods, products, instructions, or ideas contained in the material herein.

Library of Congress Cataloging-in-Publication Data
Atlas of nuclear cardiology : an imaging companion to Braunwald's heart disease / [edited by] Ami E. Iskandrian, Ernest V. Garcia. – 1st ed.
    p. ; cm.
    Nuclear cardiology
    Companion to: Braunwald's heart disease / edited by Robert O. Bonow ... [et al.]. 9th ed. c2012.
    Includes bibliographical references and index.
    ISBN 978-1-4160-6134-2 (hardcover : alk. paper)
1. Cardiovascular system–Radionuclide imaging–Atlases. I. Iskandrian, Ami E., 1941-
II. Garcia, Ernest V. III. Braunwald's heart disease. IV. Title: Nuclear cardiology.
    [DNLM: 1. Heart–radionuclide imaging–Atlases. 2. Heart Diseases–radionuclide imaging–Atlases. WG 17]
    RC670.5.R32A87 2012
    616.1'2–dc23
                                                                    2011027382

Acquisitions Editor: Natasha Andjelkovic
Developmental Editor: Bradley McIlwain
Publishing Services Manager: Patricia Tannian
Project Managers: Joanna Dhanabalan/Prathibha Mehta
Senior Project Manager: Sarah Wunderly
Design Direction: Steven Stave

Printed in China

Last digit is the print number: 9 8 7 6 5 4 3 2 1

To our wives

Greta P. Iskandrian, MD

and

Terri Spiegel

To our children

Basil, Susan, and Kristen Iskandrian

Meredith and Evan Garcia

and

To their spouses and children

Contributors

Wael AlJaroudi, MD, MS, FACC
Assistant Professor of Cardiovascular Medicine
Associate Staff, Cardiovascular Medicine
Section of Cardiac Imaging
Heart and Vascular Institute
Cleveland Clinic
Cleveland, Ohio

Ji Chen, PhD
Associate Professor of Radiology
Department of Radiology and Imaging Sciences
Emory University
Atlanta, Georgia

E. Gordon DePuey, MD
Professor of Radiology
Columbia University College of Physicians and Surgeons
Director of Nuclear Medicine
St. Luke's-Roosevelt Hospital
New York, New York

Eva V. Dubovsky, MD, PhD
Professor of Radiology
Division of Nuclear Medicine
University of Alabama at Birmingham
Birmingham, Alabama

Fabio P. Esteves, MD
Associate Professor, Radiology
Clinical Director, Nuclear Cardiology
Emory University
Atlanta, Georgia

Tracy L. Faber, PhD
Professor of Radiology
Emory University
Atlanta, Georgia

Ernest V. Garcia, PhD, FASNC, FAHA
Endowed Professor in Cardiac Imaging
Director, Nuclear Cardiology R&D Laboratory
Department of Radiology and Imaging Sciences
Emory University Hospital
Atlanta, Georgia

Fadi G. Hage, MD, FACC
Assistant Professor of Medicine
Division of Cardiovascular Diseases
University of Alabama at Birmingham
Cardiac Care Unit Director
Birmingham VA Medical Center
Birmingham, Alabama

Jaekyeong Heo, MD, FACC
Professor of Medicine
Division of Cardiovascular Diseases
Associate Director, Nuclear Cardiology
University of Alabama at Birmingham
Birmingham, Alabama

Fahad M. Iqbal, MD
Research Fellow
Nuclear Cardiology
University of Alabama at Birmingham
Birmingham, Alabama

Ami E. Iskandrian, MD, MACC, FASNC, FAHA
Distinguished Professor of Medicine and Radiology
Section Chief, Non-Invasive Cardiac Imaging
and Nuclear Cardiology
University of Alabama at Birmingham
Birmingham, Alabama

Rafael W. Lopes, MD
Section Director, Nuclear Cardiology
Hospital do Coração
HCOR
São Paulo, Brazil

Javier L. Pou Ucha, MD
Nuclear Cardiology Research Fellow
Nuclear Medicine Trainee
University Hospital Complex of Vigo
Vigo, PO, Spain

Paolo Raggi, MD, FACP, FASNC, FACC
Professor of Medicine and Radiology
Director, Emory Cardiac Imaging Center
Emory University
Atlanta, Georgia

Cesar A. Santana, MD, PhD
Director of Research and Clinical Applications
Supervising and Interpreting Physician
Doral Imaging Institute
Doral, Florida

E. Lindsey Tauxe, CNMT, FASNC
Director, Cardiology Informatics
Division of Cardiovascular Diseases
Associate Director, Nuclear Cardiology
University of Alabama at Birmingham
Birmingham, Alabama

Gilbert J. Zoghbi, MD, FACC, FSCAI
Assistant Professor of Medicine
Division of Cardiovascular Diseases
Director, Interventional Cardiology Fellowship Program
Director, Cardiac Catheterization Laboratory
Birmingham VA Medical Center
Birmingham, Alabama

Foreword

The rapid advances in cardiology during the first half of the twentieth century may be fairly ascribed to the introduction of new techniques.

Paul Wood, 1951
Diseases of the Heart and Circulation

These prophetic words of Dr. Paul Wood, the preeminent London cardiologist of the 1950s, have an even more meaningful relevance in the first half of the twenty-first century. Dr. Wood died prematurely from coronary artery disease at the age of 55, 11 years after publishing his textbook *Diseases of the Heart and Circulation*, and thus was not witness to the explosive growth of medical technology over the second 50 years of the last century. In that same period of time, coronary heart disease deaths have been cut in half.

It is unclear what role imaging has played in these improved outcomes. But it is clear that over the past 40 years, nuclear cardiology has matured, joined the mainstream of cardiology practice, and contributed, directly or indirectly, to many of the advances in care that have resulted in improved outcomes for large numbers of patients worldwide.

The editorial team of *Braunwald's Heart Disease* is delighted to present this third in a series of four imaging companions, each dedicated to one of the key cardiac imaging modalities. This companion atlas on cardiovascular nuclear medicine, expertly edited by Drs. Ami Iskandrian and Ernest Garcia, covers all of the critical technical and clinical aspects of this important field and provides a unique case-based perspective into the tremendous potential of nuclear cardiology to enhance patient diagnosis and management.

Drs. Iskandrian and Garcia and their colleagues provide succinct and practical chapters that cover image interpretation and reporting and the recognition of artifacts. They address the breadth of applications of myocardial perfusion imaging for detection and risk stratification of coronary artery disease and the integration of perfusion imaging in the management of patients who present with the acute and chronic manifestations of this disease, including imaging in patients after myocardial revascularization. The chapters on heart failure (including examples of novel imaging agents), cardiomyopathies, and structural heart disease are skillfully crafted. In light of current concerns regarding radiation exposure, the chapter on improving efficiency and reducing radiation dosage is particularly pertinent. Hybrid technologies that address both anatomic and functional imaging, discussed in the chapters on SPECT/CT and PET/CT, are also a topic of great current interest.

Diagnostic imaging in the United States has increased more rapidly than any other component of medical care in recent years, and the appropriate use of nuclear cardiology in particular is under intense scrutiny. Our challenges going forward are to attend to the issues of patient selection, clinical training, resource utilization, and cost effectiveness. The *Atlas of Nuclear Cardiology* places all of these concerns in sharp focus

We believe that this companion will be a highly valuable resource for clinicians, imaging subspecialists, and cardiovascular trainees, and that it will contribute in a significant manner to the care of the patients they serve.

Robert O. Bonow, MD
Douglas L. Mann, MD
Douglas P. Zipes, MD
Peter Libby, MD
Eugene Braunwald, MD

Preface

Nuclear cardiology remains the most widely used imaging modality in the care of patients with known or suspected cardiac diseases.

We accepted the challenge to produce an atlas of nuclear cardiology as a companion to one of the best known and widely used cardiology textbooks: *Braunwald's Heart Disease: A Textbook of Cardiovascular Medicine*. This opportunity came on the heels of our completing the fourth edition of our textbook of nuclear cardiology. The challenges were many—to produce a high-quality, factual product in a relatively short period of time that was in keeping with the high standards of the Braunwald text, to avoid duplication with our book, to use high-quality representative clinical cases that would make the book a practical and useful resource for both the novice and the expert, and to keep it contemporary.

We are very grateful to our contributors, all of whom were chosen for their expertise in nuclear cardiology, because as authors ourselves, we realize how much time and effort it takes to produce a high-quality product.

This book validates the concept that *the whole is greater than the sum of its parts*. Although each chapter can be considered an excellent reference source for a specific topic, we encourage you to read it cover to cover. We hope that you will get as much pleasure from reading it as we have in bringing it to you. As in any book with so many chapters, some degree of repetition and controversy exist. We have purposely allowed that to give the reader different perspectives and different viewpoints.

This book would not have been possible without the help of the many dedicated people who helped to generate the images and assure quality, precision, and consistency. At the University of Alabama at Birmingham, we acknowledge the contributions of Mary Beth Schaaf, RN, the secretarial help of Christalyn Cooper, and the technical support of Lindsey Tauxe.

At Emory, we thank Leah Verdes, MD, our research coordinator, and Russell Folks, CNMT, technical director of the lab, for their contributions. We also would like to thank Timothy M. Bateman, MD, Co-Director of Cardiovascular Radiologic Imaging at the Mid America Heart Institute and Professor of Medicine at the University of Missouri—Kansas City School of Medicine, for contributing Case 13-5.

We are grateful for the help of the publisher, Elsevier, and particularly want to thank Marla Sussman, Senior Developmental Editor, for her impeccable skills and attention to detail, and Sarah Wunderly, for her help during the production stage of the book.

Last but not least, we are grateful to the editors of *Braunwald's Heart Disease: A Textbook of Cardiovascular Medicine*, for entrusting us to write this companion atlas. We hope we have met the expectations of the editors and readers.

Ami E. Iskandrian
Ernest V. Garcia

Abbreviations

2D = Two-dimensional

2DE = Two-dimensional echocardiogram, echocardiography

3D = Three-dimensional

AC = Attenuation correction/Attenuation-corrected

ACS = Acute coronary syndromes

AR = Aortic regurgitation

ASA = Alcohol septal ablation

AV = Atrioventricular

B/W = Black and white

BMI = Body mass index

BMIPP = β-Methyl-p-[^{123}I]iodophenyl–pentadecanoic acid

BP = Blood pressure

CABG = coronary artery bypass graft/grafting

CAD = Coronary artery disease

CI = Cardiac index

CKD = Chronic kidney disease

CM = Cardiomyopathy

CO = Cardiac output

CRT = Cardiac resynchronization therapy

CSI = Cesium iodide

CT = Computed tomography

CZT = Cadmium-zinc-telluride

DCM = Dilated cardiomyopathy

DM = Diabetes mellitus

DSP = Deconvolution of septal penetration

EBCT = electron beam computed tomography

ECF = Extra cardiac findings

ECG = Electrocardiogram, electrocardiography

ED = Emergency department

EDV = End-diastolic volume

EF = Ejection fraction

eGFR = Estimated glomerular filtration rate

ESRD = End-stage renal disease

ESV = End-systolic volume

FBP = Filtered backprojection

FDG = fluorodeoxyglucose

FFR = Fractional flow reserve

Gd = Gadolinium

GERD = Gastroesophageal reflux disease

HCM = Hypertrophic cardiomyopathy

HF = Heart failure

HLA = Horizontal long axis

H/M = Heart-to-mediastinum ratio

HR = Heart rate

HTN = Hypertension

I-123 = Iodine-123

ICD = Implantable cardioverter defibrillator

ICM = Ischemic cardiomyopathy

IHD = Ischemic heart disease

IMA = Internal mammary artery

IV = Intravenously

keV = Kilo electron volts

LAD = Left anterior descending coronary artery

LAO = Left anterior oblique

LBBB = Left bundle branch block

LCX = Left circumflex coronary artery

L/H ratio = Lung-to-heart ratio

LIMA = Left internal mammary artery

LM = Left main coronary artery

LPO = Left posterior oblique

LV = Left ventricular/ ventricle

LVEF = Left ventricular ejection fraction

LVH = Left ventricular hypertrophy

MBF = Myocardial blood flow

mCi = millicurie

METs = Metabolic equivalents

MI = Myocardial infarction

mIBG = Metaiodobenzylguanidine

MPI = Myocardial perfusion imaging

MUGA = Multiple gated acquisition

Non-AC = Non–attenuation-corrected

NSTEMI = Non–ST-elevation MI

NYHA = New York Heart Association

OM = Obtuse marginal branch

OSEM = Ordered subset expectation maximization

PCI = Percutaneous coronary intervention

PDA = Posterior descending coronary artery
PET = Positron emission tomography
PMT = Photomultiplier tube(s)
PTCA = Percutaneous transluminal coronary angioplasty
PVCs = Premature ventricular contractions
RAO = Right anterior oblique
RCA = Right coronary artery
RNA = Radionuclide angiography
ROI = Region of interest
RRNR = Resolution recovery-noise reduction
RV = Right ventricular/right ventricle
SA = Short axis
SCD = Sudden cardiac death
SD = Standard deviation
SDS = Summed Difference Score
SPECT = Single-photon emission computed tomography

SRS = Summed Rest Score
SSS = Summed Stress Score
STEMI = ST-elevation MI
SV = Stroke volume
SVG = Saphenous vein graft
TAC = Time-activity curve
Tc-99m = Technetium-99m
TET = Treadmill exercise testing
TID = Transient ischemic dilatation
TIMI = Thrombolysis In Myocardial Infarction
Tl-201 = Thallium-201
UA = Unstable angina
VLA = Vertical long-axis
VOI = Volume of interest
WMAs = Wall motion/thickening abnormalities
WPW = Wolff-Parkinson-White

Contents

Chapter 1

Evaluating Myocardial Perfusion SPECT: The Normal Study

Ernest V. Garcia, Fabio P. Esteves, Javier L. Pou Ucha, and Rafael W. Lopes

KEY POINTS

- The first fundamental assumption of myocardial perfusion SPECT imaging is that the radiotracer is distributed in the myocardium directly proportional to the blood flow at the time of injection.

- The second fundamental assumption of myocardial perfusion SPECT imaging is that the count value in each myocardial pixel (voxel) is directly proportional to the radiotracer concentration in the myocardium that corresponds to that pixel.

- The relative differences in count values between myocardial pixels are represented in the images as a change in either brightness (in black-and-white images) or color (in color images). This is done through the use of a translation formula (translation table) that converts the number of counts to brightness or color in the image. The usual representation is the higher the number of counts the brighter the pixel.

- Following the logic in the preceding key points, the brighter the pixel, the higher the radiotracer concentration, and the higher the regional blood flow. SPECT imaging of normal subjects should then generate a uniform (homogeneous) brightness or color in the myocardial pixels.

- It would also be reasonable to assume that if the brightness of a myocardial segment is half the brightness of another segment, the first segment receives half the blood flow of the second segment.

- Some fundamental assumptions apply to the assessment of LV regional and global function from the ECG-gated tomographic slices that represent different time intervals in the cardiac cycle. The most fundamental assumption is that our eyes and the computer techniques can detect and track the LV borders throughout the cardiac cycle as a change in intensity (or color).

- In practice, our ability to detect and track the endocardial and epicardial borders throughout the cardiac cycle is limited by radiation scatter and by the spatial and contrast resolutions inherent in the imaging systems. Because of this limitation we rely on the partial volume effect concept to detect changes in myocardial thickness (i.e., changes in myocardial thickness are directly proportional to changes in brightness [or color]). The various software tools used to measure LVEF, wall motion, and wall thickening apply this concept to varying degrees.

- In practice, wall motion is assessed by tracking the apparent endocardial borders from the black-and-white images, whereas wall thickening is assessed by changes in color using color images. The normal LVEF by visual or quantitative analysis is ≥50% with some variation between software packages and specific protocols.

- Although these key points form the fundamental assumptions as to how a normal myocardial perfusion SPECT study will appear to the observer (and how it should be interpreted), these are theories that can vary significantly in everyday clinical practice because of differences in radiotracer, imaging equipment, imaging protocols, reconstruction algorithm and filters, the patient's body habitus and gender, stressors, artifacts from patient motion, display monitor, the physician's vision, and many other issues.

- Many of these variations or "exceptions" are illustrated in this book, particularly in this chapter, the chapter on image interpretation, and the chapter on image artifacts. The ability to recognize the normal variants and artifacts is what separates the expert interpreter from the novice.

BACKGROUND

Recognition of the normal patterns of myocardial count distribution, wall motion, and wall thickening are imperative to properly interpret ECG-gated myocardial perfusion SPECT studies. The normal perfusion patterns vary depending on the specific protocols used such as differences in radiopharmaceuticals, imaging equipment, count density, reconstruction algorithm and filters, stressors, artifacts such as patient motion, patient's size and gender, display monitor, and others.

Similarly, when quantitative software tools are used to assist with the interpretation, the reader should be aware of the quantitative criteria used to call a specific parameter abnormal. The more aware the reader is of the scientific principles used to generate the images and the expected normal variations, the more likely it is that the correct diagnosis will be reached. In this chapter, we will emphasize what normal myocardial perfusion SPECT studies look like.

Case 1-1   **Normal Tc-99m Perfusion Study (Nonobese Man) (Figure 1-1)**

An 84-year-old, 163-pound, 6-foot 1-inch man with hypertension, aortic insufficiency, and heart failure presented with 2-week history of atypical chest pain. Tc-99m tetrofosmin perfusion SPECT was performed using a 1-day rest/stress (12 mCi/39 mCi) protocol. The patient underwent a standard modified Bruce treadmill protocol. The resting ECG was normal. The patient exercised for 4 minutes 28 seconds, reached 88% of maximum predicted heart rate, and stopped because of fatigue. There were no ECG changes during exercise. SPECT images were acquired using a 90-degree–angled dual-head camera and a 180-degree imaging arc from the 45-degree RAO projection to the 45-degree LPO projection. Rest and poststress ECG gating were performed using eight frames per cardiac cycle.

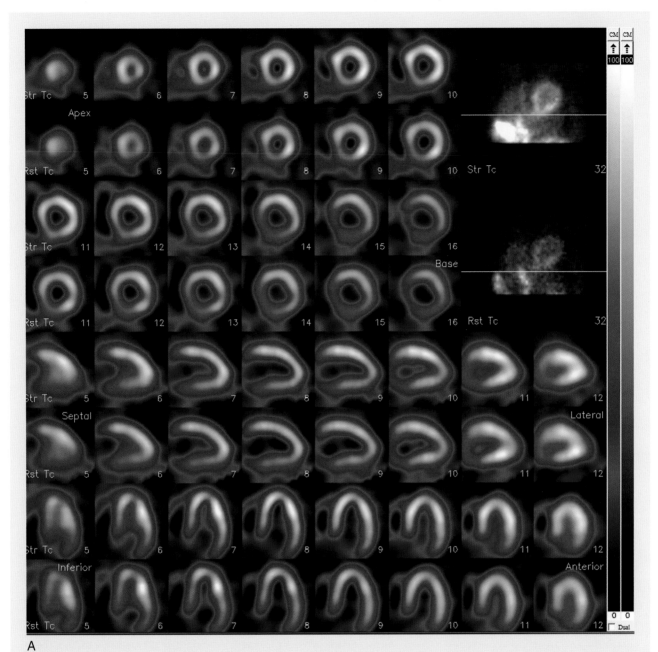

A

■ **Figure 1-1** Normal Tc-99m perfusion study (nonobese male). **A,** *Top right,* black-and-white panels are the stress and rest planar projection images demonstrating excellent image quality. Color images are the corresponding tomographic slices display with the resting results interleaved between the stress slices. Top four rows display the LV SA from apex *(top left)* to base *(bottom right).* Next two rows display the stress and rest VLA slices from the septum to the lateral wall and the last two rows show the stress and rest HLA slices from the inferior to the anterior wall. Note the high image quality and fairly homogeneous tracer uptake throughout the LV.

(Continued)

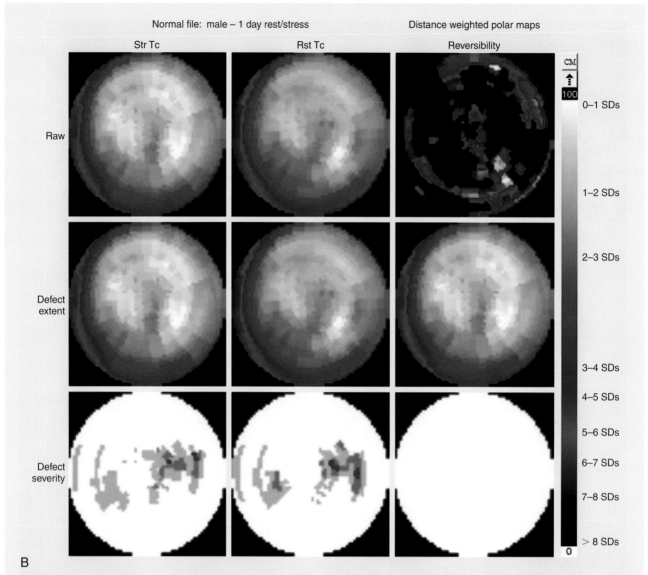

B

■ **Figure 1-1—Cont'd B,** Polar maps representation and quantification of this patient's LV tracer uptake. The three panels in the top row correspond to the stress, rest and reversibility (normalized rest-stress) LV distributions. The brighter colors represent higher counts (perfusion) and the darker colors, fewer counts as depicted by the translation table on the rightmost column. Note the relative homogeneity of the stress and rest polar maps. The middle row is the defect extent polar maps display where areas that are abnormal in comparison to the normal database are highlighted in black. Note the absence of blackout regions, indicating a normal study by quantitative analysis. The bottom row is the defect severity polar maps display where each pixel (voxel) is color coded to the number of standard deviations below the mean normal distribution with the scale shown by the translation table.

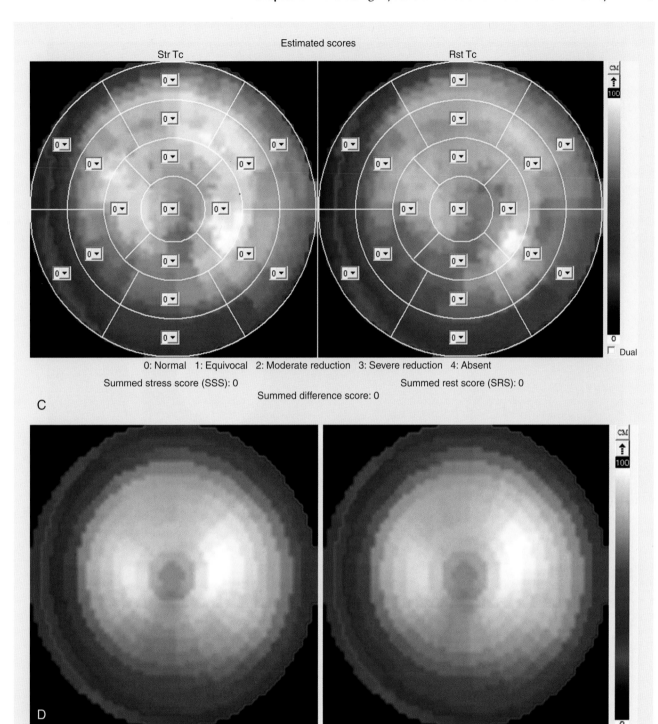

■ **Figure 1-1—Cont'd C,** Stress and rest LV myocardial perfusion polar maps with superimposed 17-segment coordinate system using the 0-to-4 score for each segment (0 = normal, 1 = mildly reduced, 2 = moderately reduced, 3 = severely reduced, 4 = absent uptake). Note that for this patient the sum of all 17 segment scores at stress *(SSS)* and at rest *(SRS)* is zero. The lower the segmental scoring the more likely the perfusion study is normal. Non-AC images are usually considered abnormal if the summed score is >4. **D,** Mean normal LV stress and rest Tc-99m myocardial perfusion distribution in males generated from a population of 30 male patients with <5% probability of CAD. Note the relatively homogeneous perfusion distribution but the somewhat reduced uptake in the inferior wall as compared to the distal septum and lateral walls. Although less discernable there is also a count reduction in the anterior wall at the 11 o'clock position seen typically when using 180-degree acquisition. The cause of this normal variant is the change in resolution of depth during a 180-degree acquisition orbit and is not seen with 360-degree acquisition.

(Continued)

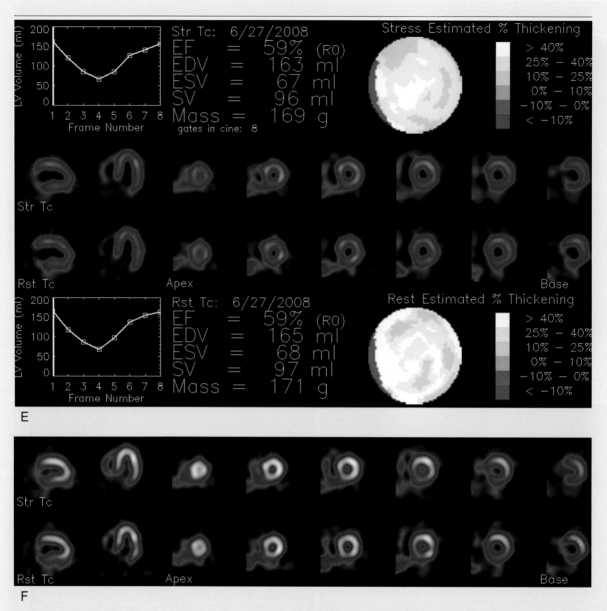

■ **Figure 1-1—Cont'd** The four rows of color images show end-dyastolic (**E**) and end-systolic (**F**) poststress *(top row)* and rest *(bottom row)*, VLA, HLA, and SA LV tomographic display of this patient's ECG-gated images. Note the normal uniform regional inward motion of the endocardial and epicardial borders from end-diastole to end-systole. Also note the normal uniform change in myocardial color from diastole to systole due to normal LV thickening. The color polar maps represent the quantification of the poststress *(top)* and rest *(bottom)* regional thickening. Note the labeled thickening scale to the right of the maps. The poststress *(top left)* and rest *(bottom left)* panels show the patient's averaged LV volume curves per cardiac cycle, LVEF, EDV, ESV, SV and LV mass. Note that both the rest and poststress LVEFs are 59%, above the 50% normal threshold for this quantitative program. These panels are accompanied by dynamic displays (Video 1-1).

COMMENTS

This is an example of a male patient with a normal perfusion study of excellent image quality. Note that the stress planar projections are of higher quality than the rest planar projections. The higher radiotracer dose injected at stress generates more counts per pixel. Despite the difference in stress and rest count density, the tomographic stress and rest images are both of high quality due to appropriate reconstruction and filtering. They exhibit high spatial and contrast resolution as depicted by the well-defined endocardial and

epicardial myocardial borders and a well-defined LV chamber. RV activity is seen in the SA and HLA slices. Note the fairly uniform count distribution throughout the LV myocardium. A mild count reduction in the inferior wall (particularly in the basal inferior segment) is consistent with diaphragmatic attenuation. The gated images show normal segmental and global LV wall motion and normal LV ejection fraction. The EDV and ESV are mildly increased, which further enhances the LV myocardium/ LV cavity contrast. For this quantitative program, EDV <171 mL and ESV <70 mL are within normal limits.

Case 1-2   Normal Tc-99m Perfusion Study (Nonobese Woman) (Figure 1-2)

A 52-year-old, 117-pound, 5-foot 1-inch woman with hypertension and family history of CAD had recurrent atypical chest pain. Tc-99m tetrofosmin myocardial perfusion SPECT was performed using a 1-day rest/stress (12 mCi/35 mCi) protocol. The patient underwent standard adenosine stress testing. The resting ECG was normal. The patient experienced no chest pain and there were no ECG changes during adenosine infusion. SPECT images were acquired using a 90-degree–angled dual-head camera and a 180-degree imaging arc from the 45-degree RAO projection to the 45-degree LPO projection. Rest and poststress ECG gating were performed using eight frames per cardiac cycle.

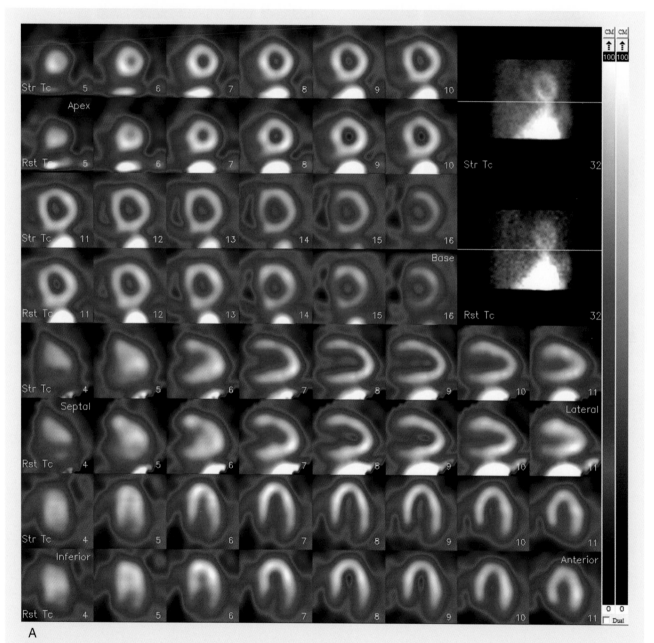

A

■ **Figure 1-2** Normal Tc-99m perfusion study (nonobese female). **A,** *Top right,* black-and-white panels are the planar projection images demonstrating excellent image quality. Note the prominent extra-cardiac activity. Color images are the corresponding tomographic slices display with the resting results interleaved between the stress slices. Top four rows display the LV SA from apex *(top left)* to base *(bottom right).* Next two rows display the stress and rest VLA slices from the septum to the lateral wall and the last two rows show the stress and rest HLA slices from the inferior to the anterior wall. Note the high image quality and fairly homogeneous tracer uptake throughout the LV.

(Continued)

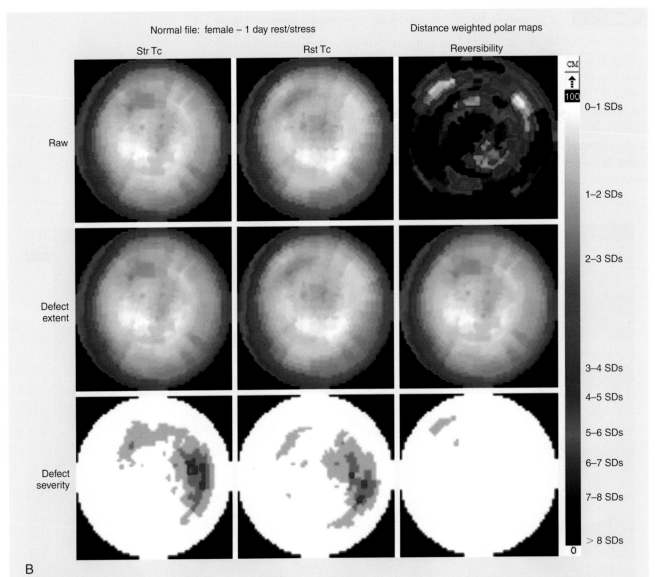

B

■ **Figure 1-2—Cont'd B,** Polar maps representation and quantification of this patient's LV tracer uptake using the same format as in Figure 1-1, *B*. Note the relative homogeneity of the stress and rest polar maps. The middle row shows the defect extent polar maps where areas that are abnormal in comparison to the normal database are highlighted in black. Note the absence of blackout regions, indicating a normal study by quantitative analysis. The bottom row is the defect severity polar maps display.

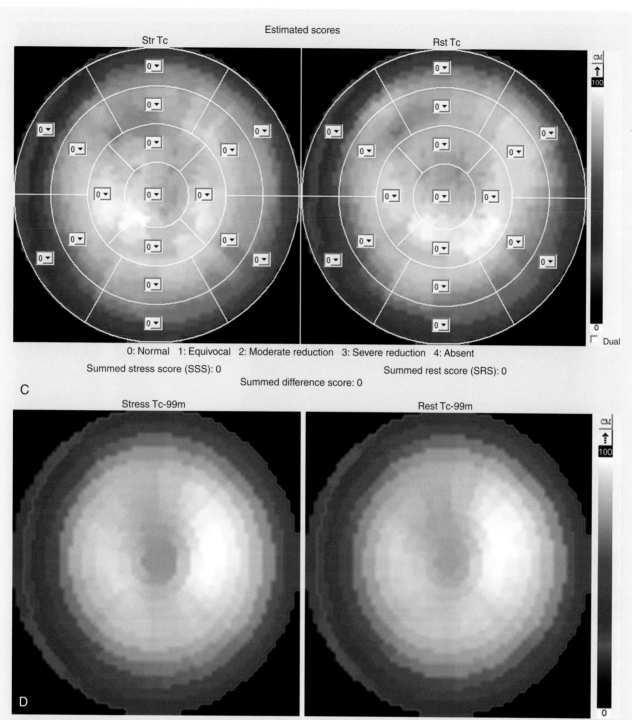

■ Figure 1-2—Cont'd C, Stress and rest LV myocardial perfusion polar maps with superimposed 17-segment coordinate system using the 0-to-4 score for each segment. Note that for this patient the sum of all 17-segment scores at stress *(SSS)* and rest *(SRS)* is zero. **D,** Mean normal LV stress and rest Tc-99m myocardial perfusion distribution in females generated from a population of 30 female patients with <5% probability of CAD. Note the relatively homogeneous perfusion distribution. Compared to the normal distributions in males (see Figure 1-1, *D*) there is less diaphragmatic attenuation of the inferior wall. Although less discernable, there is also a count reduction in the anterior wall at the 11 o'clock position often seen in normal studies when using 180-degree acquisition.

(Continued)

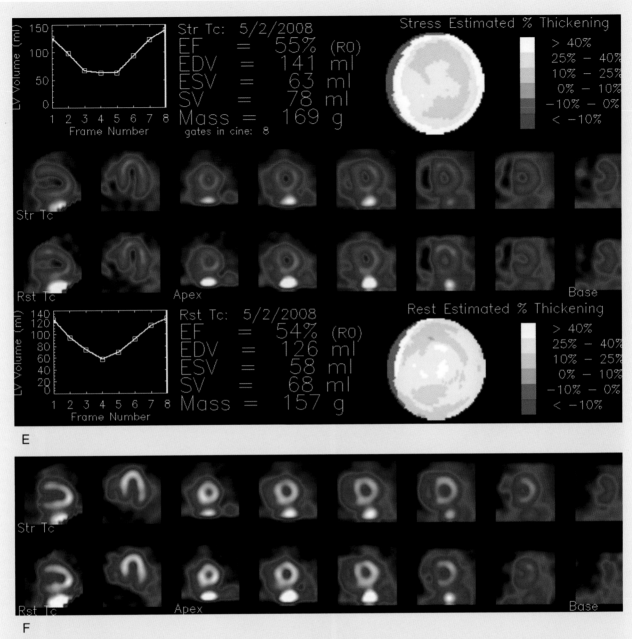

■**Figure 1-2—Cont'd** The four rows of color images show end-dyastolic (**E**) and end-systolic (**F**) stress *(top row)* and rest *(bottom row)* VLA, HLA, and SA LV tomographic display of this patient's ECG-gated images. Note the normal uniform regional inward motion of the myocardial borders from end-diastole to end-systole. Also note the significant uniform change in myocardial color from diastole to systole due to normal LV thickening. The color polar maps in **E** represent the quantification of the poststress *(top)* and rest *(bottom)* regional thickening. Note the labeled thickening scale to the right of the maps. The poststress *(top left)* and rest *(bottom left)* panels show the patient's averaged LV volume curves per cardiac cycle, LVEF, EDV, ESV, SV and LV mass. Note that both the rest and poststress LVEFs are above the 50% normal threshold for this quantitative program. These panels are accompanied by dynamic displays (Video 1-2).

COMMENTS

This is an example of a woman with a normal perfusion study of excellent image quality. Similar to Case 1, the stress planar projections are of higher quality than the rest planar projections due to the higher count density. Because of appropriate reconstruction and filtering, the tomographic stress and rest images are of similar high quality. Both the stress and rest tomographic images exhibit high spatial

and contrast resolution as depicted by the well-defined endocardial and epicardial myocardial borders and a well-defined LV chamber. Note that compared to Case 1 there is increased subdiaphragmatic uptake from stomach and bowel at rest and stress. This is normal. In fact, patients who undergo vasodilator stress testing have increased subdiaphragmatic activity compared to those who undergo exercise stress testing. Note the fairly uniform count distribution throughout the LV myocardium. A mild count deficit in the mid anterior segment is present on rest and stress images and is consistent with breast tissue attenuation. The gated images show normal segmental and global LV wall motion and normal LVEF. The EDV and ESV are normal. One reason for the high image quality in this study is reduced attenuation from soft tissue as this patient had small breasts and a BMI of 22.

| Case 1-3 | Diaphragmatic Attenuation Resolved by Attenuation Correction (Figure 1-3) |

A 54-year-old, 161-pound, 5-foot 9-inch man, smoker, with family history of CAD had atypical chest pain. Tc-99m sestamibi myocardial perfusion SPECT was performed using a 1-day rest/stress (13 mCi/38 mCi) protocol. The patient underwent standard Bruce treadmill exercise protocol. The resting ECG was normal. The patient exercised for 8 minutes 48 seconds, reached target heart rate, and stopped because of fatigue. The patient experienced no chest pain and there were no ECG changes during treadmill exercise. SPECT images were acquired using a 90-degree–angled dual-head camera and a 180-degree imaging arc from the 45-degree RAO projection to the 45-degree LPO projection. Simultaneous SPECT transmission images were acquired using a scanning Gd-153 radioactive line as the transmission source. Rest and poststress ECG gating were performed using eight frames per cardiac cycle.

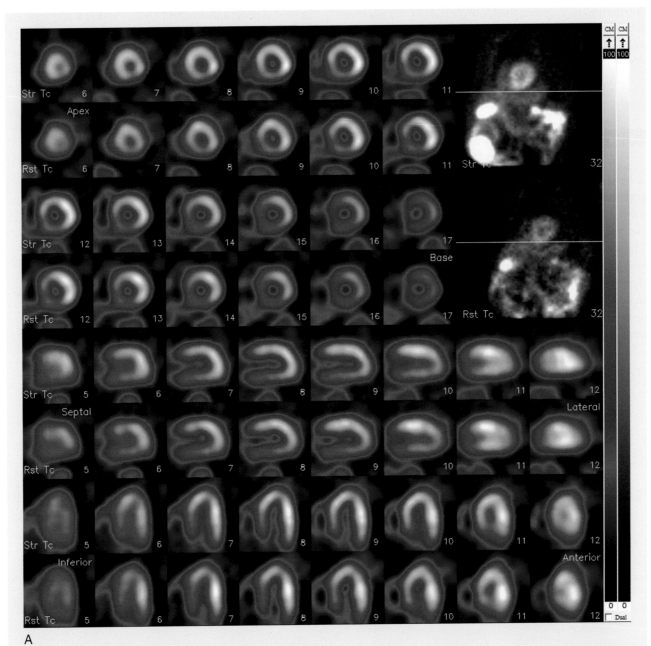

A

■ Figure 1-3 Diaphragmatic attenuation resolved by attenuation correction. **A,** Non-AC tomographic slices. Top four rows display the SA slices from apex *(top left)* to base *(bottom right)*. Next two rows display the stress and rest VLA slices from the septum to the lateral wall and the last two rows show the stress and rest HLA slices from the inferior to the anterior wall. Note in both the SA and VLA slices a fixed reduction in counts in the inferior wall.

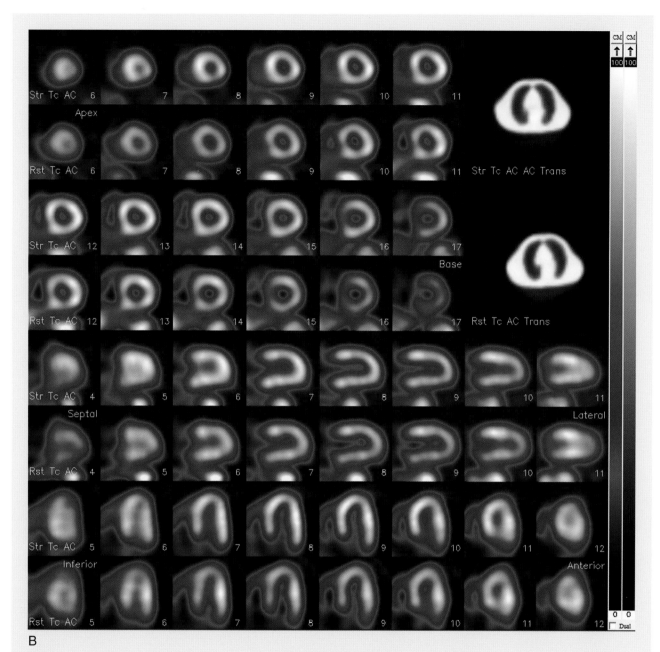

B

■ **Figure 1-3—Cont'd B,** AC tomographic slices. *Top right,* black-and-white panels show the transverse axial tomograhic transmission images generated by the Gd-163 line source and used for AC. Note that AC brings out the subdiaphragmatic activity. Color images are the corresponding AC tomographic slices display to **A.** Note the high image contrast, improved homogeneous tracer uptake throughout the LV, and increase in relative counts in the inferior and inferoseptal walls both on the rest and stress tomograms.

(Continued)

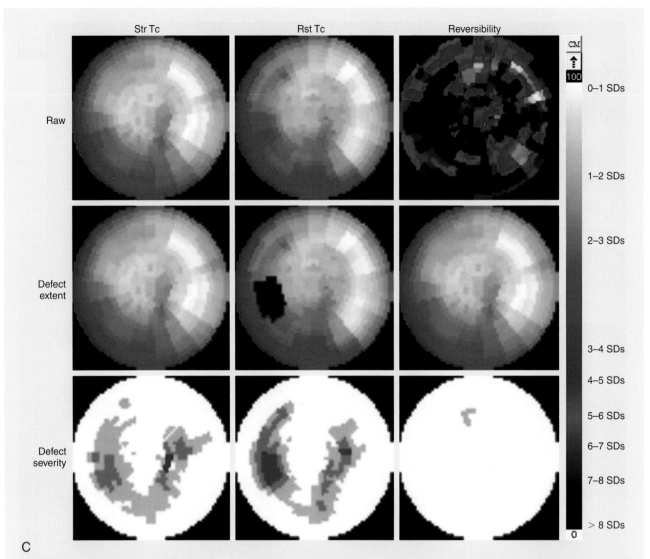

C

■ **Figure 1-3—Cont'd C,** Non-AC polar maps representation and quantification of this patient's LV tracer uptake compared to the normal database appropriate for this protocol. Note the reduction in counts in the inferior and inferoseptal walls. The middle row is the defect extent polar maps display where areas that are abnormal in comparison to the normal database are highlighted in black. Note the absence of blackout regions in the stress polar map, indicating that this degree of diaphragmatic attenuation in males is expected in normal subjects.

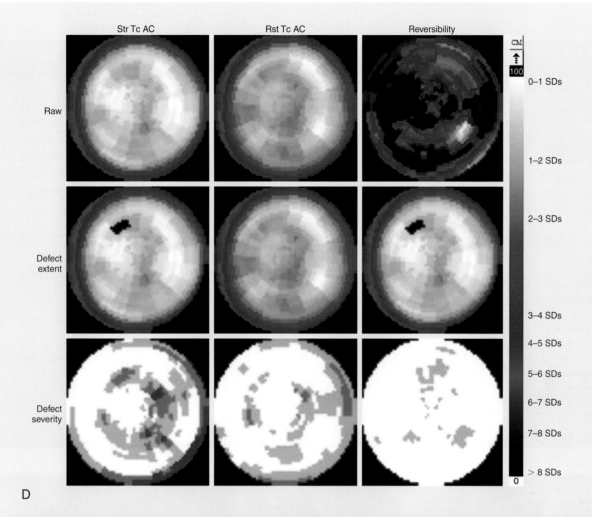

Str Tc AC	Rst Tc AC	Reversibility

Raw

Defect
extent

Defect
severity

CM
↕
100

0–1 SDs

1–2 SDs

2–3 SDs

3–4 SDs

4–5 SDs

5–6 SDs

6–7 SDs

7–8 SDs

> 8 SDs

0

D

Normal file: 1 day Rst/Str Mibi ExSPECT II AC

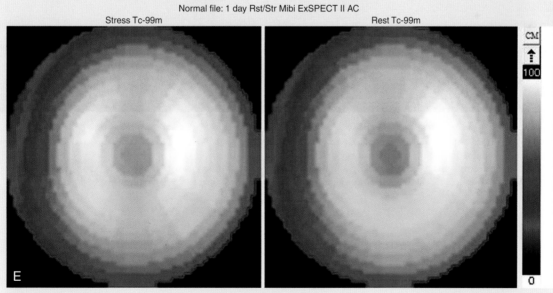

Stress Tc-99m	Rest Tc-99m

CM
↕
100

0

E

■ **Figure 1-3—Cont'd D,** AC polar maps representation and quantification of this patient's LV tracer uptake compared to the gender-independent AC normal database. Note that the reduction in counts in the inferior and inferoseptal walls has resolved. In the stress extent polar map, there is now a small but insignificant blackout region in the anteroseptal wall which encompasses 1% of the LV myocardium. Only defects involving ≥3% of the LV myocardium are considered abnormal by this quantitative program. **E,** Mean normal LV stress and rest gender-independent AC Tc-99m myocardial perfusion distribution in patients with <5% probability of CAD. Note the homogeneous perfusion distribution. Compared to the normal distributions in males (Figure 1-1, D) there is no diaphragmatic attenuation of the inferior wall. Although less discernable, there is still a mild count reduction in the anterior wall at the 11 o'clock position.

(Continued)

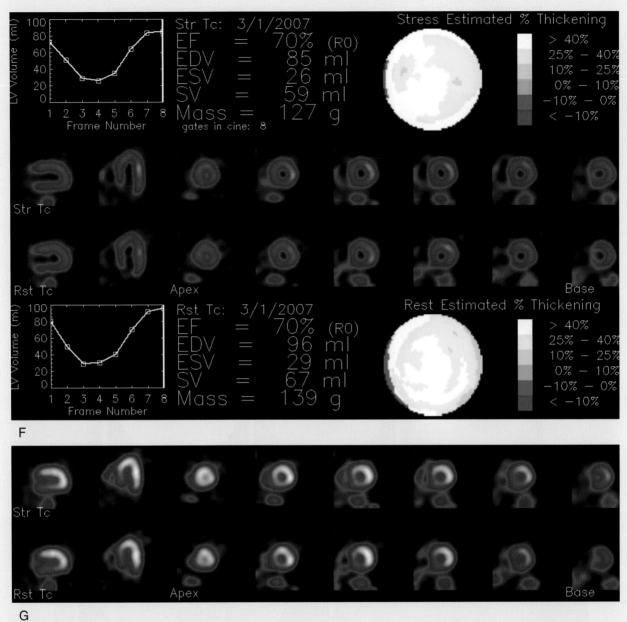

■ Figure 1-3—Cont'd The four rows of color images show end-dyastolic **(F)** and end-systolic **(G)** stress *(top row)* and rest *(bottom row)*, VLA, HLA and SA LV tomographic display of this patient's ECG-gated images. Typically ECG-gated tomograms are not corrected for attenuation. Note the normal wall motion and wall thickening in this patient's LV. Also note that both the rest and poststress LVEFs are above the 50% normal threshold for this quantitative program. These panels are accompanied by dynamic displays (Video 1-3).

COMMENTS

This is an example of a male patient with a perfusion study that shows a mild but discernable inferior wall reduction in counts on stress and rest images caused by diaphragmatic attenuation. Note that the gender-matched normal database quantification accounts for this relative count reduction in males and does not highlight this area as abnormal in the extent polar maps. Also note that when attenuation correction is applied the regional myocardial uptake in both the tomographic slices and the polar maps becomes more homogeneous and the reduction in counts in the inferior wall resolves.

Case 1-4	**Diaphragmatic Attenuation Resolved by Prone Imaging (Figure 1-4)**

A 55-year-old, 170-pound, 5-foot 8-inch man with hypertension and hypercholesterolemia had intermittent atypical chest pain. Tc-99m sestamibi myocardial perfusion SPECT was performed using a 2-day stress/rest (27 mCi/ 25 mCi) protocol. The patient underwent standard Bruce treadmill exercise protocol. The resting ECG was normal. The patient exercised for 9 min 30 seconds, reached target heart rate, and stopped because of fatigue. The patient experienced no chest pain and there were no ECG changes during treadmill exercise. SPECT stress and rest images were acquired using a 90-degree–angled dual-head camera and a 180-degree imaging arc from the 45-degree RAO projection to the 45-degree LPO projection. After each supine imaging session the SPECT acquisition was repeated with the patient in the prone position. Poststress and rest ECG gating were performed using eight frames per cardiac cycle.

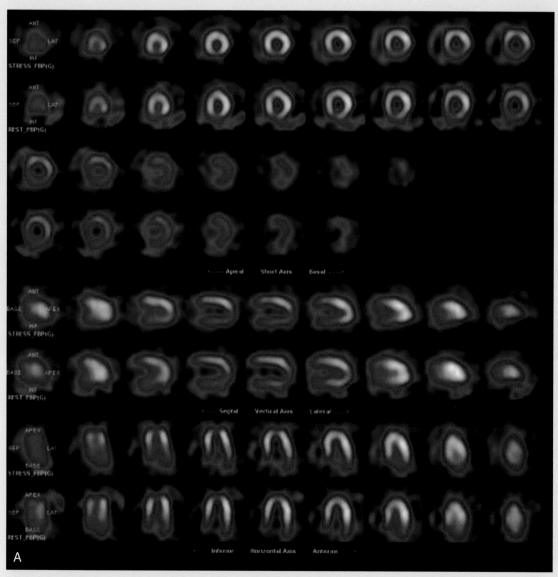

■**Figure 1-4** Diaphragmatic attenuation resolved by prone imaging. **A,** Supine tomographic slices. Note that both the SA and VLA slices demonstrate a fixed reduction in counts in the inferior wall.

(Continued)

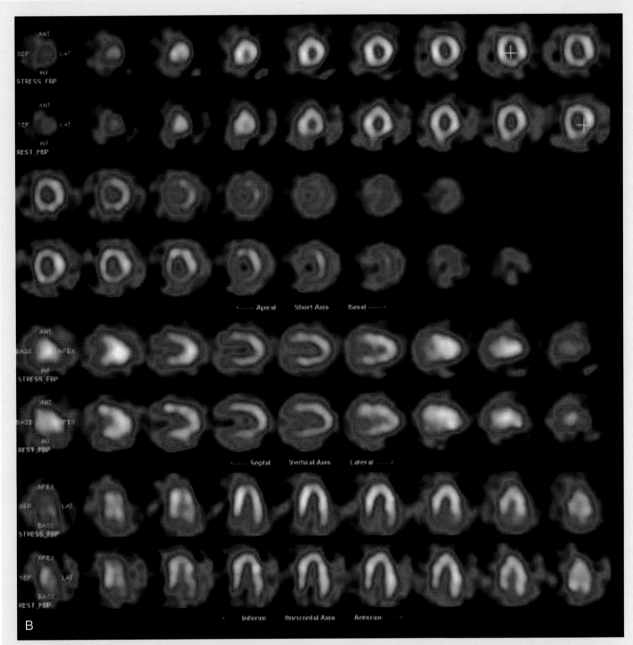

■**Figure 1-4—Cont'd B,** Prone tomographic slices. Note that prone imaging improves the uniformity of tracer uptake throughout the LV in this patient and increases the relative counts in the inferior wall on both the rest and stress tomograms.

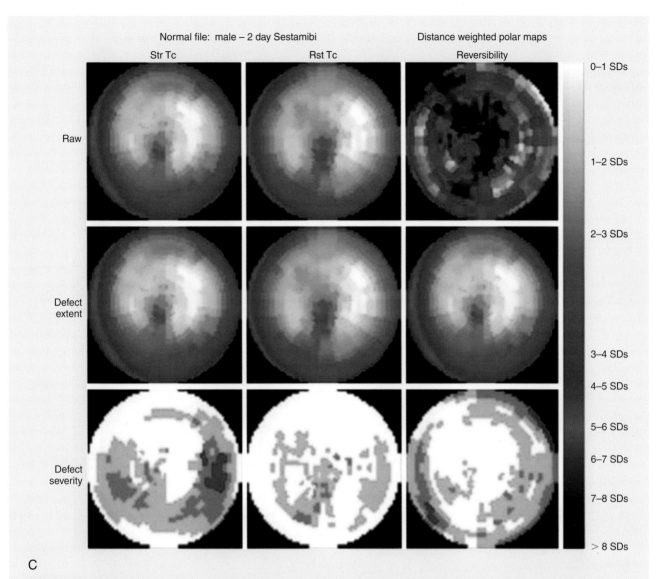

C

■ **Figure 1-4—Cont'd C,** Polar maps representation and quantification of this patient's LV tracer uptake in the supine position compared to the gender-matched normal database. Note the reduction in counts in the inferior wall from apex to base. The middle row is the defect extent polar maps display where areas that are abnormal in comparison to the normal database are highlighted in black. Note the absence of blackout regions, indicating that this moderate degree of diaphragmatic attenuation in males is expected in normal subjects.

(Continued)

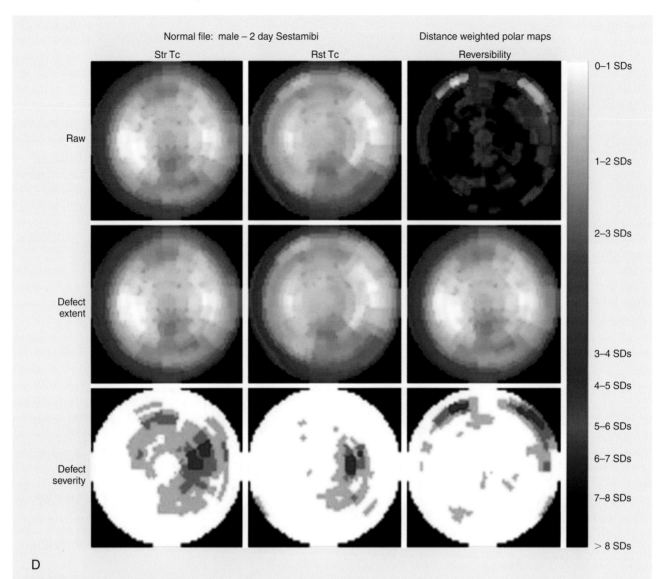

D

■ **Figure 1-4—Cont'd D,** Polar maps representation and quantification of this patient's LV tracer uptake with the patient imaged in the prone position. Note that the reduction in counts in the inferior wall has resolved.

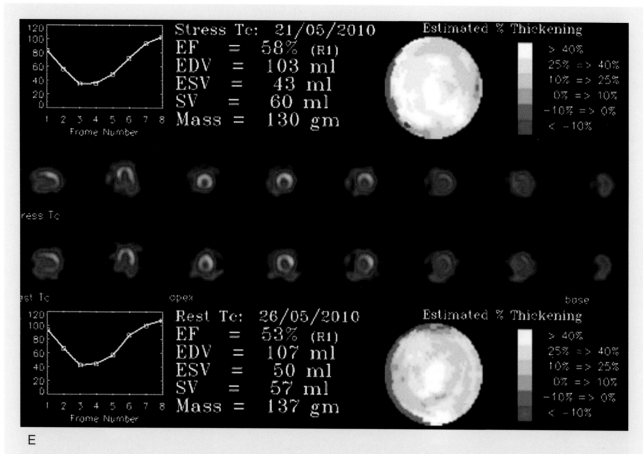

■ **Figure 1-4—Cont'd** The two rows of color images are the end-systolic poststress *(top)* and rest *(bottom)*, VLA, HLA, and SA LV tomographic display of this patient's ECG-gated images with the patient imaged supine. Typically ECG-gated tomograms are not corrected for attenuation. Note that both the rest and poststress LVEFs are above the 50% normal threshold for this quantitative program.

COMMENTS

This is an example of a male patient with a perfusion study that shows a mild but discernable fixed inferior wall reduction in counts due to diaphragmatic attenuation. Note that the gender-matched normal database quantification accounts for this count reduction in the inferior wall and does not highlight this area as abnormal in the extent polar maps. Also note on the prone study that the regional myocardial uptake in both the tomographic slices and the polar maps becomes more homogeneous and the reduction in counts in the inferior wall resolves. It is worth mentioning that a count reduction in the anteroseptal wall may develop on prone imaging because of sternal attenuation. Therefore imaging only in the prone position is not recommended.

Case 1-5   **Breast and Diaphragmatic Attenuation Resolved by Attenuation Correction (Figure 1-5)**

A 59-year-old, 202-pound, 5-foot 5-inch woman had hypertension, diabetes, and end-stage renal disease. She was referred for myocardial perfusion SPECT imaging for cardiac risk stratification prior to renal transplant. Tc-99m sestamibi myocardial perfusion SPECT was performed using a 1-day rest/stress (10 mCi/32 mCi) protocol. The patient underwent standard adenosine stress testing. The resting ECG was normal. The patient experienced no chest pain and there were no ECG changes during stress. SPECT images were acquired using a 90-degree–angled dual-head camera and a 180-degree imaging arc from the 45-degree RAO projection to the 45-degree LPO projection. Simultaneous SPECT transmission images were acquired using a scanning Gd-153 radioactive line as the transmission source. Rest and poststress ECG gating were performed using eight frames per cardiac cycle.

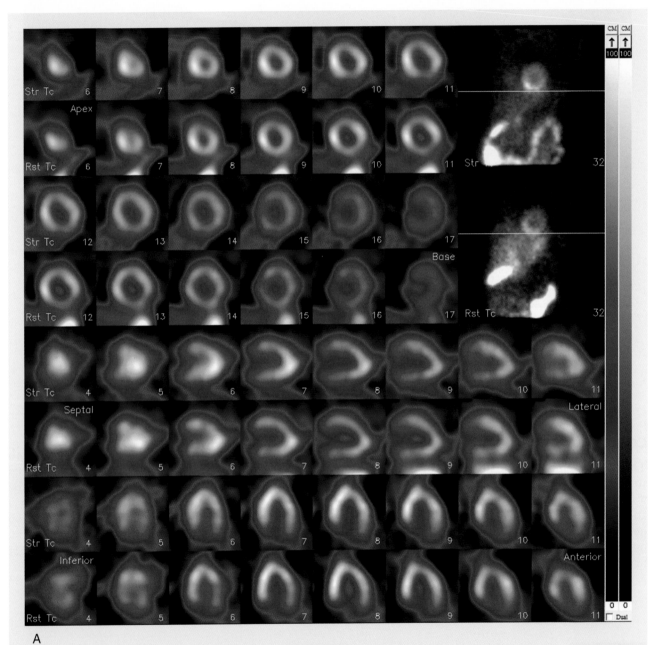

A

■ **Figure 1-5** Breast and diaphragmatic attenuation resolved by attenuation correction. **A,** Uncorrected planar projections and tomographic slices using the same format as in Figure 1-3, *A*. Note the reduction in counts across the anterior, lateral, and inferior walls indicative of soft tissue attenuation from breast and diaphragm. There is mild vertical (*y*-axis) patient motion on stress images. Note in the tomographic slices a fixed reduction in counts in the anteroseptal, lateral, and inferior walls.

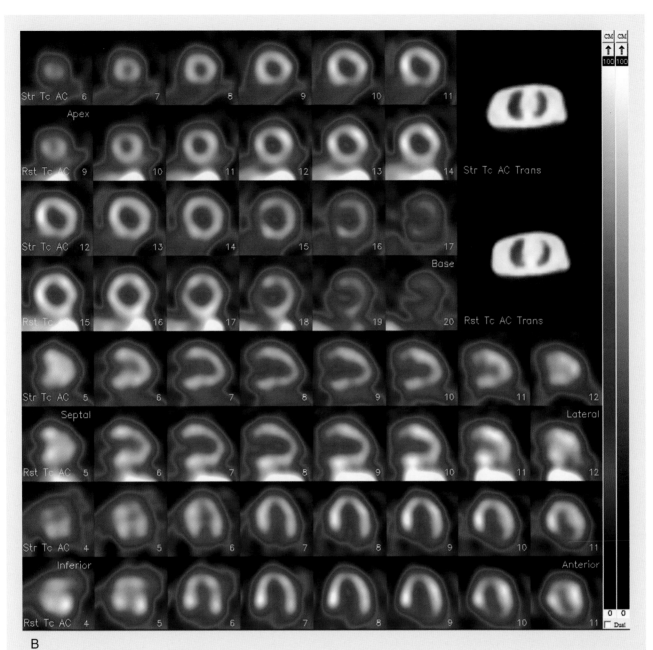

B

■ **Figure 1-5—Cont'd B,** AC tomographic slices. *Top right,* black-and-white panels show the transverse axial tomographic transmission images generated by the Gd-163 line source and used for AC. Note that AC brings out the subdiaphragmatic activity. Color images are the corresponding AC tomographic slices display to **A.** Note the high image contrast, improved homogeneous tracer uptake throughout the LV, and increase in counts in the regions shown as attenuated in **A.** This improvement is evident in both the rest and stress tomograms.

(Continued)

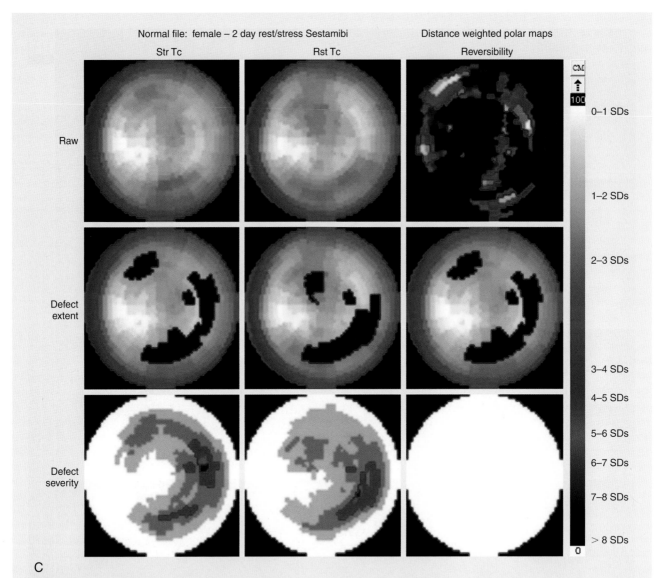

C

■ **Figure 1-5—Cont'd C,** Non-AC polar maps representation and quantification of this patient's LV tracer uptake compared to the female gender-matched normal database. Note the reduction in counts in the anteroseptal, inferior, and lateral walls in both the stress *(top left)* and rest *(top middle)* polar maps. In the middle row is the corresponding stress and rest defect extent polar maps display where areas that are abnormal in comparison to the normal database are highlighted in black. Note the blackout regions indicating that this degree of soft tissue attenuation is above the expected in normal females.

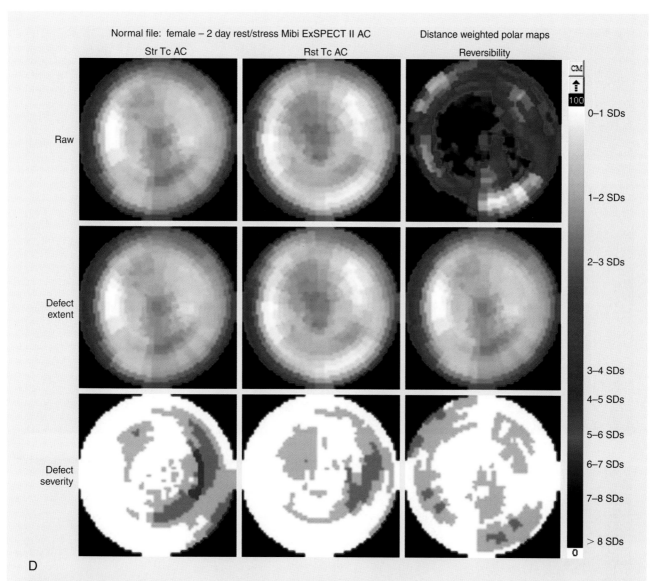

■ Figure 1-5—Cont'd D, AC polar maps representation and quantification of this patient's LV tracer uptake compared to the gender-independent AC normal database. Note that the blackout regions in the extent polar maps have resolved.

(Continued)

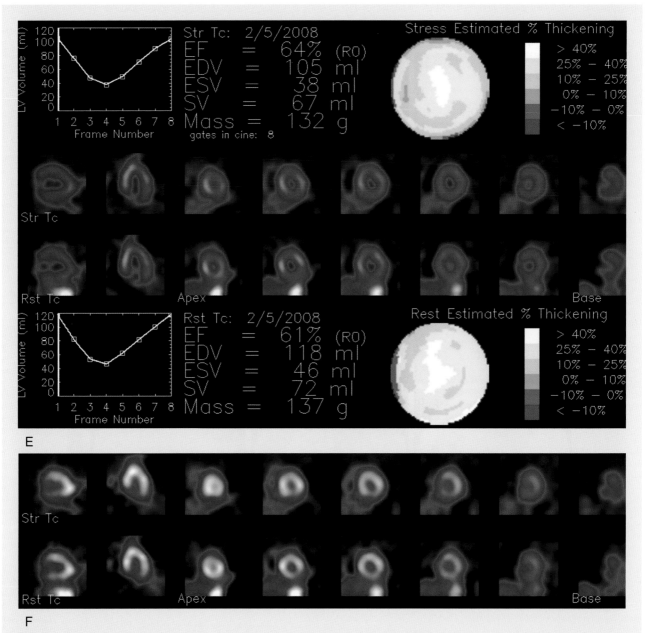

Figure 1-5—Cont'd The four rows of color images are end-diastolic **(E)** and end-systolic **(F)** poststress *(top)* and rest *(bottom)*, VLA, HLA, and SA LV tomographic display of this patient's ECG-gated images. Typically ECG-gated tomograms are not corrected for attenuation. Note the normal wall motion and wall thickening in this patient's LV. Also note that both the rest and poststress LVEFs are above the 50% normal threshold for this quantitative program. These panels are accompanied by dynamic displays (Video 1-4).

COMMENTS

This is an example of a female patient with a perfusion study that shows a moderate anterior, lateral, and inferior wall reduction in counts in both the stress and rest studies due to soft tissue attenuation (breast and diaphragm). Although the count reduction due to breast attenuation is usually seen in the anterior and anterolateral walls it can extend to any wall depending on the size, shape, position, and density of the breasts. Moreover, large breasts that are positioned differently between stress and rest (such as in bra-on/bra-off scenario) can mimic inducible myocardial ischemia. Note from the black-and-white planar projections the breast shadow across most of the LV in this patient. The stress extent polar map shows that the gender-matched normal database quantification does not account for the moderate reduction in counts from soft tissue attenuation and does highlight the anteroseptal, inferior, and lateral walls as abnormal in both the stress and rest polar maps. The ECG-gated images show uniformly normal wall motion and wall thickening of the LV myocardium, suggesting that the fixed regional count reduction in the perfusion images is likely due to breast and diaphragm attenuation and not due to an infarct.

Note that when attenuation correction is applied, the regional myocardial uptake in both the tomographic slices and the polar maps becomes much more uniform. The reduction in counts in the anteroseptal, inferior, and lateral walls is significantly reduced and the blackout regions in the extent polar maps disappear when compared to a gender-independent AC normal database.

| Case 1-6 | Normal Dual-Isotope Study (Woman With Small LV and Artificially High LVEF) (Figure 1-6) |

A 49-year-old, 150-pound, 5-foot 5-inch woman, smoker, had atypical chest pain and no prior cardiac history. Dual-isotope myocardial perfusion SPECT was performed using 3 mCi of Tl-201for rest imaging and 22 mCi of Tc-99m sestamibi for stress imaging. The patient underwent a modified Bruce treadmill exercise stress protocol. The resting ECG was normal. The patient exercised for 6 minutes 25 seconds, reached target heart rate, and stopped because of fatigue. The patient experienced no chest pain and there were no ECG changes during treadmill exercise. SPECT images were acquired using a 90-degree–angled dual-head camera and a 180-degree imaging arc from the 45-degree RAO projection to the 45-degree LPO projection. ECG gating of the poststress study was performed using eight frames per cardiac cycle.

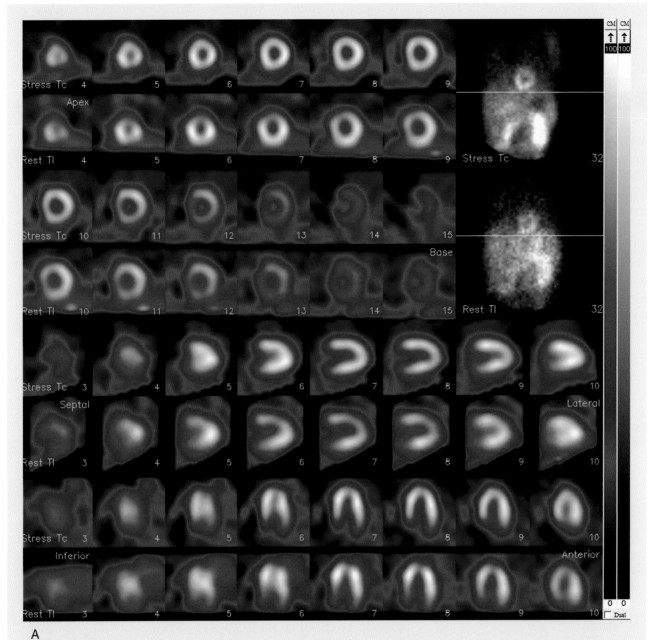

A

■ **Figure 1-6** Normal dual-isotope study (female with small LV size and artificially high LVEF). **A,** Color images are the tomographic slices display with the resting results interleaved between the stress slices. Top four rows display the LV short axis from apex *(top left)* to base *(bottom right)*. Next two rows display the stress and rest VLA slices from the septum to the lateral wall and the last two rows show the stress and rest HLA slices from the inferior to the anterior wall. Note the high image quality and homogeneous tracer uptake throughout the LV, and a count reduction of the anterior wall seen in the resting SA and VLA Tl-201 slices due to the higher attenuation of the Tl-201 lower energy photons as compared to Tc-99m. The small LV size is responsible for increased scatter into the LV cavity, falsely lowering the ESV and yielding an artificially high LVEF.

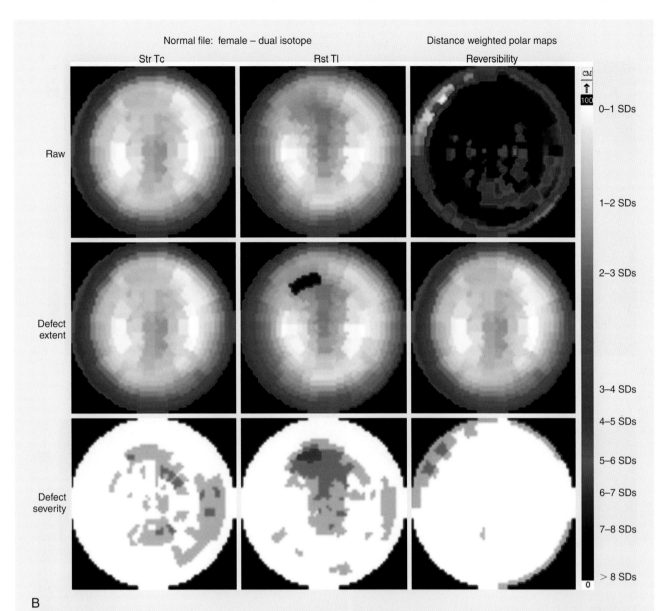

Normal file: female – dual isotope

Distance weighted polar maps

Str Tc   Rst Tl   Reversibility

Raw

Defect extent

Defect severity

0–1 SDs
1–2 SDs
2–3 SDs
3–4 SDs
4–5 SDs
5–6 SDs
6–7 SDs
7–8 SDs
> 8 SDs

B

■ **Figure 1-6—Cont'd B,** Polar maps representation and quantification of this patient's LV tracer uptake. Note the relative homogeneity of the stress polar maps and a small count reduction in the anteroseptal region due to mild breast attenuation. The middle row is the defect extent polar maps display where the small anteroseptal count reduction at rest is blacked out to highlight a significant difference when compared to the gender-matched normal database. Since the stress perfusion distribution is normal, the entire study is considered normal.

(Continued)

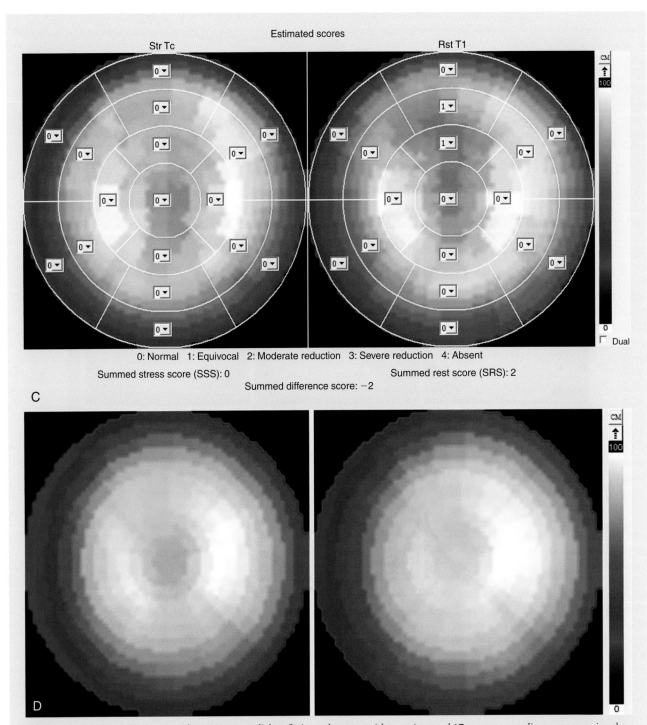

Estimated scores

Str Tc

Rst T1

0: Normal   1: Equivocal   2: Moderate reduction   3: Severe reduction   4: Absent

Summed stress score (SSS): 0

Summed rest score (SRS): 2

Summed difference score: −2

C

D

■ **Figure 1-6—Cont'd C,** Stress and rest LV myocardial perfusion polar maps with superimposed 17-segment coordinate system using the 0-to-4 score for each segment. Note that for this patient the sum of all 17-segment scores at stress *(SSS)* is 0 but at rest *(SRS)* is 2 due to breast attenuation seen in the Tl-201 rest images. **D,** Mean normal LV dual-isotope myocardial perfusion distribution in females generated from a population of 30 female patients with <5% probability of CAD. Note the fairly homogeneous perfusion distribution.

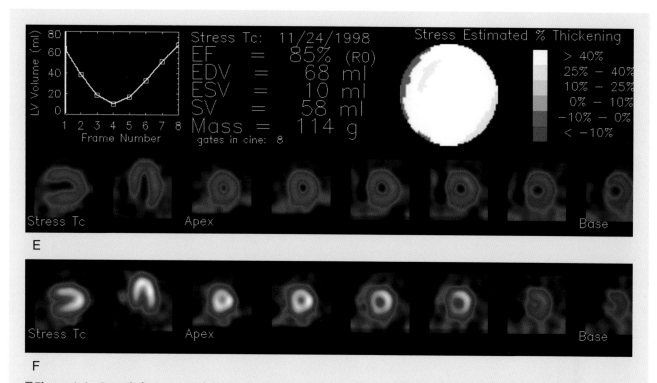

■ Figure 1-6—Cont'd The two rows of color images show end-diastolic (**E**) and end-systolic (**F**) poststress VLA, HLA, and SA LV tomographic display of this patient's ECG-gated images. Note the normal uniform regional inward motion of the endocardial and epicardial borders from end-diastole to end-systole. Also note the significant uniform change in myocardial color from diastole to systole due to normal LV thickening. The LV chamber appears small, at least in part due to photon scatter. This phenomenon falsely decreases the ESV and consequently falsely increases the poststress LVEF calculated at 85%. These panels are accompanied by dynamic displays (Video 1-5).

COMMENTS

This is an example of a woman with a normal dual-isotope perfusion study of excellent image quality. Note that the stress planar projections are of higher quality than the rest planar projections due to the higher radiotracer dose injected at stress and the lower attenuation and scatter of Tc-99m compared to Tl-201. For these same reasons the tomographic Tc-99m stress images are of somewhat higher quality than the Tl-201 tomographic rest images. Note the uniform count distribution throughout the LV myocardium at stress, which is consistent with homogeneous relative perfusion and no significant coronary obstructions. Note also a count reduction in the anteroapical and mid anteroseptal walls seen in the resting SA and VLA Tl-201 slices caused by the higher attenuation of the Tl-201 lower energy photons compared to Tc-99m. This same area is blacked out in the rest extent defect polar map. The gated images reveal a small LV that is responsible for increased scatter into the LV cavity, particularly at end-systole, yielding an artificially high LVEF.

Case 1-7   **Normal Stress/Rest-Reinjection Tl-201 Study (Figure 1-7)**

A 49-year-old, 154-pound, 5-foot 8-inch man with two episodes of unexplained syncope in the last 3 weeks. The risk factors for CAD included hypertension and hypercholesterolemia. Stress imaging was performed using 3 mCi of Tl-201. Three hours later, following the reinjection of 1 mCi of Tl-201, rest imaging was performed. The patient underwent standard adenosine stress testing. The resting ECG was normal. The patient experienced no chest pain and there were no ECG changes during pharmacologic stress. SPECT images were acquired using a 90-degree–angled dual-head camera and a 180-degree imaging arc from the 45-degree RAO projection to the 45-degree LPO projection. Poststress and rest ECG gating was performed using eight frames per cardiac cycle.

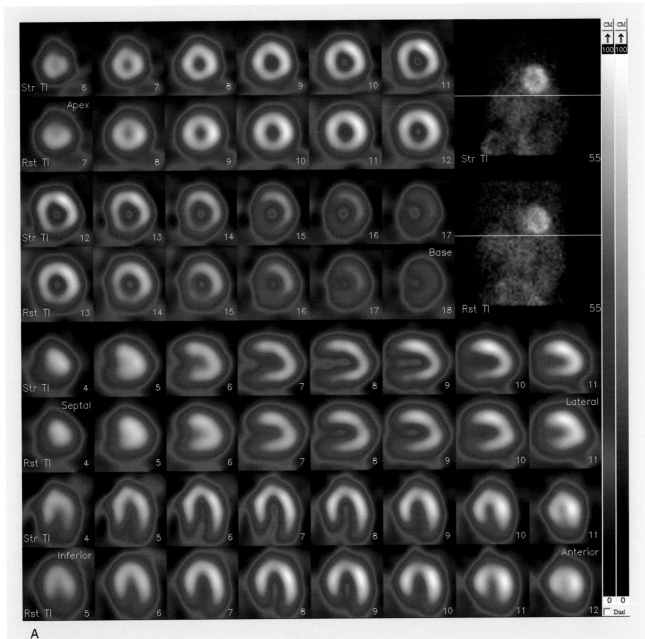

A

■ **Figure 1-7** Normal stress/rest-reinjection Tl-201 study. **A,** *Top right,* black-and-white panels are the stress *(top)* and redistribution *(bottom)* Tl-201 planar projection images demonstrating adequate image quality. Color images are the corresponding tomographic slices display with the rest/redistribution results interleaved between the stress slices. Note the fairly uniform tracer myocardial distribution for both the stress and redistribution images. There is a mild count reduction in the base of the inferior wall, which is consistent with diaphragmatic attenuation. The cavity and endocardial/epicardial definition is not as good quality as the Tc-99m examples shown in this chapter.

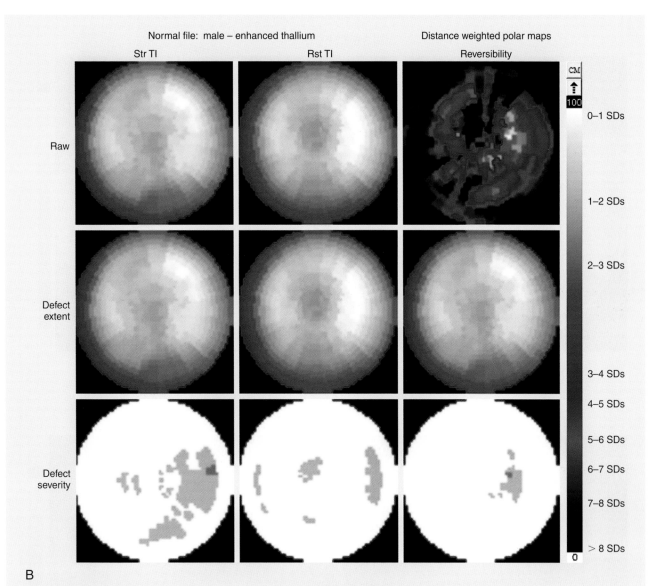

Normal file: male – enhanced thallium

Distance weighted polar maps

Str Tl   Rst Tl   Reversibility

Raw

Defect
extent

Defect
severity

0–1 SDs
1–2 SDs
2–3 SDs
3–4 SDs
4–5 SDs
5–6 SDs
6–7 SDs
7–8 SDs
> 8 SDs

B

■ **Figure 1-7—Cont'd B,** Polar maps representation and quantification of this patient's LV tracer uptake. Note the relative homogeneity of the stress and redistribution polar maps. The middle row is the defect extent polar maps display where areas that are abnormal in comparison to the normal database are highlighted in black. Note the absence of blackout regions, indicating that the mild count reduction in the inferior wall is within normal expected limits.

(Continued)

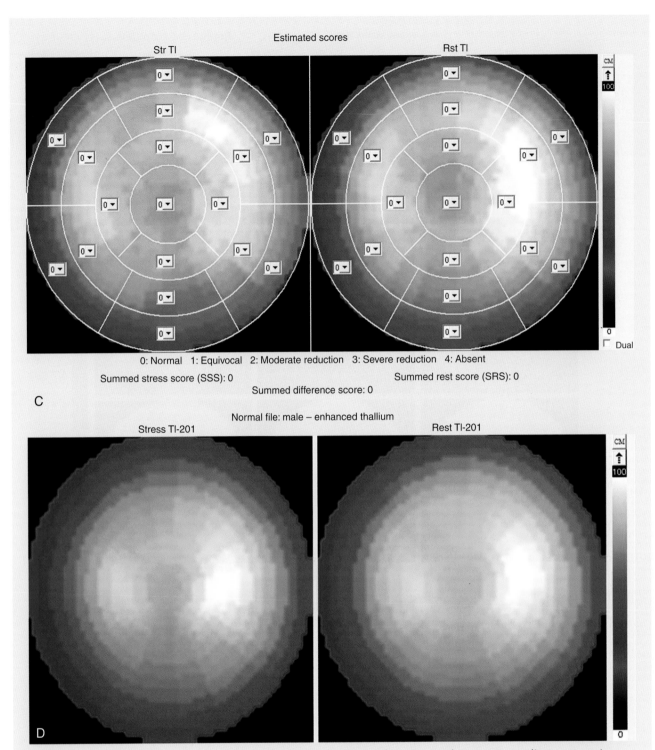

0: Normal   1: Equivocal   2: Moderate reduction   3: Severe reduction   4: Absent

Summed stress score (SSS): 0   Summed rest score (SRS): 0

Summed difference score: 0

■ **Figure 1-7—Cont'd C,** Stress and rest LV myocardial perfusion polar maps with superimposed 17-segment coordinate system using the 0-to-4 score for each segment. Note that for this patient the sum of all 17-segment scores at stress (SSS) and rest (SRS) is zero. **D,** Mean normal LV stress and rest Tl-201 myocardial perfusion distribution in males generated from a population of 30 male patients with <5% probability of CAD. Note the uniform perfusion distribution but the somewhat increased uptake in the lateral wall due to reduced attenuation of the free wall. Although less discernable, there is also a mild count reduction in the anterior wall.

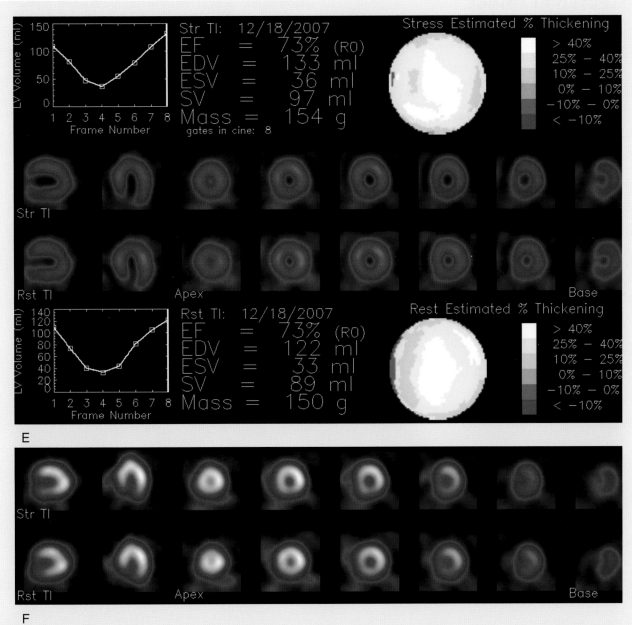

■ **Figure 1-7—Cont'd** The four rows of color images show end-diastolic **(E)** and end-systolic **(F)** poststress *(top)* and rest *(bottom)*, VLA, HLA, and SA LV tomographic display of this patient's ECG-gated images. Note the normal uniform regional inward motion of the endocardial and epicardial borders from end-diastole to end-systole, and the normal uniform change in myocardial color from diastole to systole due to normal LV thickening. The color polar maps represent the quantification of the poststress *(top)* and rest *(bottom)* regional thickening. Note the labeled thickening scale to the right of the maps. The poststress *(top left)* and rest *(bottom left)* panels show the patient's averaged LV volume curves per cardiac cycle, LVEF, EDV, ESV, SV, and LV mass. Note that both the rest and poststress LVEFs are 73%, above the 50% normal threshold for this quantitative program. These panels are accompanied by dynamic displays (Video 1-6).

COMMENTS

This is an example of a male patient with a normal perfusion study of excellent image quality. Note that the Tl-201 planar projections and tomographic slices are not as high quality compared to the Tc-99m images shown in the other normal cases. In particular, compared to Tc-99m studies, the LV cavity appears smaller due to the increased photon scatter. Note also the uniform count distribution throughout the LV myocardium at rest and stress. Both the rest and stress LVEF are 73%. LVEF measured from Tl-201 studies are usually higher than those from Tc-99m studies due to the artificially smaller ESV from increased photon scatter.

SELECTED READINGS

DePuey EG: Artifacts in SPECT myocardial perfusion imaging. In DePuey EG, Garcia EV, Berman DS, et al: editors: *Cardiac SPECT*, Philadelphia, 2001, Lippincott Williams and Wilkins, pp 231–262.

Garcia EV, Galt JR, Faber TL, et al: Principles of nuclear cardiology. In Dilsizian V, Narula J, editors: *Atlas of Nuclear Cardiology*, ed 3, Philadelphia, 2009, Current Medicine Group LLC, pp 1–36.

Garcia EV, Santana C, Grossman G, et al: Pitfalls and artifacts in cardiac imaging. In Vitola JV, Delbeke D, editors: *Nuclear Cardiology & Correlative Imaging: A Teaching File*, New York, 2004, Springer-Verlag LLC, pp 345–377.

Iskandrian AE, Garcia EV: Practical issues: Ask the experts. In Iskandrian AE, Garcia EV, editors: *Nuclear Cardiac Imaging: Principles and Applications*, ed 4, New York, 2008, Oxford University Press, pp 703–718.

Wackers F.J.Th., Bruni W, Zaret BL: Display and analysis of SPECT myocardial perfusion images. In *Nuclear Cardiology: The Basics—How to Set Up and Maintain a Laboratory*, Totowa, NJ, 2004, Humana Press, pp 97–125.

Chapter 2

Interpretation, Reporting, and Guidelines

Ami E. Iskandrian, Jaekyeong Heo, and E. Lindsey Tauxe

KEY POINTS

- Image interpretation is not the same as "pattern recognition" as it requires knowledge of tracer kinetics, instrumentation, protocols, cardiac physiology, etc., skills that are acquired from years of experience and commitment. The board certification in nuclear cardiology, just like other boards, is a test of minimum competency; we should strive to do better, consistently!

- The reader should recognize normal variations that might be patient, gender, and tracer specific.

- The reader should be familiar with the capabilities of the software suites illustrated in Chapter 1.

- Attention should be paid at every step to quality measures such as indication, acquisition, interpretation, reporting, and personal communication of results. If perfected, the results will enhance patient management. It is the main reason why nuclear cardiology has remained the imaging procedure of choice over almost four decades at our institution.

- The images should be reviewed before the patient leaves the laboratory and repeated, if necessary, if the quality is suboptimal because of excessive motion or subdiaphragmatic activity. There is a tremendous difference between an equivocal study and a poor-quality study. This is the only way that the entire team will realize that there are no short cuts to quality (and yes, someone has to stay late to repeat the images!). If done a few times, the message will resonate with the individual team members and the department!

- Interpretation should be systematic and should include a review of the raw images and the use of quantitative techniques and attenuation correction, if available.

- When reading serial studies, the report should be concise, devoid of jargon, and should be prepared with the primary care provider in mind rather than the imaging specialist. A friendly, and timely, telephone call in selected cases will go a long way toward improving communication.

- To maintain competence, the reader should be familiar with available guidelines, appropriateness criteria, and new developments in the field.

- The reader should be cognizant of incidental findings that may have a major impact on patient care.

- Reports should not be relied on; the current images should be compared side-by-side to prior studies.

INTERPRETATION OF THE IMAGES

On a consistent basis, there is no substitute for good quality images, but quality is more than just pretty images; it includes appropriate indications, acquisition, interpretation, and reporting. We shall address all these issues.

Rotating images: There is, like in many other things, more than one way to do the right thing. What follows is our own approach based on over three decades of experience. A good place to start (always) is to review the rotating images, both the stress and rest (if there is a rest study); we find the gray scale to be most useful. Reset the intensity so the brightness is just right. In some patients the diagnosis is made from these images alone, such as a hiatal hernia or a lung tumor (see Chapter 16). The most common things to pay attention to are cardiac motion, breast shadow, arm position, and hot spots.

Motion can be in any of the three axes (x, y, and z). The y-axis motion (up and down) is the easiest to recognize and to correct, if not excessive. The z-axis motion (forward-backward) cannot be seen but is inferred when there is evidence of motion on the slices (overlapping walls or hurricane sign; see Chapter 3) but no motion in the x- or y-axes (side-by-side). Some programs automatically correct for motion but that is never a substitute for reviewing the raw images. It is important to review the images before the patient leaves the laboratory, because in some patients correction is not feasible and the best way is to repeat the acquisition (as painful as it may be!). One caveat: if the images are normal despite motion, then they are likely to be normal. It is when the images are abnormal that concern arises as to whether the abnormality is real or due to motion. Motion can also affect the LVEF measurement.

The **breast shadow** is quite variable as it can cover the entire cardiac silhouette, the anterior wall, the lateral wall, the septum, or any combination of the above. A variation in the breast shadow between stress and rest studies can occur. This can have a profound effect on the images, producing both fixed and reversible artifactual defects. When the breast shadow covers the entire cardiac silhouette, an inferior abnormality can be produced because of diaphragmatic attenuation superimposed on uniform attenuation. We have not used prone imaging to differentiate real defects from those due to diaphragmatic attenuation but when used it can prove very useful. Remember, however, that prone imaging might introduce artifacts in the anterior wall and therefore both supine and prone images should be acquired.

The left arm position is usually on the top of the head but in patients who cannot do so, the arm is left at the side of the body, potentially creating lateral wall attenuation. It is important in these patients to have the arm in the same position in both sets of images (stress and rest) (Figure 2-1).

The presence of "hot spots," either within the heart (such as a prominent papillary muscle) or outside the heart (such as the liver or more likely a bowel loop), can produce downscaling in adjacent areas and also impact the quantitative analysis as the activity is back-projected into the cardiac ROI.

Orthogonal views: Next, the non-gated perfusion slices are reviewed in the SA, HLA, and VLA projections. We use both the "cool" color and gray scales. The color scale makes it easier to recognize milder abnormalities, whereas gray scale makes it easier to recognize reversibility. It is amazing how much more activity can be appreciated on the gray scale compared to the color scale! This is one more reason why quantification is important (Figure 2-2).

The crucial step when looking at the images is to be sure they are properly aligned and scaled. Scaling is the "Achilles' heel" of proper interpretation and it cannot be learned from books, including this one! It requires experience and knowledge as it is affected by cardiac and extracardiac activity. If the images are too bright, perfusion defects are missed; if the opposite, artifactual defects are created, defects appear larger, or defects are changed from fixed to reversible or vice versa (Figure 2-3). Using the dual control button, adjust each set of images such that the brightest areas on the stress and rest images match in intensity, no more and no less. You may need to use the "expanded mode" in one or both sets if the images are too bright. Adjust by changing the upper scale and leaving the lower scale at 0 all the time!

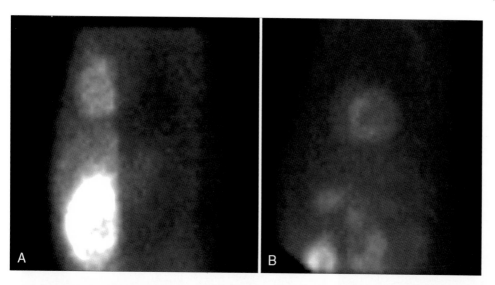

■**Figure 2-1** Planar views of rotating images showing the left arm alongside the body **(A)** and above the head (conventional) **(B)**. The presence of the arm alongside the body could produce lateral attenuation artifacts. The dynamic images for both cases are shown in Video 2-1, A, B.

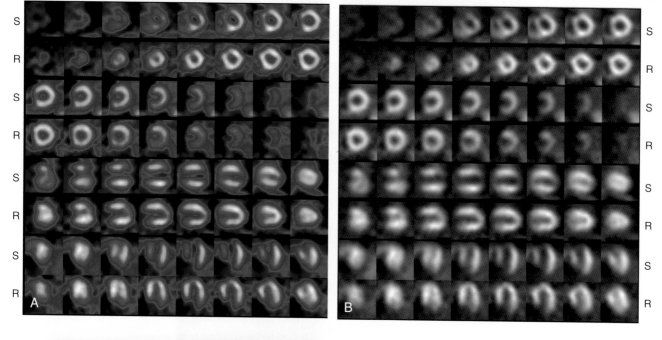

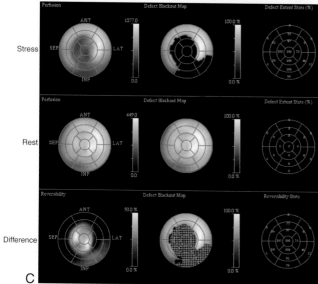

■**Figure 2-2** Perfusion abnormality on stress *(S)* and rest *(R)* gated SPECT sestamibi images in color (cool) **(A)** and in gray scale **(B)**. The gray scale shows more residual activity than the color scale because the low activity is depicted in the blue range, which is not readily appreciated by the human untrained eyes. It can, however, be mastered by experience. The polar maps show some activity in the defect zone as depicted in the gray scale perfusion images **(C)**.

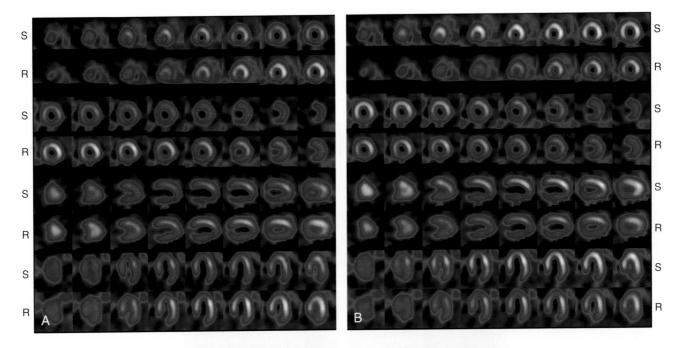

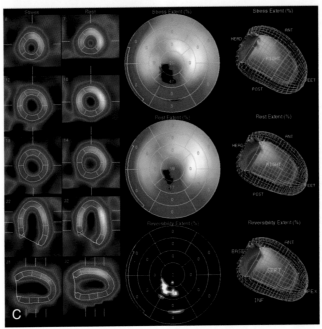

■ **Figure 2-3** Perfusion abnormality by *(S)* and rest *(R)* gated SPECT sestamibi imaging. **A,** Defect appears reversible. **B,** Same defect appears fixed. Polar maps are not affected by a change in the color scale **(C)**.

The **four steps** for reading images in every patient:

1. Are the images normal or abnormal?
2. If abnormal, where is the abnormality (one-, two-, or three-vessel territory)?
3. What is the size of the abnormality (small, medium, or large)?
4. What is the nature of the abnormality (reversible, fixed, or mixed)?

Our trainees are drilled on this exercise day in and day out. The practice has paid off as we have had a 100% passing rate on the Nuclear Cardiology Board Certification Examination for the past 10 years (all first attempts).

Site, size, severity, and reversibility: The vascular territory of the LAD includes the anterior wall, septum, and apex (9 segments of the 17-segment model) (Figure 2-4). The RCA territory includes 3 segments

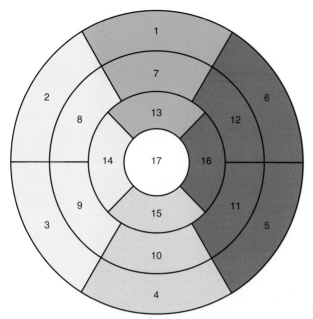

■ **Figure 2-4** The segmentation model used to generate 17 segments: the 6 basal (1-6), 6 mid (7-12), and 4 distal (13-16), and the apex (17). These are further divided as follows: 3 anterior (1, 7, 13); 2 anteroseptal (2, 8); 2 inferoseptal (3, 9); 3 inferior (4, 10, 15); 2 inferolateral (5, 11); 2 anterolateral (6, 12); and one each distal lateral (16), distal septal (14), and apical (17). As can be seen, the basal segments appear larger than the distal segments.

(± apex) and the LCX territory includes 5 segments (± apex). There are a few caveats:

1. The apex is shared by all three vessels; for example, RCA disease causing an inferior defect that can involve the apex. Such a defect should not be called RCA plus LAD disease just because the apex is involved.

2. The apex is not a point but a segment just like the other segments. But when it is just a dimple, avoid labeling it as a defect as this is due to apical thinning; it is a common source of "false positive" scans.

3. There is an overlap between the vascular territories. Thus, some LAD defects can extend to the anterolateral wall and some LCX defects can extend to the base of the anterior wall. The same applies for the overlap between the LAD and RCA (the inferior and the inferoseptal segments) and between the LCX and the RCA (the inferior and inferolateral segments). As a general rule, if the overlap involves more than half of a different vascular territory, call it two-vessel disease, otherwise it is an extension.

4. In LAD disease, the defect is more severe distally than at the base (one exception is in patients with prior CABG; see Chapter 8). This is another hint as to whether the LAD is involved in a patient with an LCX abnormality and only a basal anterior wall abnormality.

5. In patients with disease limited to the diagonal branch of the LAD (not uncommon especially after LAD stenting, if these branches are jailed; see Chapter 8), the defect is localized to distal and mid anterolateral segments (between 12 and 2 o'clock). These defects

sometimes are seen only in the SA tomograms. Otherwise, in general, we prefer to see the defect in at least two orthogonal planes.

6. Isolated small septal defects are rare but can be due to a septal branch being jailed after stenting of the LAD or to muscular bridging. If the defect involves most of the septum, however, pay careful attention to the inferior wall. Disease involving both the LAD and RCA tends to produce inferior and septal perfusion abnormalities (i.e., they spare the anterior wall) (Figure 2-5). The reason is that the septum has a dual blood supply from the LAD and RCA and, therefore, is more severely affected than the anterior wall. For the same reason, disease of the LAD and LCX tends to involve the anterior and lateral walls but spare the septum (Figure 2-6). This pattern may potentially represent left main disease as there is no other specific pattern for LM disease. Always be aware of this possibility as ostial LM stenosis could be easily missed on coronary angiography.

7. There is considerable variability in the extent of perfusion abnormalities in patients with CAD that cannot be entirely explained by variations in coronary anatomy (Figure 2-7). It is likely the single most important reason that perfusion imaging provides such powerful prognostic information. In patients undergoing coronary interventions, injection of the tracer during transient coronary occlusion by balloon inflation shows a similar variability in the extent of myocardium at risk (Figure 2-8). It should be noted that although catheter-based methods can be used to assess coronary physiology (whether a stenosis is significant), they do not provide information on the area at risk or the extent of perfusion defects.

8. Attenuation-corrected images should be reviewed side-by-side with the uncorrected images. Obviously, one needs to assure that the quality of the transmission images is acceptable regardless of whether a line source or CT is used for correction. We do not recommend reading only the corrected images at this stage.

9. The size and severity of a perfusion abnormality can be assessed visually. Size is graded as small, moderate, or large, and severity as mild, moderate, or severe. One needs to adjust for the severity of a defect based on the presence of attenuation artifacts in the same segments. For example, the inferior defect may look more severe in men because the true abnormality is superimposed on an attenuation artifact in the same location. The quantitative methods are more robust, however, than visual methods for assessing size and severity (see below).

10. The nature of the perfusion abnormality is defined as reversible (ischemia), fixed (scar), or mixed (subendocardial scar). As will be discussed in Chapter 15, this definition of scar is not precise. The assessment of reversibility, either presence or absence, is more difficult than appreciated, and, in general, reversibility is under-reported. Again some caveats:

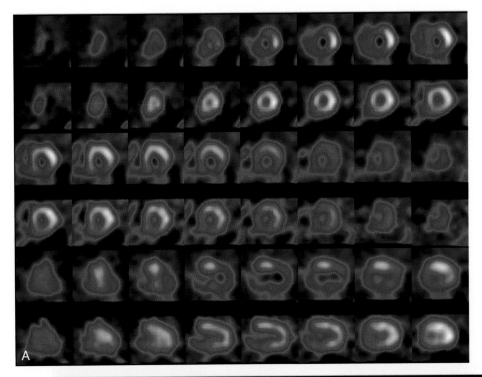

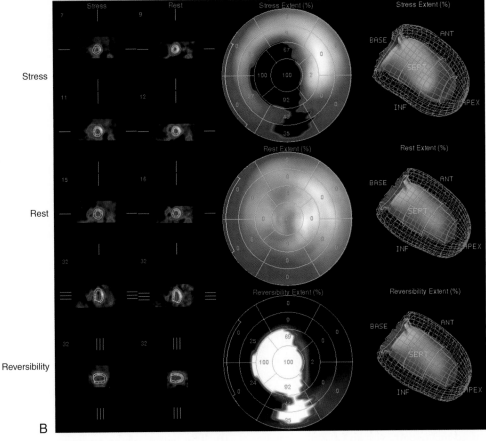

■ **Figure 2-5** Perfusion abnormality in a patient with LAD and RCA disease. **A,** There is a perfusion abnormality involving the septum and inferior wall; the anterior wall abnormality is less conspicuous than the septal abnormality. The septum has a dual blood supply from both these vessels and is therefore more affected than the anterior wall. The TID of 1.3 means the summed LV size is 30% larder on the stress than on the rest images. **B,** The polar maps are shown.

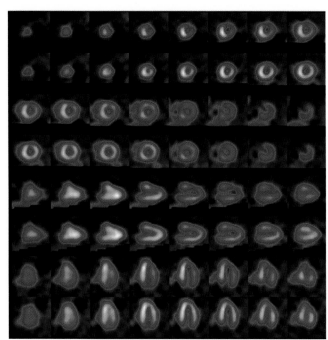

■ **Figure 2-6** Perfusion abnormality in a patient with LAD and LCX disease. There is a perfusion abnormality involving the anterior wall and lateral wall but sparing the septum. The septum is less affected because the septal perforator branches from the posterior descending branch of the RCA supply the posterior septum.

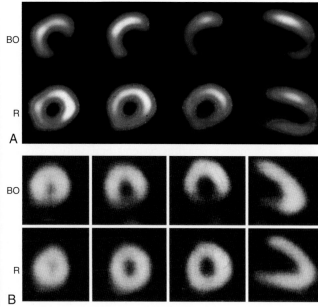

■ **Figure 2-8** Variation in the size of a perfusion defect in two patients (**A** and **B**) with LCX disease. The tracer was injected during transient balloon occlusion (BO) in the cardiac catheterization laboratory during planned angioplasty for severe stenosis. The rest images (R) were normal in both patients. There is a marked difference in the size of the area at risk in these two patients despite comparable coronary angiographic findings.

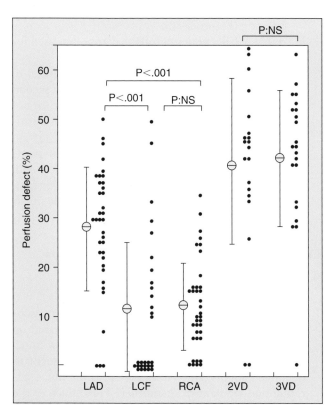

■ **Figure 2-7** Variation in the size of the perfusion abnormality during exercise in patients with isolated one-, two-, or three-vessel disease. The defect size was measured by planimetry of planar images. (*Modified from* Circulation *1983;67:983.*)

A. The color scale is not as reliable as the gray scale in detecting reversibility of a mild nature. It requires more training, but if perfected it can be just as useful. So, use the gray scale , at least in the beginning.

B. Perfusion defects in some areas that are prone to attenuation artifacts will never appear completely normal on the rest study. Therefore, we tend to label such segments as showing "partial redistribution," implying there is an element of scarring. As a rule, if the motion on the gated images is normal, call it reversible.

C. The reason why segments appear fixed or reversible is not entirely related to the segment in question but rather to the remote and normal zones. If the hyperemic MBF is not as high in the normal area (either because the stress is not adequate, as with submaximal exercise or microvascular disease), then the relative MBF ratio (maximum/rest in the abnormal zone divided by maximum/rest in the normal zone) is not big enough and the defect appears fixed. That is why it is important to pay attention to the type of stress when comparing serial tests in the same patient in which one study shows reversible defects and the second study shows fixed defects.

Once again, proper scaling and alignment of the images and attention to extracardiac activity are essential for accurate interpretation.

Quantitative analysis: It should be clear that the best we can do at present with SPECT imaging is semiquantitative analysis. True quantitative analysis is possible with PET as it allows measurement of absolute MBF (in cc/g/min). One day the same could be possible with SPECT with attenuation correction and rapid acquisition protocols using newer imaging systems and software (see Chapter 18). Until then, quantitative analysis can be done in one of two ways:

1. Visual scoring: a score (e.g., 0 = normal, 1 = mild decrease, 2 = moderate decrease, 3 = severe decrease, and 4 = absent activity) is assigned to each segment of the 17-segment model of the stress and rest images. The total score at stress is called the summed stress score (SSS) and reflects the extent and severity of abnormality (regardless of location). The total score at rest is called the summed rest score (SRS) and reflects the extent of fixed defects. The difference between the SSS and SRS is called the summed difference score (SDS), which reflects reversible defects. The larger the SSS, SRS, and SDS, the greater the total abnormality, scar, and ischemia, respectively.

2. Automated analysis: this is computer-derived and is done in one of three ways:

   A. SSS, SRS, and SDS as described above but the scores are computer-generated based on some threshold of activity in each segment. For example, 0 = >80%, 1 = 70%-80%, 2 = 60%-70%, 3 = 50%-60%, and 4 = <50%.

   B. Polar maps: These are circumferential profiles of individual slices but encompass the entire LV ROI. Each point depicts activity vs. angular location. The profiles are compared to a database of normal controls and any pixel (or *voxel* to be more precise) that falls outside a predefined range is tagged as abnormal. The number of abnormal pixels is expressed as a ratio to the total number of pixels within the ROI. For example, if there are a total of 600 pixels and 200 pixels are tagged as abnormal, then the total abnormality is 33%. Again this number is independent of the location of the abnormality. It is also possible to assess the severity of the abnormality by the number of standard deviations (SDs) that each pixel deviates from normal. Finally, it is possible to determine the reversibility (or lack thereof) by determining the change in activity from stress to rest in each pixel in comparison to a normal control or to show interval changes (either worsening or improvement) (Figure 2-9). In the example used above, half of the defect is severe and half is mild-to-moderately abnormal and the reversibility is complete in 25%, partial

in 50% and absent in 25% (amazing indeed is the wealth of information obtained).

   C. Three commercial software suites can be used to perform polar map analysis: Cedar Sinai's Autoquant, Michigan/Baylor's 4DM, and the Emory tool box. These programs differ from each other in terms of database, number and selection of slices, threshold for defining an abnormality, and the number of abnormal pixels required before a vascular territory is tagged as abnormal. It is preferable not to mix programs, especially when evaluating changes on serial studies. Other institutions have local programs based on the same concept but these are not commercially available. Most of our work has been with the 4DM program. The polar maps can be viewed without comparing the data to a normal database (so called "raw" polar maps), or in comparison to a normal file ("normalized" polar maps). The normalized maps are used to generate size, severity, and reversibility.

   D. The Yale program uses the same principles of circumferential profile analysis but on selected slices—one distal apical, one at mid region, and one at the base of the LV. The polar maps often displayed alongside the images with profiles from the normal database. These profiles have been in common use since the days of planar thallium imaging (Figure 2-10).

   E. Table 2-1 illustrates cutoffs that are often used for defect sizing.

   F. Polar maps and the Yale program, in addition to providing quantitative data, act as friendly second readers to alert the primary reader of subtle (or not so subtle) abnormalities that were missed or misinterpreted for one reason or another.

   G. The computer programs do not adjust for poor-quality studies, hot spots, or other artifacts and, therefore, should be used with reader oversight. Nevertheless, we find polar maps invaluable in our clinical and research studies.

Comparison Between SSS and Polar Maps

Both have strengths and limitations:

1. Both have served the field well in terms of diagnosis and risk assessment. However, the SSS based on visual analysis is subjective. For example, how much of a segment must be involved for that segment to be judged abnormal? Where exactly is the line separating one segment from another? How much of the segment should show improvement before judging it reversible? Obviously, these problems are multiplied when two sets of images are acquired at different times, as the image quality may not be the same in both sets.

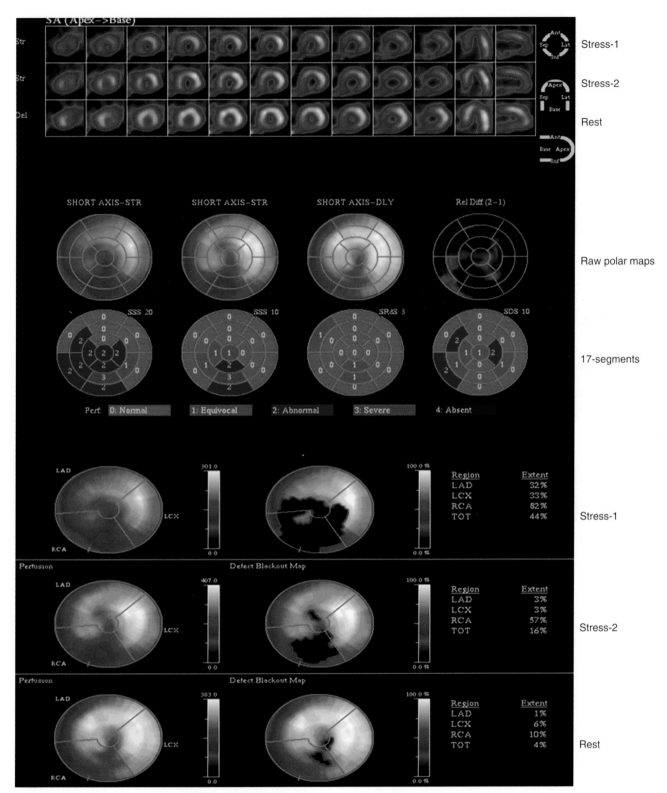

■**Figure 2-9** The use of automated methods to measure defect size and severity using polar maps and 17-segment model in a patient who had two separate studies. The defect size is clearly less extensive on stress study 2. The rest study suggests that the defect is almost totally reversible.

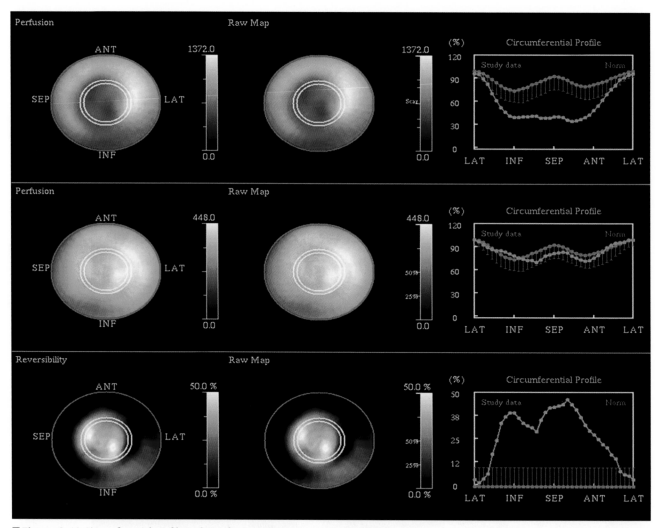

■**Figure 2-10** Circumferential profile analysis of stress and rest images. The profiles show the stress curve and the rest curve in comparison to normal database (mean ± SD). The stress profile is below the normal limit in the anterior wall, septum, and inferior wall. The rest profile is within normal limits. The bottom profile shows the extent of reversibility.

TABLE 2-1 Definitions of Defect Size

	DEFECT SIZE		
	SMALL	MODERATE	LARGE
Summed stress score	<4	4-8	>8
Abnormal segments	1-2	3-5	≥6
Involved vessels	≤1	1-2	2-3
Polar maps			
% of LV (4DM)	<10%	10-20%	>20%
% of LV (Autoquant)	<5%	5-10%	>10%

2. With polar maps, these issues are not as great a problem because the method is based on pixels rather than segments. But there are other problems such as defining the ROI, especially at the apex and the base. Also, the use of one value (given in SD of the normal mean, 2.5 is often used) across all regions may mask some defects. One can readily examine the effect of different SDs on defect size (Figure 2-11). It is possible to use a different SD for each segment, but it is not as easy or reproducible. In patients with marked septal hypertrophy, such as patients with hypertension on dialysis or those with hypertrophic cardiomyopathy, the program may signal lateral wall abnormality because in normal subjects the lateral wall has the highest activity. Finally, as mentioned earlier, the automated polar maps do not recognize or adjust for motion artifacts or extracardiac activity.

Assessment of gated images: It must be clear that the way we acquire images is by gating them to the R-wave on the ECG using 8 or 16 frames per R-R cycle. After acquisition, the gated images are summed together to produce the non-gated perfusion images that are used to analyze the presence or absence of perfusion defects. This is done because the individual gated frames (end-diastolic and end-systolic) have low counts and too much noise to be useful for image analysis. The gated images are used to study regional and global function.

We recommend reviewing not only the three-dimensional images but also the individual slices. The three-dimensional images are acceptable in normal hearts or uniformly abnormal hearts but are not reliable for assessing regional dysfunction. The slices need to be reviewed with and without the contours and in both color and gray scales. The gray scale (or alternatively the "thermal" scale) is good for motion while the color scale is better for wall thickening. A scoring system could be used to assess motion and thickening; 0 = normal, 1 = mild hypokinesia or decreased thickening, 2 = moderate, 3 = severe, 4 = akinesia/dyskinesia or lack of any thickening. In some patients with severe hypertrophy and with some software

programs, the EF appears low because the contours do not track the endocardial border but rather the mid wall, which has less thickening. One can easily see cavity obliteration and yet the EF is calculated to be abnormal. In such cases just ignore the number and report what you see: cavity obliteration! The time-activity curve and polar plots of motion and thickening are helpful. In our laboratory, we have established a range of normal values for LV volumes (indexed to body surface area) and use them to define the degree of enlargement based on SD from the mean (mild, moderate, and severe). There are gender differences in LV volumes; in men, mild, moderate, and severe LV enlargements correspond to end-diastolic volume index of 74–87, 88–100, and >100 ml/m^2, respectively. The corresponding numbers in women are 56–65, 66–75, and >75 ml/m^2.

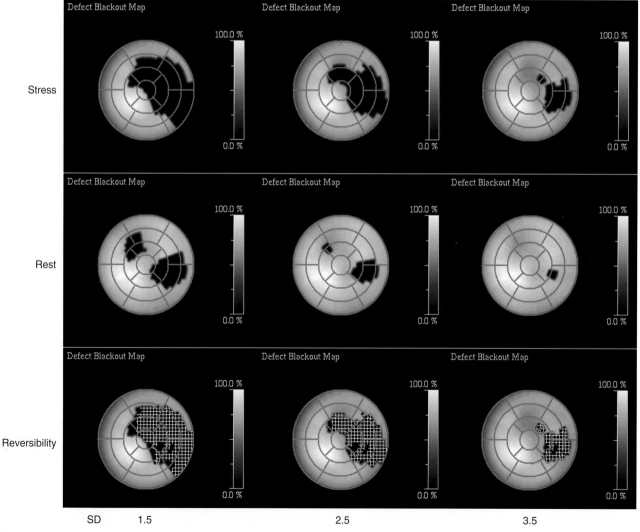

■ Figure 2-11 Effect of changing the standard deviation (SD) on defect size using polar maps in the 4DM program. Increasing the SD from 1.5 to 2.5 and 3.5 gradually decreases the defect size.

Integration of perfusion and function: The gated SPECT images provide precise registration for simultaneous assessment of perfusion and function. Either could be normal or abnormal (and the abnormality of varying degrees of severity). The function is a load-dependent measurement and could be affected by other factors besides scar or ischemia. Patients with dilated cardiomyopathy are a good example of this—the perfusion is normal but the function is abnormal. In patients with CAD, the following points are worth considering:

1. Color scale is preferred for wall thickening and gray scale for motion. Wall thickening is a more sensitive marker of regional dysfunction than wall motion, a theme well recognized by 2DE.
2. The perfusion pattern appears worse in cases of dilated LV and reduced EF due to partial volume effect. Thus, areas of natural attenuation, such as apical thinning and the inferior wall in men or the anterior wall in women, will appear even more attenuated.
3. There is a time delay between tracer injection and image acquisition. The perfusion image is a snapshot at the time of tracer injection, whereas the wall motion/thickening represents events at the time of image acquisition (almost 1 hour in most laboratories, including ours).
4. The presence of a reversible perfusion abnormality in poststress images is often associated with normal regional function. The presence of regional dysfunction is referred to as poststress stunning. Thus, the presence of a normal wall motion/thickening in poststress images does not differentiate between attenuation and ischemia though it is helpful in differentiating between scar and attenuation.
5. It is possible to have a small (often mild) fixed perfusion abnormality with normal regional function.
6. There is discordance between EF and perfusion defect size because the function could be supernormal (hyperdynamic) but the perfusion could only be normal. (Figure 2-12). This is an important reason why perfusion and EF provide complementary prognostic information.

Other Measurements

1. The three-dimensional display does not allow assessment of RV size and function. This is, however, possible when reviewing the gated slices. The measurements are purely qualitative at present but still quite useful. Incidental findings of RV dysfunction in patients with shortness of breath might be an indication for pulmonary thromboembolism. In patients with pulmonary hypertension, activity in the RV appears to be as much or even greater than LV activity. Transient increases in RV activity during stress have been described in LM disease, arguably due to diffuse LV ischemia, but we have not found this sign to be helpful.

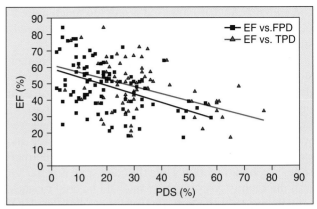

■ **Figure 2-12** The relationship between LV EF and perfusion defect size (total: TPD and fixed: FPD) obtained with automated 4DM polar maps method. The correlation is modest in a group of patients with CAD. *(Modified from* Q J Nucl Med Mol Imaging *[in press].)*

2. Lung activity is often evaluated in thallium studies but not with Tc-labeled tracers (sestamibi or tetrofosmin). In general, lung activity is lower with Tc-labeled tracers (lower lung-heart ratio). However, in patients with clearly higher lung activity during stress than rest imaging, this would suggest a transient increase in LV filling pressure similar to thallium-201.
3. Increased tracer activity in the lungs reflects elevation in LV filling pressure. As such it is not a specific marker of CAD or ischemia and could be seen in any condition with high filling pressures. We have seen, however, examples of increased lung thallium activity in patients with noncardiogenic pulmonary edema. It seems that pulmonary edema, whether associated with high or normal LV filling pressure, could produce increased tracer lung uptake as long as there is transudation of fluid at the time of tracer injection.
4. Transient ischemic dilatation (TID) indicates a larger LV cavity during stress than rest. This observation is based on reviewing the non-gated perfusion images. The reason for the disparity is the low counts in the subendocardial zone during stress but not rest. It can be seen with exercise or pharmacologic stress, and we have seen it on rest 4-hour redistribution thallium images as well. It can be measured quantitatively by measuring the LV volumes from the non-gated images. The actual end-diastolic volume could be unchanged between stress and rest although in some patients it is also increased. The threshold for defining TID is higher when using hybrid imaging with rest thallium and stress Tc-labeled tracer (1.2 versus 1.1). Visually, it can be divided into mild, moderate, or severe. We have seen examples where there is regional TID at the site of a perfusion defect (usually the apex), which is clearly visible and yet the global TID ratio is normal. TID is better appreciated on gray scale than on color scale. When present with perfusion defects it indicates severe ischemia and a reminder to review the images more closely. We do not believe that isolated TID

(no perfusion defects and normal EF) is a marker of poor outcome. The reasons for such isolated findings are not clear but could be related to the use of a different camera for stress and rest images, variation in detector position, or hydration status.

5. Poststress stunning is defined as transient wall motion/ thickening abnormality detected on stress but not (or less severe) on rest images. It signifies severe ischemia and is seen in areas with perfusion defects (most defects especially those during vasodilator stress testing represent flow heterogeneity rather than ischemia). If it is severe and extensive, the EF might be lower as well. This is one more reason why the rest and stress images need to be gated. The other is that, for one reason or another, one of the two measurements has technical problems with gating and, therefore, is not accurate.

Discordant results: When interpreting the images, we routinely review the clinical presentations and ECG results as well. Discordant results should make you pay close attention but should not alter your interpretation to make it "fit." Some have suggested that the images should be read without any other information, then the clinical presentation should be reviewed together with ECG responses and the probability (definitely normal, probably normal, equivocal, probably abnormal, and definitely abnormal) is readjusted by one point, up or down, depending on the clinical information. We do not use probability; the study is read as either normal or abnormal.

Reporting: The report should be concise, informative, and devoid of jargon. The report is not a data entry form with endless segmental scores for perfusion and function. These elements are useful for a database and research. The American Society of Nuclear Cardiology has recommendations as well. As much useful information should be included as necessary, but remember that physicians do not like to read long reports! The report should have a narrative summary of pertinent findings. Examples of these are in Appendices 2-1 through 2-4. There is no substitute for picking up the phone and talking directly to the treating physician in at least some cases. We do it routinely.

Guidelines and Appropriateness

A number of guidelines on "how to" are available on ASNC website. The appropriateness criteria in nuclear imaging have been updated since the initial publication. These criteria categorize indications for testing as appropriate (scores 7, 8, and 9), uncertain (scores 4, 5, and 6) or inappropriate (scores 1, 2, and 3). Of the 66 scenarios studied, 33 were judged to be appropriate, 25 inappropriate, and 8 uncertain. Many reports have examined local adherence to these criteria. In one multicenter study, 13% of the studies were deemed inappropriate, 14% uncertain, and 7% could not be classified, leaving only 66% of the studies as appropriate. These criteria obviously have implications in reimbursement by third party payers, including Medicare. We believe that any guidelines or criteria are simply just that, and reasonable people may disagree on their implications or implementations. It is hard to believe that any imaging person would know a patient as well as the treating physician who has ordered the test. There could be subtle changes in symptoms that only a seasoned physician can appreciate. That is not to say that there are no inappropriate uses (and yes, self-referral and greed) but the distinction is not always black and white; this does not begin to address those indications that are in the uncertain category.

Case 2-1   **Normal Study**

A 53-year-old man with atypical angina of 6 months' duration is referred for stress MPI. His risk factors include diabetes, hypertension, and smoking. The physical findings were unremarkable except for obesity (weight 245 pounds) and hypertension. Because of severe knee arthritis, he underwent vasodilator stress testing with regadenoson. The ECG showed T-wave changes at baseline and during stress (negative for ischemia). The SPECT images were of good quality (Figure 2-13).

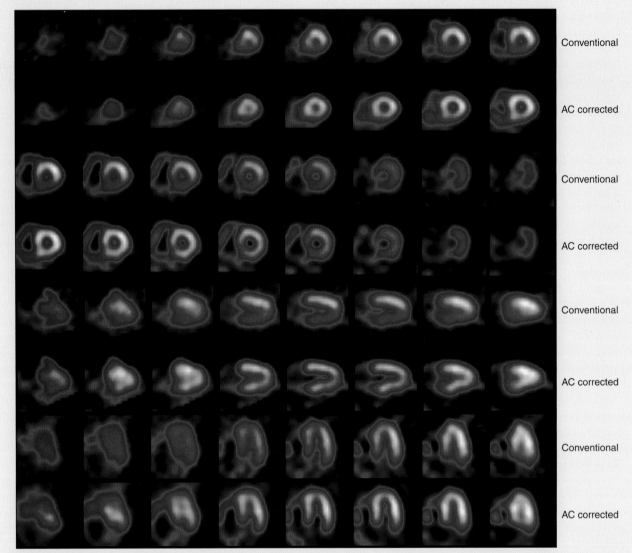

■ **Figure 2-13** Stress images without *(top)* and with attenuation correction *(bottom)* in a patient with atypical angina. There is mild inferior attenuation that is normalized by attenuation correction.

COMMENTS

The images are normal by visual and quantitative analysis and the regional and global LV functions are normal. The reader should remember that there are 2 sets of images (gated and non-gated) for rest and 2 sets (gated and non-gated) for stress. These 2 sets should not be mixed together because erroneous conclusions could be drawn on the presence and nature of perfusion defects. Also,

basal septal abnormality is a normal finding attributable to the membranous septum. Slight inferior abnormality is common and is seen on the stress and rest images due to diaphragmatic attenuation. The attenuation correction program nicely corrects this abnormality. Finally, the presence of normal motion and thickening in the inferior wall suggests the abnormality is due to attenuation artifact and not due to scar.

| Case 2-2 | **Abnormal Study** |

A 59-year-old woman presents with exertional dyspnea after an acute myocardial infarction a year earlier. She did not receive fibrinolytic therapy or coronary intervention at that time because of late arrival. She has no angina but did not have angina prior to the infarction either.

She is on appropriate medical therapy. Physical examination reveals enlarged heart but no evidence of volume overload. The ECG shows an old anterior myocardial infarction with Q-waves in V_1 to V_5. She exercised for 5 minutes and stopped because of shortness of breath. There were no ischemic ST changes. The SPECT sestamibi images are shown in Figure 2-14.

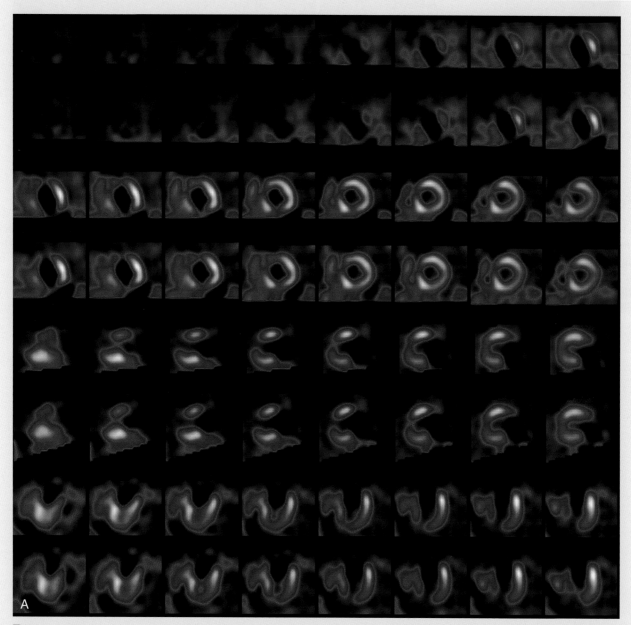

■ **Figure 2-14** Stress and rest gated SPECT sestamibi images **(A)**. There is a large fixed abnormality involving the distal anterior wall, septum, lateral wall, and apex. Although the defect involves the anterior wall, septum, apex, inferior wall, and lateral wall, it is still due to single-vessel LAD disease. There is evidence of LV aneurysm with divergence of the walls and black-hole sign. The LV cavity is dilated. The defect involves 56% of the LV myocardium. The 3D images at end-diastole and end-systole are shown in **B**. There is severe LV dysfunction. The dynamic images are shown in Video 2-2, A, B, for both the 3D and selected slices, respectively.

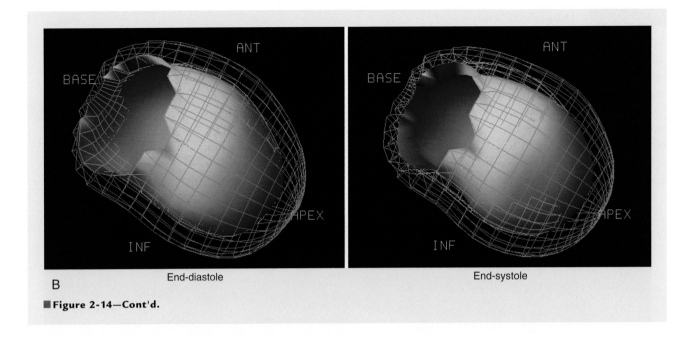

B   End-diastole   End-systole

■ **Figure 2-14—Cont'd.**

COMMENTS

The images show extensive scarring with evidence of aneurysm formation. In the days before gating, two signs were used for aneurysm detection; (1) parallel or diverging walls in the VLA or HLA projections as the LV loses the ellipse shape, and (2) black-hole sign, where the apex looks as if it is devoid of any activity and is of a similar intensity as the background. The reason is that there is a scatter of activity from the normal segments, especially during systole where the counts are higher. In the absence of any wall thickening, there is no scatter and, hence, no activity. With gating, it is easy to see dyskinesia. The aneurysm is three-dimensional and affects all adjacent walls and therefore may look like three-vessel disease but should be attributed to LAD disease alone.

Case 2-3   Stress Only Images

A 39-year-old man was referred for exercise testing because of lack of energy, fatigue, and shortness of breath on exertion. He had stenting of the RCA 1 year ago using a drug-eluting stent and is still on clopidogrel treatment. He exercised for 8 minutes on the Bruce protocol and stopped because of shortness of breath. He achieved his target heart rate. There were no ST changes. The SPECT images were acquired using a 12 mCi dose of Tc-99m sestamibi, 1 hour after the termination of exercise (Figure 2-15).

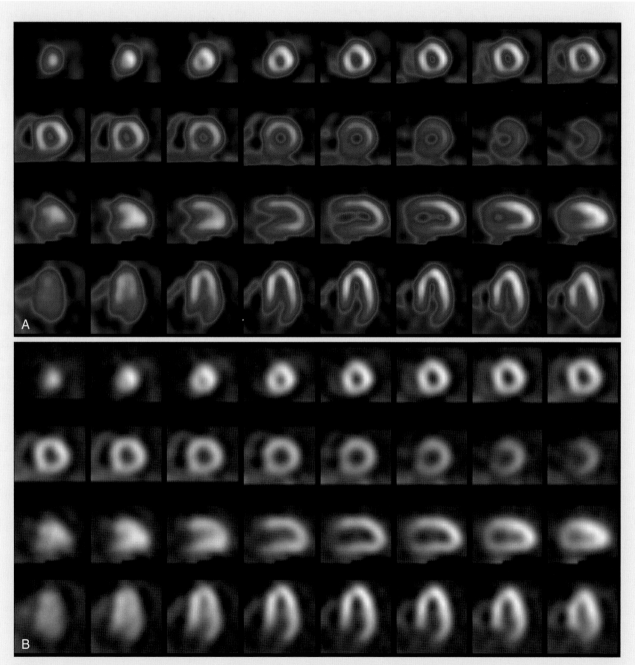

■**Figure 2-15** Normal stress-only images, in a color scale **(A)** and gray scale **(B)**. The polar maps and volume curve were also normal. The images are normal without attenuation correction, which indicates that attenuation correction is not a prerequisite for stress-only imaging.

COMMENTS

The stress images were reviewed and, because they were unequivocally normal, no rest study was acquired. Stress-only imaging provides convenience to the patient, decreases the radiation dose, and improves the laboratory throughput. We have used this option for more than 10 years. Patients with normal stress-only images have the same outcome as patients with normal images based on stress and rest studies. The images are normal without attenuation correction, which indicates that attenuation correction is not a prerequisite for stress-only imaging. Further, this patient had established CAD, which indicates stress-only imaging is not limited to low-risk patients.

Appendix 1

Summary of Stress ECG Report

The ECG response is negative for ischemia, or
The ECG response is positive for ischemia, or
The ECG response is non-diagnostic for ischemia because of baseline ECG abnormality, or
The ECG response is non-diagnostic for ischemia because of sub-maximal heart rate response (this is only with exercise or dobutamine).

Appendix 2

Summary of an Abnormal Gated SPECT Myocardial Perfusion Imaging Study

There is a large perfusion abnormality in the anterior wall, septum, and apex involving 30% of the LV myocardium. This abnormality is mostly reversible (25% ischemia and 5% scar).
There is regional wall motion and thickening abnormality in the poststress images involving the anterior wall but not in the rest images consistent with poststress stunning.
The LV EF is 69% in the rest images and 55% in the poststress images. There is transient LV dilatation consistent with a large ischemic burden.
Compared to the study performed on February 20, 2009, there has been considerable worsening of the perfusion pattern.
The right ventricular size and function are normal.

Appendix 3

Summary of a Normal Gated SPECT Myocardial Perfusion Imaging Study

The stress/rest (or stress) myocardial perfusion images are normal. The left ventricular size and function are normal with EF of 65%.
The right ventricular size and function are normal.

Appendix 4

Summary of a Viability Report Using Rest/Delayed Thallium and Stress Sestamibi

The initial thallium images show a large perfusion abnormality in the distal anterior wall and septum, the apex, and most of the inferior wall and inferolateral area. The abnormality involves 60% of the myocardium. Most of the abnormality is of moderate severity.
The 4-hr delayed images reveal redistribution in the anterior wall and septum.
The stress sestamibi images reveal much more severe and extensive abnormality.
The LV is moderately dilated with EF of 25% with abnormal motion and thickening, especially in the areas with perfusion defect.
The lung thallium uptake is increased consistent with elevated LV filling pressure.
The right ventricular size and function are normal.
These findings are consistent with 3-vessel disease and considerable viable myocardium and evidence of hibernation and the likelihood of benefit from coronary revascularization if target vessels are adequate.

SELECTED READINGS

DePace NL, Iskandrian AS, Nadell R, et al: Variation in the size of jeopardized myocardium in patients with isolated left anterior descending coronary artery disease, *Circulation* 67:988–994, 1983.

Hendel RC, Berman DS, Di Carli MF, et al: ACCF/ASNC/ACR/ AHA/ASE/SCCT/SCMR/SNM 2009 Appropriate Use Criteria for Cardiac Radionuclide Imaging: A Report of the American College of Cardiology Foundation Appropriate Use Criteria Task Force, the American Society of Nuclear Cardiology, the American College of Radiology, the American Heart Association, the American Society of Echocardiography, the Society of Cardiovascular Computed Tomography, the Society for Cardiovascular Magnetic Resonance, and the Society of Nuclear Medicine, *J Am Coll Cardiol* 53: 2201–2229, 2009.

Henzlova MJ, Cerqueira MD, Mahmarian JJ, et al: Stress protocols and tracers, *J Nucl Cardiol* 13:e80–e90, 2006.

Iskandrian AE: Stress-only myocardial perfusion imaging: a new paradigm, *J Am Coll Cardiol* 55:231–233, 2010.

Iskandrian AE, Garcia EV, editors: *Nuclear Cardiac Imaging: Principles and Applications*, ed 4, New York, 2008, Oxford University Press.

Iskandrian AE, Garcia EV, Faber T, et al: Automated assessment of serial SPECT myocardial perfusion images, *J Nucl Cardiol* 16:6–9, 2009.

Iskandrian AS, Lichtenberg R, Segal BL, et al: Assessment of jeopardized myocardium in patients with one-vessel disease, *Circulation* 65:242–247, 1982.

Ogilby JD, Iskandrian AS, Untereker WJ, et al: Effect of intravenous adenosine infusion on myocardial perfusion and function. Hemodynamic/angiographic and scintigraphic study, *Circulation* 86:887–895, 1992.

Shaw LJ, Iskandrian AE: Prognostic value of gated myocardial perfusion SPECT, *J Nucl Cardiol* 11:171–185, 2004.

Tilkemeier PL, Cooke CD, Ficaro EP, et al: American Society of Nuclear Cardiology information statement: standardized reporting matrix for radionuclide myocardial perfusion imaging, *J Nucl Cardiol* 13:e157–e171, 2006.

Zaret BL, Beller GA, editors: *Clinical nuclear cardiology: state of the art and future directions*, ed 4, Philadelphia, 2010, Mosby.

Chapter 3

Image Artifacts

E. Gordon DePuey

KEY POINTS

- Correct energy window position of the pulse height analyzer should be verified for each detector prior to SPECT acquisition.

- Maximal myocardial counts should be identified (usually by the computer) and the image display normalized to that value. In order to avoid normalization errors, appropriate time should be allowed for the radiotracer to be excreted from the liver. To avoid duodenogastric reflux of radiotracer, the patient should be instructed to drink water (at least 8 ounces) following radiotracer injection.

- The Ramp filter artifact occurs commonly with filtered backprojection tomographic reconstruction. Iterative reconstruction (ordered subset expectation maximization, [OSEM]) is useful to reduce this artifact. In order to avoid the Ramp filter artifact appropriate time should be allowed for the radiotracer to be excreted from the liver. This is particularly important for pharmacologic stress studies.

- Findings most consistent with photon attenuation by the left hemidiaphragm are an elevated left hemidiaphragm noted in planar projection images, a fixed inferior defect that appears to taper from the mid to basal portion of the ventricle, and normal wall motion and wall thickening.

- Findings most consistent with photon attenuation by the breasts are: a dense anterolateral breast "shadow" noted in planar projection images, a fixed anterolateral defect somewhat more severe in resting images, and normal wall motion and wall thickening. However, breast attenuation artifacts can vary depending on size and shape of the breast.

- In women with breast implants, which are more dense than soft tissue, associated attenuation artifacts extent tend to be smaller, more discrete, and more marked than breast attenuation artifacts caused by actual breasts.

- Attenuation correction, gated imaging, and prone imaging are helpful in interpreting studies with breast and/or diaphragmatic tissue attenuation.

- In patients with LVH, although there is generalized hypertrophy of the left ventricle, septal hypertrophy may be more marked. Therefore SPECT images demonstrate a relative increase in tracer concentration in the septum. Because tomograms are normalized to the region of myocardium with the highest count density, the septum appears relatively normal, and the remainder of the myocardium demonstrates relatively decreased count density. This is especially true in patients with end-stage renal disease who are on dialysis.

- Partial dose infiltration is one of several causes of suboptimal myocardial count density. To avoid "equivocal" interpretations of low count density scans, repeat imaging is appropriate.

- Incorrect ECG gating can occur for a number of reasons including: loose ECG leads, arrhythmias, or any cause of variability in the detected R-R time window.

Artifacts and normal variants are a significant source of false-positive interpretations of myocardial perfusion SPECT. By anticipating and recognizing such findings, the astute technologist and interpreting physician can increase test specificity in the diagnosis of coronary artery disease and avoid unnecessary catheterization of normal patients.

Case 3-1   Off-Peak Detector (Figure 3-1)

A 60-year-old man had atypical chest pain and no prior cardiac history. Technetium-99m sestamibi myocardial perfusion SPECT was performed using a single-day rest (9 mCi)/stress (32 mCi) protocol. The resting ECG was normal. The patient experienced no chest pain and there were no electrocardiographic changes during treadmill exercise. SPECT images were acquired using a 90-degree–angled dual-head camera and a 180-degree imaging arc from the 45-degree LPO projection to the 45-degree RAO projection. Therefore images from the 45-degree LPO projection to the 45-degree LAO projection, acquired with detector No. 1, are of good spatial resolution, whereas those images from the 45-degree LAO projection to the 45-degree RAO projection, acquired with detector No. 2, are of poor spatial resolution.

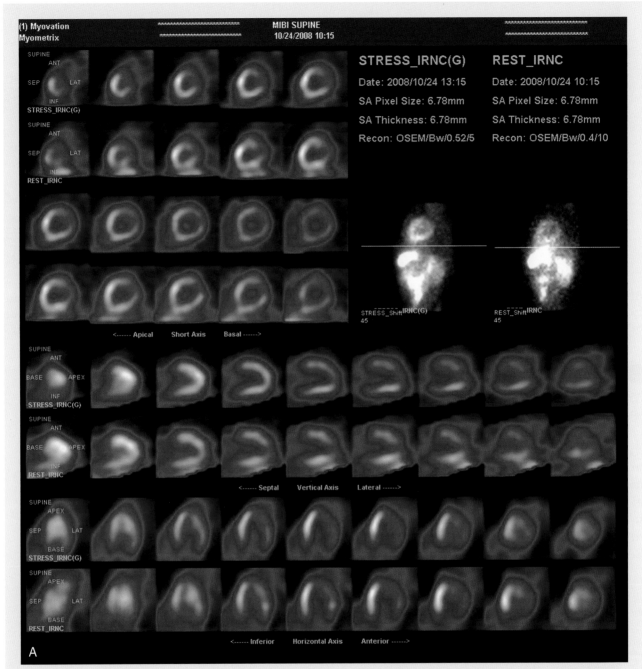

■**Figure 3-1 A,** Planar projection images from detector No. 1 *(top right grey level images)* from both the poststress and resting acquisitions demonstrate good spatial resolution. In the left lateral projection, the left ventricle is well defined with a good target-to-background ratio.

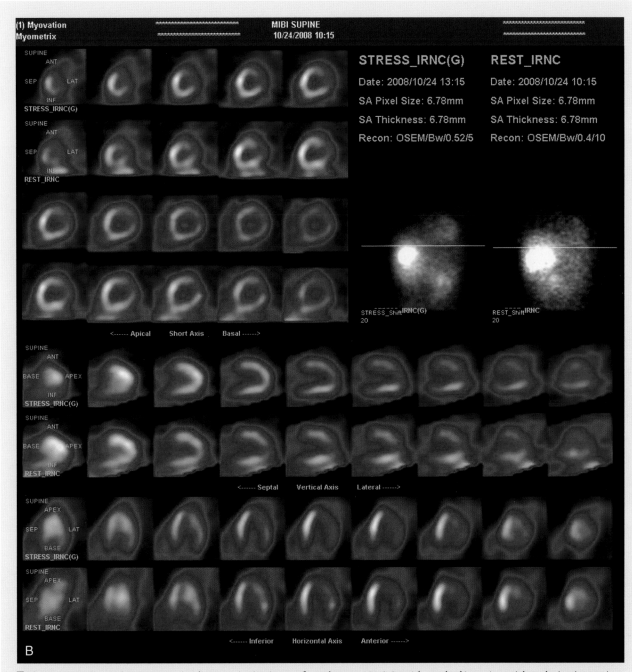

■ Figure 3-1—Cont'd B, However, in planar projection images from detector No. 2 *(top right grey level images)*, spatial resolution is poor in both the poststress and resting images. In the anterior view, the left ventricle is poorly defined and there is poor delineation of extracardiac structures. These findings are characteristic of incorrect camera energy peaking. It appears that the energy peak is too low, detecting primarily low energy, scattered photons.

(Continued)

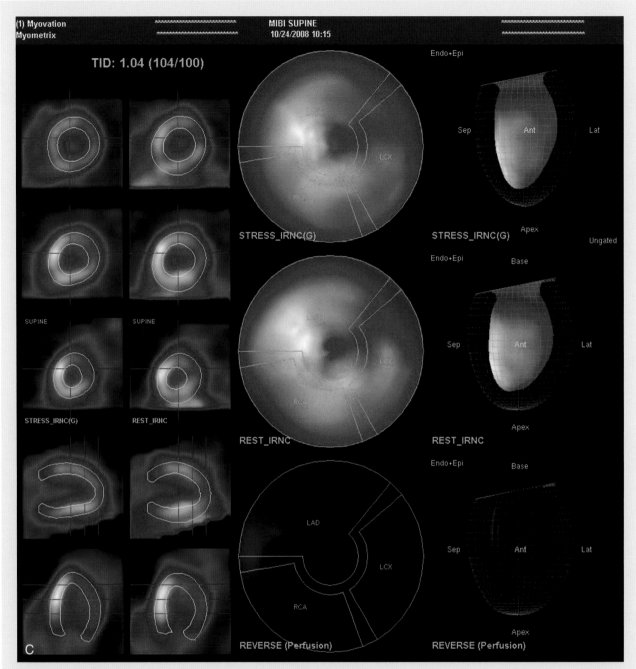

■ **Figure 3-1—Cont'd C,** In reconstructed tomographic images and polar plots, there is a moderately extensive, moderately severe fixed defect in the lateral wall of the left ventricle. However, gated poststress tomograms demonstrate normal global and regional wall motion, including that of the lateral wall. **C** is accompanied by dynamic displays (Video 3-1).

COMMENTS

The fixed lateral wall defect is likely secondary to SPECT reconstruction, which includes projection images of poor spatial resolution during one half of the acquisition. Considering the patient's history and normal regional LV function, lateral wall myocardial scarring is very unlikely. Prior to SPECT acquisition, correct energy window position of the pulse height analyzer should be verified. A 10%-15% symmetrical window should be centered on the 140-keV technetium-99m photopeak. For most cameras the selected energy window is automatically applied simultaneously to both detectors. In this case, however, there was a camera software error that failed to apply the selected energy window to detector No. 2.

| Case 3-2 | Normalization Error (Figure 3-2) |

A 56-year-old woman with risk factors for CAD and atypical chest pain underwent a single-day, low-dose (9 mCi)/high-dose (32 mCi) technetium-99m sestamibi scan. During treadmill exercise the patient experienced no chest pain and there were no ECG abnormalities.

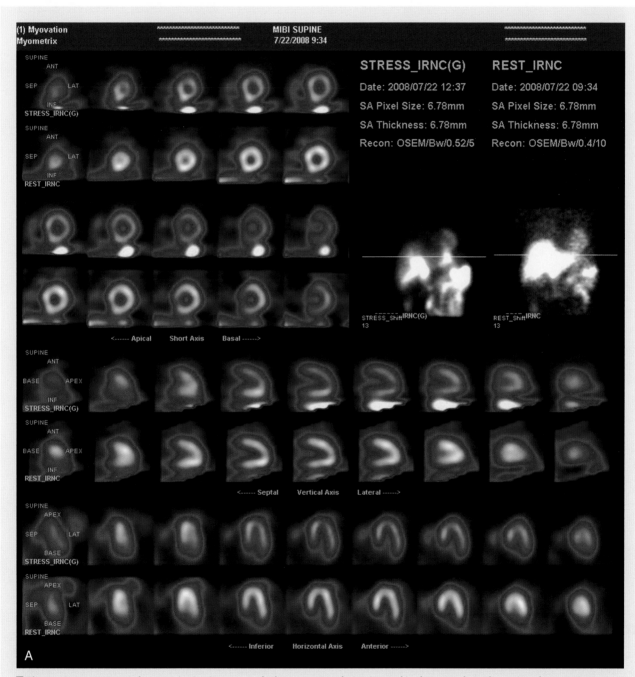

■ **Figure 3-2 A,** In stress planar projection images, marked tracer accumulation is noted in the stomach. In the resting planar projection images, although there is moderate tracer concentration in the liver, no accumulation is noted in the stomach. The LV cavity of both the planar projections and oblique tomograms also appears larger at stress than at rest (transient ischemic dilatation). However, these artifactual findings are due to incorrect normalization of the stress images to the intense tracer concentration in the stomach (activity excreted from the liver via the biliary tract into the duodenum with reflux into the stomach), rendering the LV myocardium relatively less intense and making the LV cavity appear larger at stress.

(Continued)

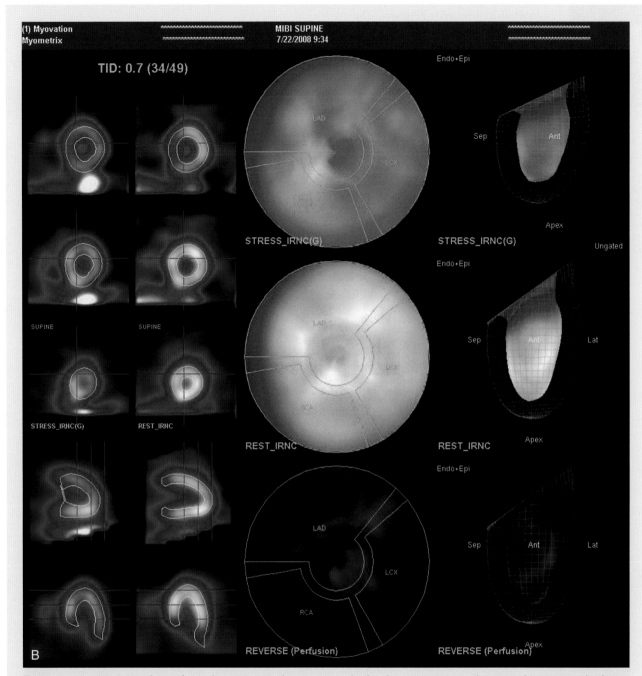

■ **Figure 3-2—Cont'd B,** This artifact is also apparent in the reconstructed polar plots. In reconstructed tomographic images and polar plots, it appears that there is a generalized decrease in tracer concentration in the myocardium in the stress images compared to the resting images, mimicking "stress-induced global ischemia."

COMMENTS

The various commercially available software programs used to process myocardial perfusion SPECT normalize reconstructed tomograms by different means. Preferably, maximal myocardial counts should be identified and the images normalized to that value. If instead the image is normalized to the entire frame or reconstructed volume, the maximal pixel counts in the entire frame will be chosen for normalization. If that pixel is outside of the myocardium (i.e., the stomach, bowel, or liver), the myocardium will be assigned a lower intensity value, as in the present case example. To correctly view and interpret reconstructed tomograms under these circumstances, the interpreting physician must arbitrarily increase the intensity of the images in which the normalization error occurred. This must be done carefully to avoid obscuring (overintensifying) actual perfusion abnormalities. In order to avoid normalization errors, appropriate time should be allowed for the radiotracer to be excreted from the liver. To avoid duodenogastric reflux of radiotracer, the patient should be instructed to drink water (at least 8 ounces) after radiotracer injection.

Case 3-3   Compton Scatter Image Degradation (Figure 3-3)

A 60-year-old woman had multiple risk factors for CAD and atypical angina. The patient underwent dual-isotope myocardial perfusion SPECT, receiving 3.5 mCi of thallium-201 at rest and subsequently 30.0 mCi of technetium-99m sestamibi during dipyridamole pharmacologic stress. The stress tomographic images are slightly suboptimal for interpretation due to Compton scatter into the inferoapical region. The resting images are inadequate for interpretation due to marked Compton scatter into the inferior wall.

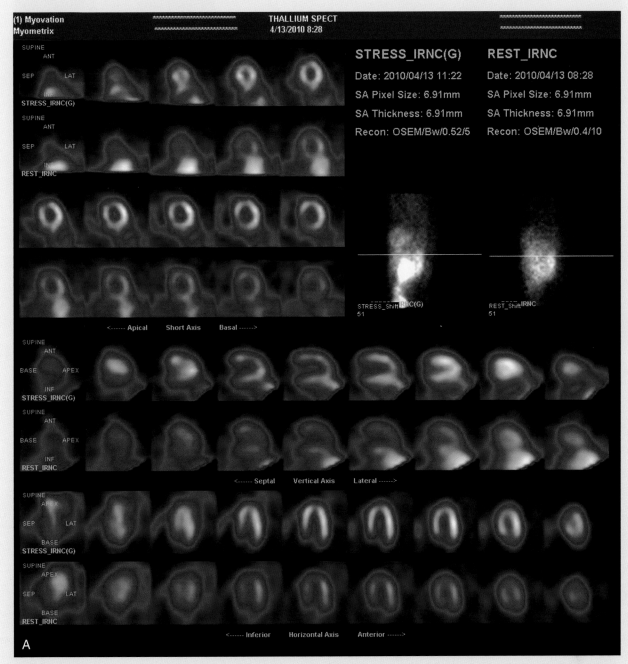

■ **Figure 3-3 A,** Both the stress and rest planar projection images demonstrate considerable subdiaphragmatic radiotracer concentration. In the reconstructed tomographic images, there is moderate subdiaphragmatic tracer concentration in the technetium-99m sestamibi stress images, probably localized to the stomach. In the resting thallium-201 reconstructed images, subdiaphragmatic tracer concentration is much more marked and extensive, also most likely localized to the stomach. The subdiaphragmatic activity appears to "overlap" the inferior wall of the left ventricle, resulting in a relative increase in count density in the inferior wall.

(Continued)

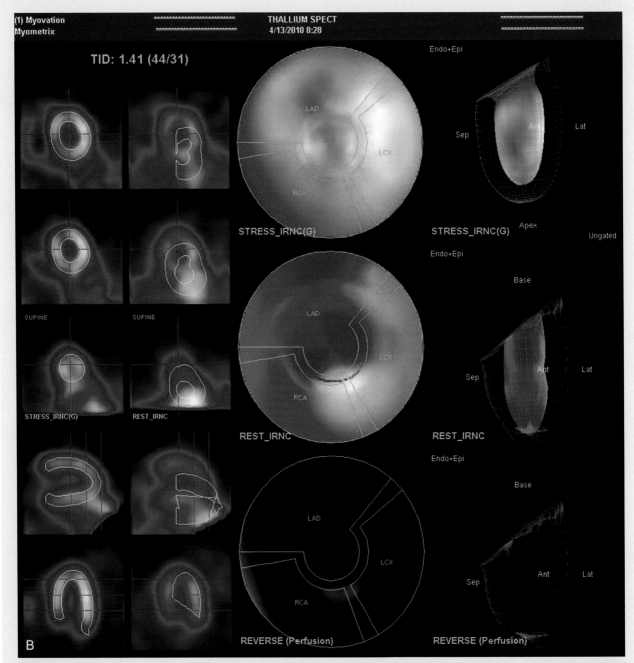

■ **Figure 3-3—Cont'd B,** The resting polar plot is incorrectly normalized to the intense "overlapping" subdiaphragmatic activity. Error is also introduced in quantitative endocardial edge detection, which "misinterprets" the subdiaphragmatic activity as the inferior wall of the left ventricle.

COMMENTS

The phenomenon shown in Figure 3-3 is due to Compton scatter of photons emanating from subdiaphragmatic activity. In the process of Compton scattering, these scattered photons have not lost enough energy to be eliminated by the energy windows positioned over the 68- to 80-keV Hg-201 mercury x-ray of thallium-201 or the 140-keV photon of technetium-99m, respectively. Therefore, as the scattered photons pass through the parallel-hole collimator, they are accepted by the pulse height analyzer and superimposed upon the inferior wall of the LV.

Because reconstructed myocardial tomograms are normalized to the area of greatest count density, in this case they are normalized to the artifactually intense inferior wall, resulting in a relative decrease in count density in the contralateral anterior wall. In this particular case example, this artifact is more marked in the resting thallium-201 tomograms than in the stress technetium-99m sestamibi tomograms.

To avoid normalization errors and endocardial edge-tracking errors, as present in this case example, appropriate time should be allowed for the radiotracer to be excreted from the liver. To avoid duodenogastric reflux of radiotracer, the patient should be instructed to drink water (at least 8 ounces) after radiotracer injection.

Case 3-4   Ramp Filter Artifact (Figure 3-4)

A 62-year-old man had multiple risk factors for CAD and nonanginal chest pains. The patient had no history of prior MI, and his resting ECG was normal. The patient underwent a single-day, low-dose (9 mCi)/high-dose (32 mCi) technetium-99m sestamibi scan. During dipyridamole pharmacologic vasodilatation, the patient experienced no chest pain and there were no ECG abnormalities.

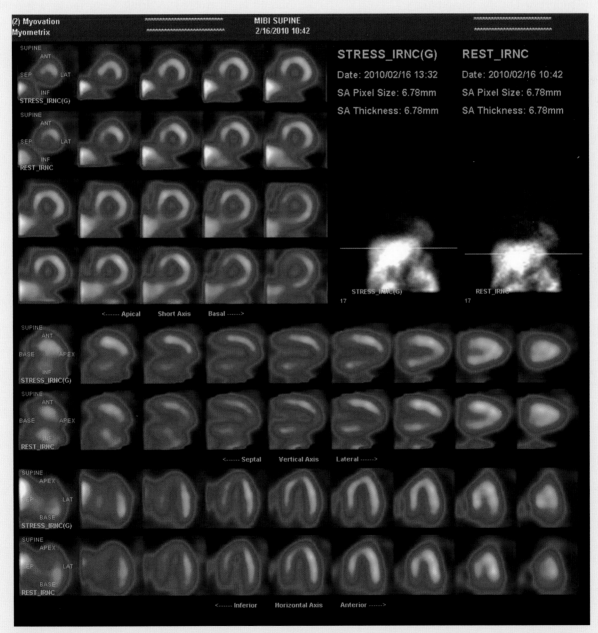

■ **Figure 3-4** In both the stress and rest planar projection images, there is considerable radiotracer accumulation in the liver. The right hemidiaphragm is mildly elevated, with the superior portion of the right lobe of the liver in the x-plane of the inferior wall of the left ventricle. In this plane, there is a fixed inferoapical perfusion defect. Video 3-2 shows gated tomographic images demonstrating normal LV wall motion and wall thickening, including that of the inferoapical portion of the left ventricle in the distribution of the fixed perfusion defect described above.

COMMENTS

In this case example the fixed inferoapical defect is most likely secondary to a Ramp filter artifact. After the process of filtered backprojection used to reconstruct planar projection images into tomograms, the Ramp filter is routinely applied to minimize/eliminate the "star artifact" caused by reconstruction of a finite number of projection images. By this means the Ramp filter suppresses counts immediately adjacent to "hot" objects/structures. The Ramp filter operates primarily in the x-plane. Therefore counts in the inferoapical wall of the LV in the same x-plane as the intense activity in the dome of the right lobe of the liver are suppressed by the Ramp filter.

The Ramp filter artifact occurs commonly with filtered backprojection tomographic reconstruction. Iterative reconstruction (ordered subset expectation maximization, [OSEM]) is useful to minimize the Ramp filter artifact. However, although in the present case example images were reconstructed using OSEM, the Ramp filter artifact is still present.

To avoid the Ramp filter artifact, appropriate time should be allowed for the radiotracer to be excreted from the liver. This is particularly important for pharmacologic stress studies, for which poststress radiotracer concentration is more marked than with exercise. To avoid duodenogastric reflux of radiotracer into the stomach, which also may lie in the x-plane of the inferior wall, the patient should be instructed to drink water (at least 8 ounces) after radiotracer injection.

Case 3-5   **Diaphagmatic Attenuation (Figure 3-5)**

A 45-year-old man with atypical angina underwent a single-day, low-dose (9 mCi)/
high-dose (32 mCi) technetium-99m sestamibi scan. During peak treadmill exercise,
the patient experienced no chest pain and there were no ECG abnormalities.

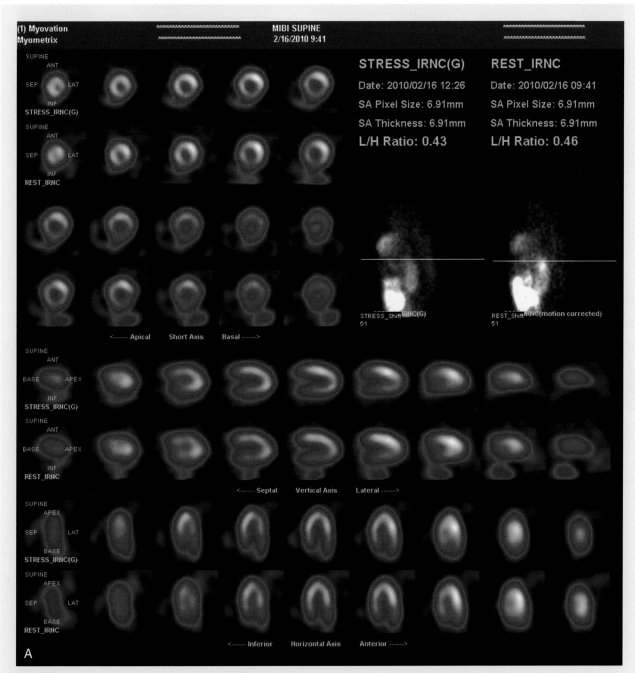

■ **Figure 3-5 A,** In planar projection images viewed in the left lateral/left posterior oblique view, the left hemidiaphragm is noted to be
moderately elevated, evidenced by a curvilinear "shadow" partially "eclipsing" the inferior wall of the left ventricle. Tomographic images
demonstrate a fixed, moderately severe decrease in tracer concentration in the basal one third/one half of the inferior wall of the left ventricle.
Note that the inferior wall appears to "taper" from the mid to basal portions of the ventricle. Findings are identical in the stress and rest
projection images and polar plots.

(Continued)

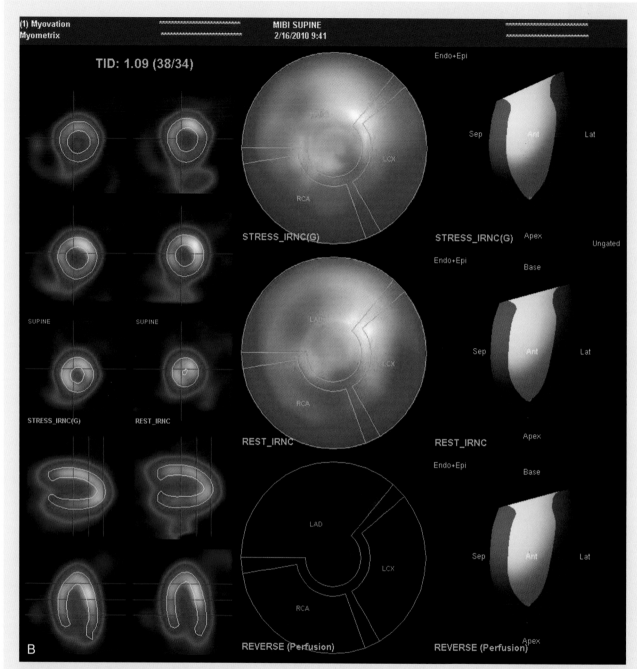

Figure 3-5—Cont'd B, Polar plots also demonstrate a progressive decrease in tracer concentration from the mid to basal portion of the inferior wall in the stress and rest images.

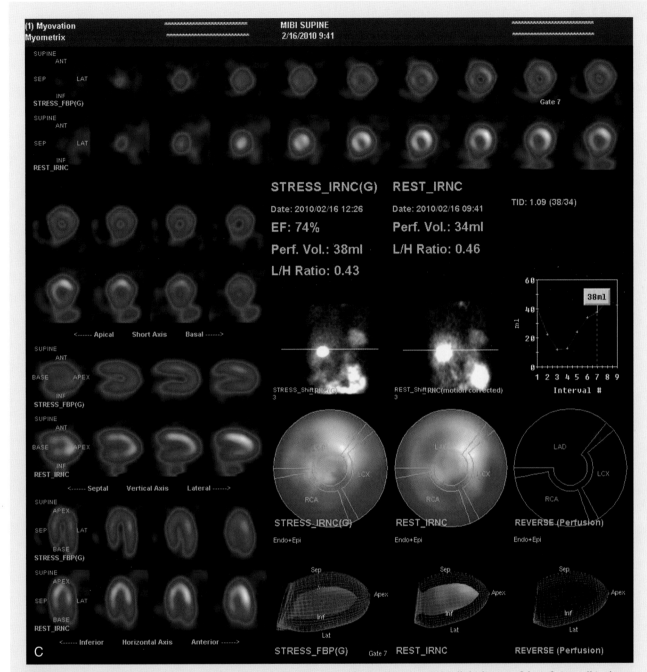

■ **Figure 3-5—Cont'd C,** Gated tomographic images demonstrate normal LV wall motion and wall thickening of the inferior wall in the distribution of the fixed inferior defect. **C** is accompanied by a dynamic display (Video 3-3).

COMMENTS

A combination of an elevated left hemidiaphragm noted in planar projection images, a fixed inferior defect that appears to taper from the mid to basal portion of the LV, and normal wall motion and wall thickening are findings most consistent with photon attenuation by the left hemidiaphragm (see Figure 3-5). Attenuation correction, upright imaging, and prone imaging are additional means to differentiate diaphragmatic attenuation from myocardial scarring as the cause of a fixed inferior defect.

Case 3-6   Breast Attenuation (Figure 3-6)

A 67-year-old woman with multiple coronary risk factors but no history of chest pain or prior MI underwent a single-day, low-dose (9 mCi)/high-dose (32 mCi) technetium-99m sestamibi scan. During peak treadmill exercise the patient experienced no chest pain and there were no ECG abnormalities.

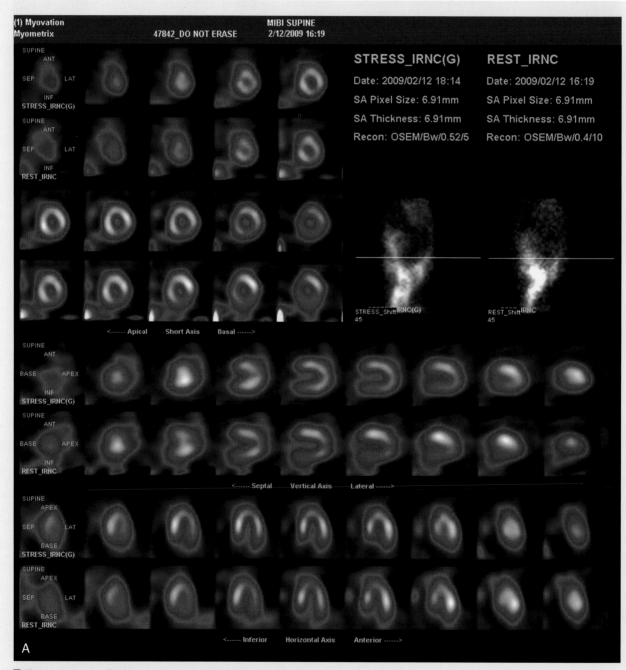

■ **Figure 3-6 A,** In planar projection images viewed in the left lateral/left posterior oblique view, a "shadow" from the patient's dense, pendulous left breast is noted partially "eclipsing" the inferior/inferoposterior wall of the left ventricle as well as the adjacent structures of the abdomen. Note that findings are identical in the stress and rest projection images. Tomographic images demonstrate a fixed, moderate decrease in tracer concentration in the inferolateral wall of the left ventricle. This finding is particularly abnormal in a female. Normally, in women, due to the usual anterior location of the breast, the count density of the anterior wall is equivalent to or somewhat less than that of the inferior/inferolateral wall.

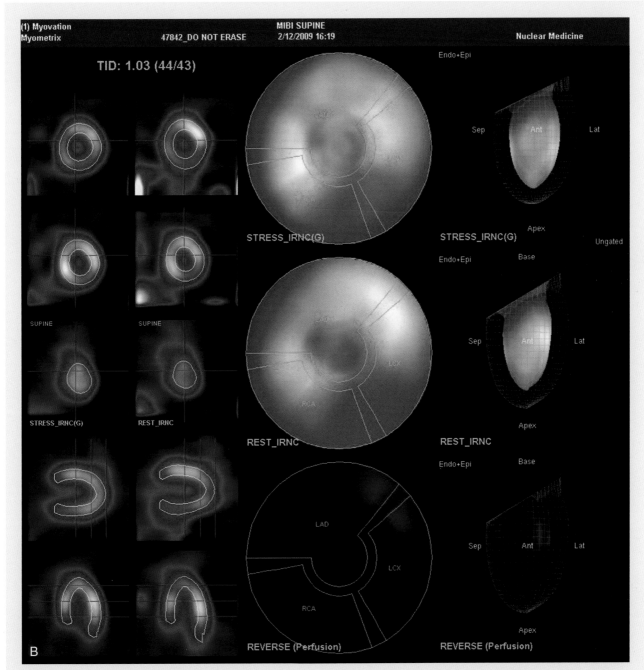

■ Figure 3-6—Cont'd B, Polar plots also demonstrate a fixed, moderately severe inferolateral defect. Upon careful inspection of these images, the inferolateral defect is slightly more marked in the resting images than in the poststress images. This pattern of "pseudo-reverse distribution" is characteristic of attenuation artifacts in low-dose rest/high-dose stress single-day protocol is performed with Tc-99m–labeled radiopharmaceuticals.

(Continued)

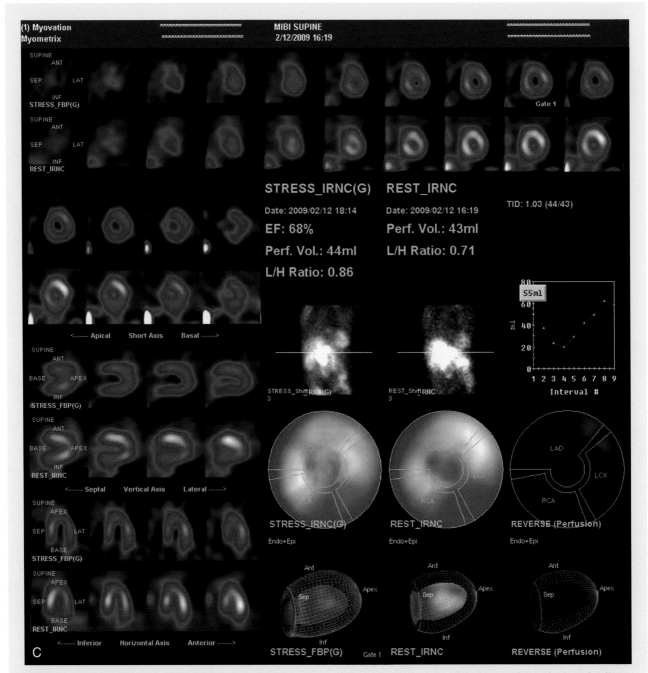

■ **Figure 3-6—Cont'd C,** Gated tomographic images demonstrate normal LV wall motion and wall thickening of the inferolateral wall in the distribution of the fixed defect. **A** and **C** are accompanied by dynamic displays (Video 3-4).

COMMENTS

A combination of a dense inferolateral breast "shadow" noted in planar projection images, a fixed inferolateral defect somewhat more severe in resting images, and normal wall motion and wall thickening are findings most consistent with breast photon attenuation artifact (see Figure 3-6). Breast attenuation artifacts are most commonly localized to the anterior/anterolateral wall. However, in women with large, pendulous breasts, inferolateral artifacts, as noted in this case example, are common. Of note, with semisitting and upright imaging, the breasts become more pendulous,

so inferior/inferolateral attenuation artifacts are encountered more commonly.

The planar projection images, displayed in endless-loop cinematic format, should always be inspected to ascertain the position of the left breast, its consistency in position in the stress versus rest images, and degree of associated photon attenuation.

Attenuation correction is helpful to minimize/eliminate the effect of breast attenuation. Gated imaging is helpful to differentiate breast attenuation artifact from myocardial scarring as the cause of a fixed defect.

Case 3-7   **Breast Implants (Figure 3-7)**

A 56-year-old woman had multiple coronary risk factors but no history of chest pain or prior MI. The patient had received bilateral breast implants five years previously. The patient underwent a single-day, low-dose (9 mCi)/high-dose (32 mCi) technetium-99m sestamibi scan. During peak treadmill exercise, the patient experienced no chest pain and there were no ECG abnormalities.

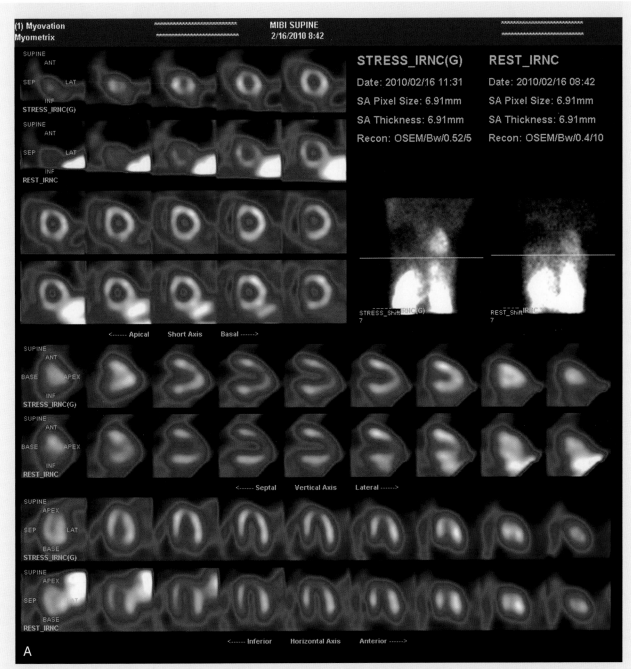

■ **Figure 3-7 A,** In planar projection images viewed in the left lateral/left posterior oblique view, a discrete, round "shadow" from the patient's left breast implant is noted partially "eclipsing" the anterior wall of the left ventricle. In addition, a similar round "shadow" is noted over the right chest wall. Note that findings are identical in the stress and rest projection images. Tomographic images demonstrate a fixed, moderate decrease in tracer concentration in the anterior wall of the left ventricle.

(Continued)

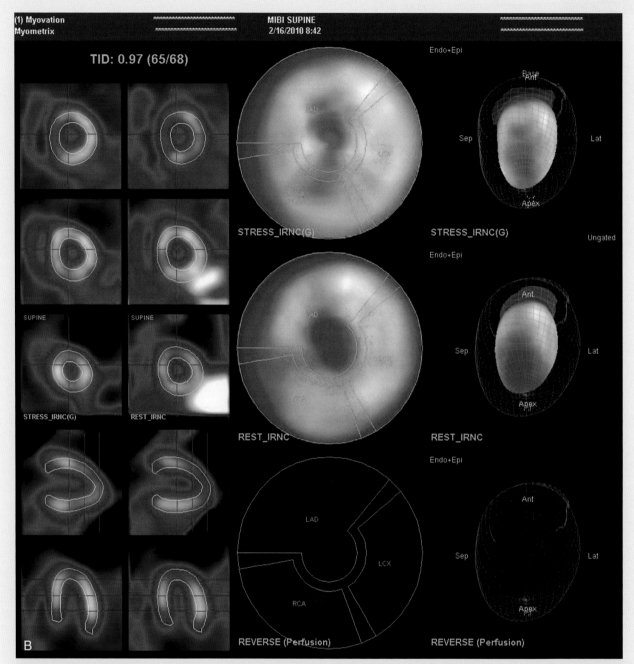

■**Figure 3-7—Cont'd B,** Polar plots also demonstrate a fixed, localized, moderately severe anterior defect. Gated tomographic images demonstrate normal LV wall motion and wall thickening, including that of the anterior wall in the distribution of the fixed defect. Dynamic displays accompany these figures (Video 3-5).

COMMENTS

A combination of a dense, round, anterior "shadow" caused by the breast implant noted in planar projection images, a fixed anterior perfusion defect, and normal wall motion and wall thickening are findings most consistent with a photon attenuation artifact secondary to a breast implant or prosthesis (see Figure 3-7). Physiologic breast attenuation artifacts are most commonly localized to the anterior/anterolateral wall. However, in women with breast implants, which are more dense than soft tissue, associated attenuation artifacts tend to be smaller, more discrete, and more marked than breast attenuation artifacts caused by actual breasts. Patients should always be questioned prior to imaging about a history of breast implants or prostheses.

Attenuation correction is helpful to differentiate breast attenuation artifact from myocardial scarring as the cause of a fixed defect. Gated imaging is also helpful to differentiate breast attenuation artifact from myocardial scarring as the cause of a fixed defect.

Case 3-8 Small Breasts (Figure 3-8)

A 73-year-old woman had atypical chest pain and multiple risk factors for CAD.
The patient is 5 foot 6 inches tall, 116 pounds, with a bra cup size of 36A.
The patient underwent a single-day, low-dose (9 mCi)/high-dose (32 mCi)
technetium-99m sestamibi scan. She performed treadmill exercise using the Bruce
protocol, and achieved 90% of her age-predicted maximum heart rate with no chest
pain and no ECG changes.

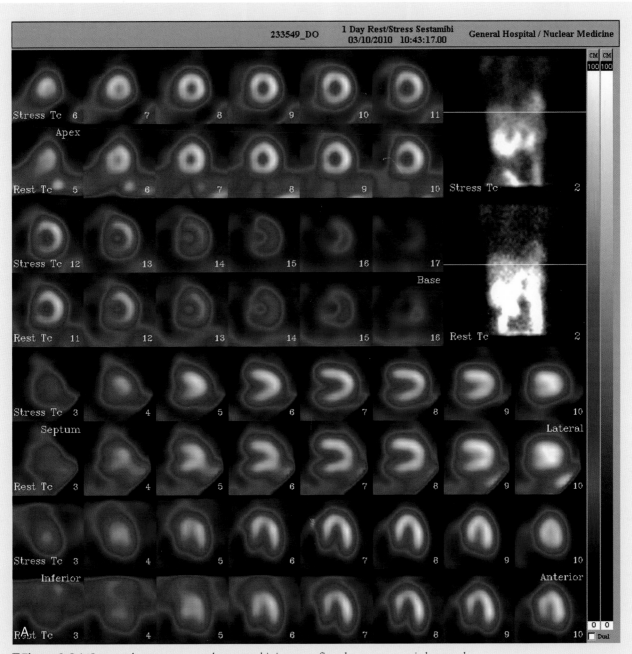

■ **Figure 3-8 A,** Stress and rest reconstructed tomographic images at first glance appear entirely normal.

(Continued)

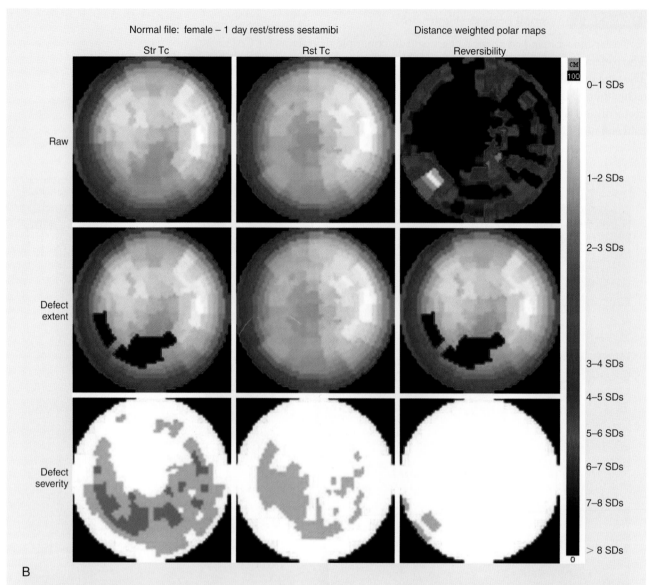

B

■ **Figure 3-8—Cont'd B,** However, by quantitative analysis (Emory Toolbox) of reconstructed polar plots, whereby patient data are compared to normal female files, an inferior perfusion abnormality is evident.

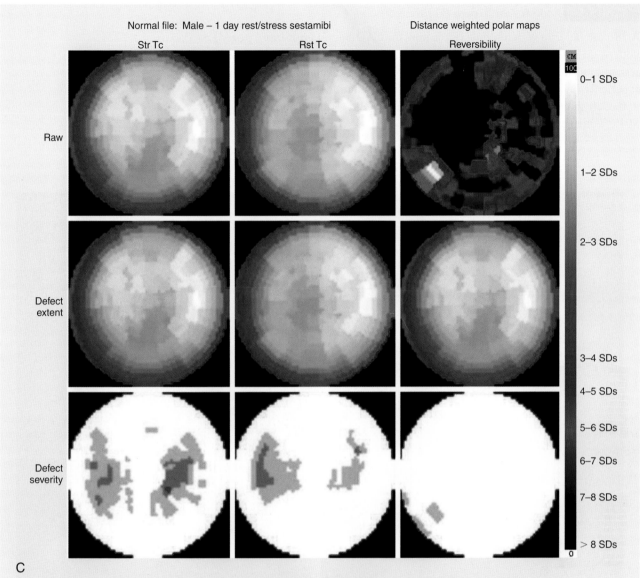

Normal file: Male – 1 day rest/stress sestamibi   Distance weighted polar maps

Str Tc   Rst Tc   Reversibility

Raw

Defect extent

Defect severity

0–1 SDs
1–2 SDs
2–3 SDs
3–4 SDs
4–5 SDs
5–6 SDs
6–7 SDs
7–8 SDs
> 8 SDs

C

■ **Figure 3-8—Cont'd C,** Considering the patient's lack of breast attenuation, data were compared instead to the normal *male* file. Quantitatively the scan is normal, and the inferior quantitative defect is no longer present. Poststress gated imaging (not shown) demonstrated normal wall motion and systolic LV function.

COMMENTS

With a mild fixed inferior defect and associated normal wall motion and thickening, the scan was interpreted as normal. Quantitative analysis compares patient data to gender-matched normal limits. For the various commercially available quantitative analysis software programs, normal female files are derived from women with "average"-sized breasts (bra cup about B–C). Due to physiologic breast attenuation in these subjects, normal female files anticipate some degree of anterior wall attenuation by the left breast, counterbalancing inferior wall attenuation by the left hemidiaphragm. Therefore, in normal female files, anterior and inferior wall count densities are approximately equivalent, or the anterior wall may have slightly lower count density than the inferior wall.

However, for women with very small breasts, such as the patient in this case example, or for women who have undergone left mastectomy, there is minimal attenuation of anterior counts. Therefore, anterior wall count density is greater than that of the inferior wall, which is physiologically attenuated by the left hemidiaphragm. Because of the relative decrease in inferior count density in these patients, the inferior wall is determined to be "abnormal" by quantitative analysis.

Therefore, for women who have undergone left mastectomy, patient data should be compared to a normal *male* file instead of a normal female file. In general, for women with small breasts, a normal female file is still used for quantitative analysis, but the interpreting physician should be aware of the potential for "false-positive" quantitative results in the inferior wall in such patients.

| Case 3-9 | Left Arm Down (Figure 3-9) |

A 78-year-old man with multiple risk factors for CAD but no prior history of MI underwent a single-day, low-dose (9 mCi)/high-dose (32 mCi) technetium-99m sestamibi scan. During dipyridamole pharmacologic vasodilatation, the patient experienced no chest pain and there were no ECG abnormalities. Due to arthritis in the left shoulder, the patient was unable to elevate the left arm above the head for SPECT image acquisition.

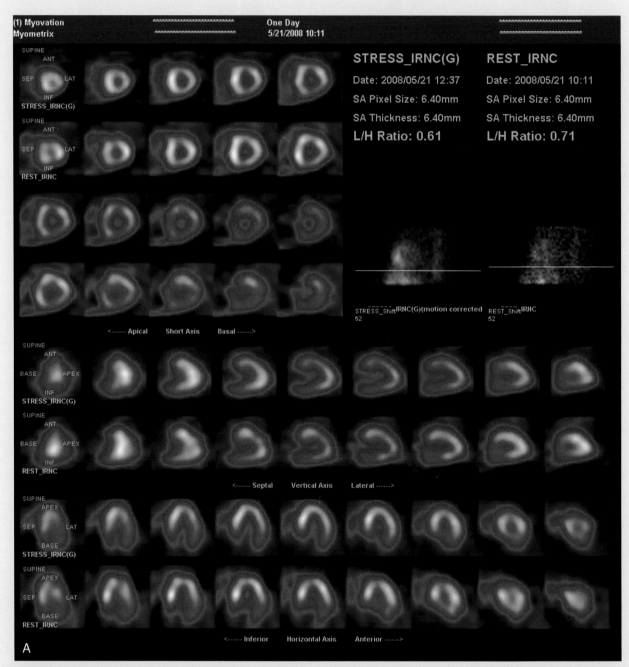

■ **Figure 3-9 A,** In both the stress and rest planar projection images, a vertical left arm "shadow" is noted, "eclipsing" the basal lateral and inferior wall of the left ventricle. Note that the position of the left arm is consistent in the stress and rest images. In tomographic short-axis and vertical long-axis images, a moderate-to-severe fixed defect is noted in the basal inferior wall.

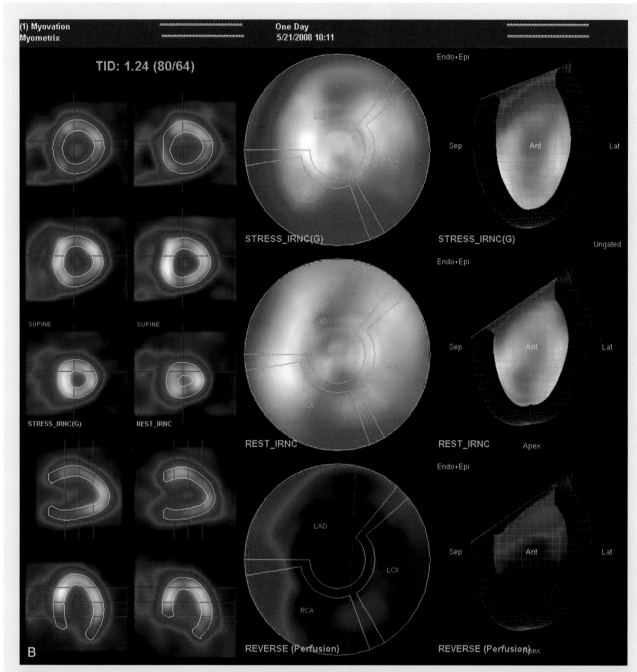

■ Figure 3-9—Cont'd B, The defect is also clearly delineated in the polar maps. Gated tomographic images demonstrate normal regional LV wall motion and wall thickening of the basal inferior wall. **A** and **B** are accompanied by dynamic displays (Video 3-6).

COMMENTS

Since the fixed basal inferior perfusion defect with normal regional and wall thickening is in the distribution of the overlying left arm, the finding was attributed to an attenuation artifact, and the scan was interpreted as normal.

SPECT imaging with the left arm down at the patient's side is discouraged due to attenuation artifacts, as noted in this case example. If the patient is indeed unable to elevate the left arm, if possible, the left arm should be positioned as posteriorly as possible to minimize attenuation of the left ventricle. Importantly, the position of the left arm should be consistent for stress and rest SPECT image acquisitions. The arm should never be positioned over the left chest wall. If the left arm cannot be elevated or positioned posteriorly and if attenuation correction is not available, planar imaging is recommended as an alternative to SPECT.

Case 3-10   **RV Insertion Site (Figure 3-10)**

A 55-year-old woman with multiple risk factors for CAD but no prior history of
MI underwent a single-day, low-dose (9 mCi)/high-dose (32 mCi) technetium-99m
sestamibi scan. During dipyridamole pharmacologic vasodilatation, the patient
experienced no chest pain and there were no ECG abnormalities.

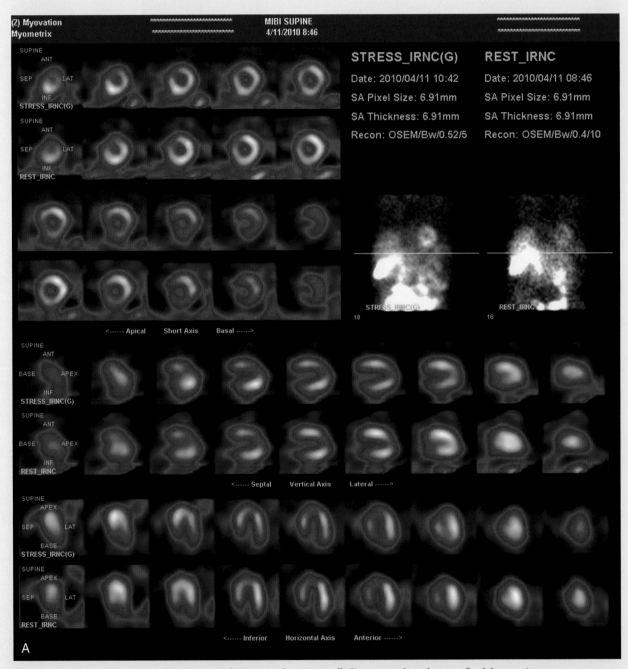

■ **Figure 3-10 A,** In the stress and rest tomographic images, there is a small, discrete, moderately severe focal decrease in tracer
concentration in the distal anteroseptal wall of the left ventricle. A corresponding abnormality is noted in the vertical long-axis tomograms.
Otherwise, tracer distribution is normal. Viewing the planar projection images in endless-loop cinematic format, the patient's left breast is
noted to overlay the anterior and anterolateral walls of the left ventricle; therefore, the fixed anteroseptal defect cannot be attributed to breast
attenuation.

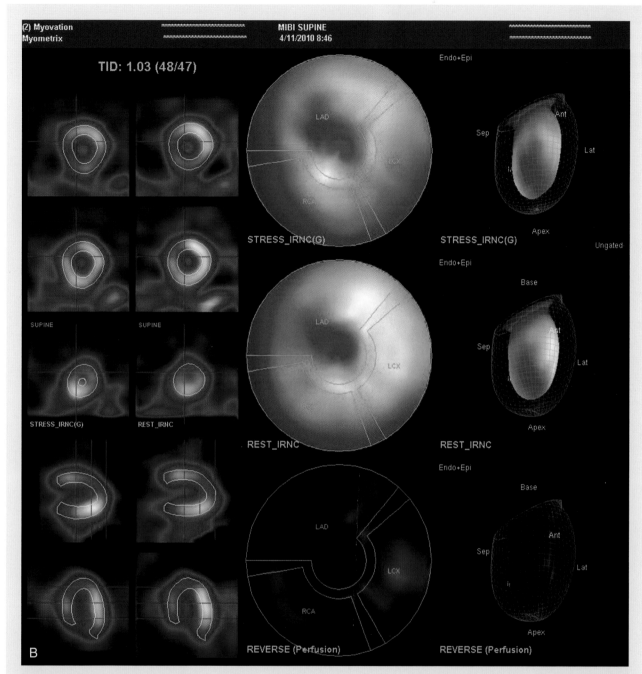

■ **Figure 3-10—Cont'd B,** The fixed defect is demonstrated clearly on polar maps and three-dimensional reconstructed tomographic images. Gated tomographic imaging demonstrates normal wall motion and wall thickening, including that of the anteroseptal wall. **A** and **B** are accompanied by dynamic displays (Video 3-7).

COMMENTS

The scan was interpreted as normal. The discrete, fixed anteroseptal defect was attributed to a normal variant at the site of the insertion of the anterior free wall of the right ventricle.

This finding, often termed the "11 o'clock defect," represents a common normal variant. The cause of the perfusion defect, however, is not known. "Cleftlike" localized defects are frequently observed at 11 o'clock and 7 o'clock in the short-axis tomograms immediately adjacent to the sites of insertion of the anterior and inferior free walls of the right ventricle, respectively. Although it is not entirely possible to exclude myocardial scarring as a cause of these defects, is less likely in the presence of normal regional wall motion. Moreover, the "11 o'clock defect" is not likely be due to a breast attenuation artifact since the breasts usually lie anterolaterally when female patients are in the supine position.

Case 3-11   LV Hypertrophy With "Hot" Septum (Figure 3-11)

A 52-year-old man had a long-standing history of hypertension and renal insufficiency. There was no prior history of MI. The patient underwent a single-day, low-dose (9 mCi)/high-dose (32 mCi) technetium-99m sestamibi scan. During peak treadmill exercise, the patient experienced no chest pain. The resting ECG demonstrated LV hypertrophy and nonspecific ST-T wave abnormalities. No S-T segment depression beyond baseline was present during treadmill exercise.

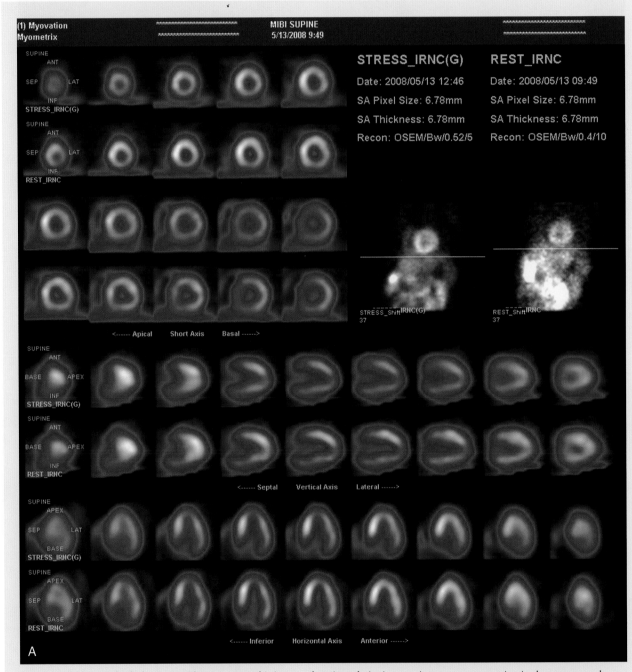

■ **Figure 3-11 A,** In both the stress and rest tomographic images, there is a relative increase in tracer concentration in the septum, and consequently a corresponding relative decrease in concentration throughout the remainder of the left ventricle, most notably in the lateral wall. Viewing the planar projection images in endless-loop cinematic format, no significant attenuation by left lateral chest wall soft tissue is present. Therefore the apparent fixed lateral defect cannot be attributed to chest wall soft tissue attenuation.

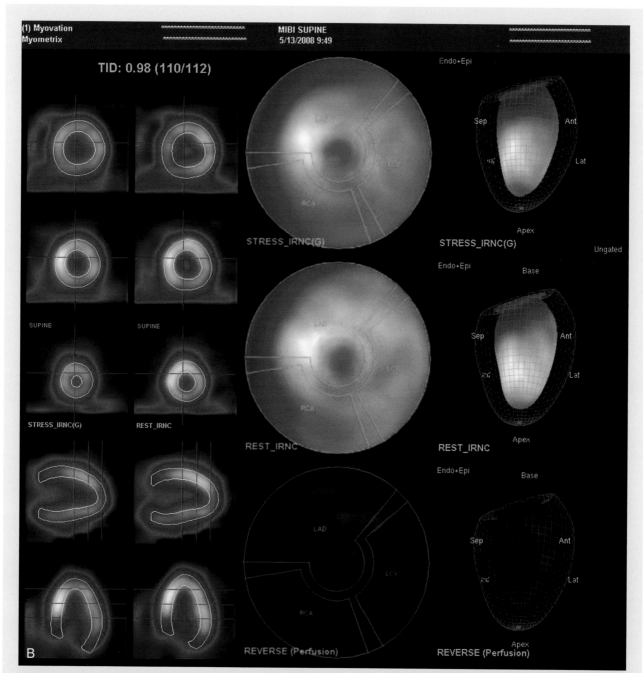

■ **Figure 3-11—Cont'd B,** The localized increase in tracer concentration in the septum ("hot" septum) and contralateral apparent fixed lateral defect are demonstrated clearly on polar maps and three-dimensional reconstructed tomographic images.

(Continued)

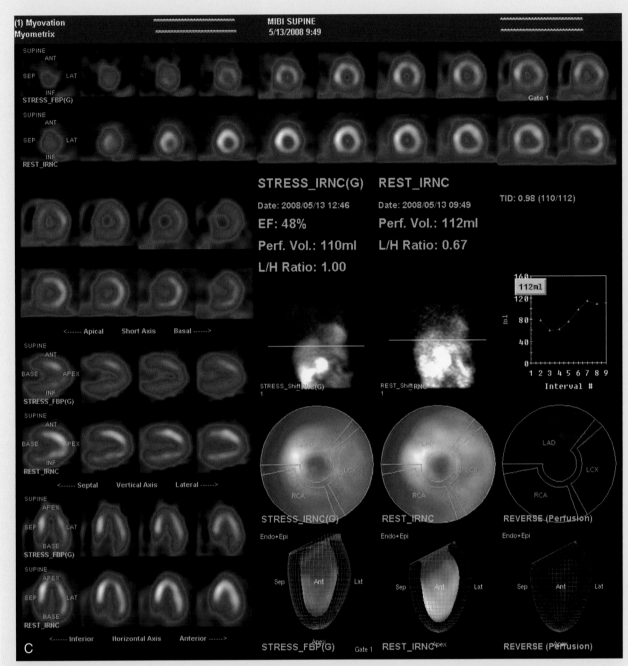

■ **Figure 3-11—Cont'd C,** Gated tomographic images demonstrate mild LV dilatation and mild, diffuse hypokinesis. However, no regional wall motion abnormalities are present, particularly in the anterior, lateral, and inferior walls where tracer concentration was noted to be relatively decreased. LV ejection fraction is 48%. **A** and **C** are accompanied by dynamic displays (Video 3-8).

COMMENTS

The findings are most consistent with LV hypertrophy and a mild nonischemic cardiomyopathy. Commonly in patients with LV hypertrophy, although there is generalized hypertrophy of the LV, septal hypertrophy may be more marked. Therefore, SPECT images demonstrate a relative increase in tracer concentration in the septum. Because tomograms are normalized to the region of myocardium with the highest count density, the septum appears relatively normal, and the remainder of the myocardium demonstrates relatively decreased count density. These findings could be consistent with scarring involving the entire myocardium, sparing only the septum. If this were present, however, there would very likely be associated LV dilatation and regional wall motion abnormalities. However, in this patient there was only mild LV dilatation and no regional dysfunction, favoring an increase in septal count density due to myocardial hypertrophy rather than an abnormal decrease in tracer concentration in the remainder of the left ventricle. Other scan findings associated with LV hypertrophy are prominence of the papillary muscles and generalized thickening of the LV myocardial wall.

Case 3-12   **Dose Infiltration (Figure 3-12)**

A 45-year-old woman with multiple CAD risk factors and atypical chest pain had an exercise treadmill stress technetium-99m sestamibi scan (25 mCi). The patient experienced no chest pain during exercise, and there were no ECG changes. Because the initial stress scan was inadequate (see figure legend), a repeat test was performed the next day. The patient experienced no chest pain during exercise and there were no ECG changes.

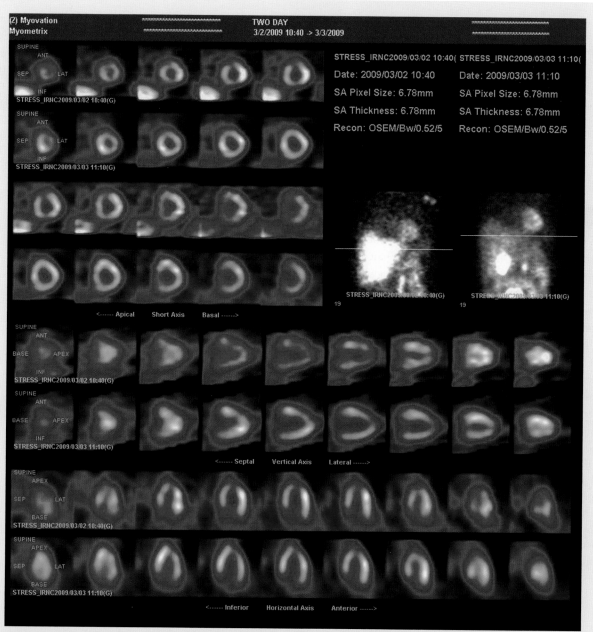

■ **Figure 3-12** Gray level images, *left*. In the planar projection images, focal areas of tracer concentration are noted in the left axilla, consistent with partial infiltration of the radiopharmaceutical dose, which was injected intravenously in the left antecubital fossa and migrated to axillary lymph nodes via lymphatic channels. The overall stress planar projection image count density is low. Tomograms, *top row*. The resulting reconstructed SA, VLA, and HLA tomograms demonstrate low count density, poor-quality stress images. Due to suboptimal image quality, anterior and apical reversible defects are questioned. Poststress gated tomographic images are of very low count density and were judged to be uninterpretable. Gray level images, *right*. Planar projection images no longer demonstrate findings consistent with dose infiltration. Stress planar projection image count density is adequate. Tomograms, *bottom row*. The resulting reconstructed tomograms demonstrate adequate count density and were interpreted as normal. Poststress gated tomographic images are of adequate count density and acceptable quality and were interpreted as normal. This figure is accompanied by dynamic displays (Video 3-9).

The planar projection images in Figure 3-12 exhibit focal areas of tracer concentration in the left axilla, consistent with partial infiltration of the radiopharmaceutical dose. Both poststress static and gated myocardial images are of low count density and deemed technically inadequate. Therefore, stress imaging was repeated the next day. Again, an exercise treadmill stress technetium-99m sestamibi scan (with an additional 25 mCi) was performed. The patient experienced no chest pain during exercise and there were no ECG changes.

COMMENTS

Due to the poor-quality poststress tomograms and questioned abnormalities described in Figure 3-12, the scan was interpreted as "equivocal" for stress-induced ischemia. Repeat poststress imaging the following day with no dose infiltration was normal (see Figure 3-12). Partial dose infiltration is one of several causes of suboptimal myocardial count density. To avoid "equivocal" interpretations of low count density scans, repeat imaging if appropriate.

Case 3-13   Faulty ECG Gating: Loose Leads (Figure 3-13)

A 75-year-old man had multiple risk factors for CAD and nonanginal chest pain. The patient underwent a single-day, low-dose (9 mCi)/high-dose (32 mCi) technetium-99m sestamibi scan. During dipyridamole pharmacologic vasodilatation, the patient experienced no chest pain. The baseline ECG was normal with the patient in normal sinus rhythm. During and after dipyridamole infusion, there were no ECG abnormalities and no arrhythmia. The poststress sinogram shown in Figure 3-13 demonstrates rejection of counts from many heartbeats during many of the planar projection images. In this case example, the heartbeats rejected were not due to cardiac arrhythmia but instead to a loose ECG lead. Similarly, the poststress planar projection images displayed in endless-loop cinematic format likewise demonstrated "flashing" due to relatively decreased count density in some, but not all, projections. In this case example, such "flashing" also was not due to a cardiac arrhythmia but instead was due to the loose ECG lead.

Of note, because the resting acquisition was not gated in this patient, similar findings are present in neither the resting sinogram nor the resting planar projection images displayed in endless-loop cinematic format.

The poststress images were reacquired after the ECG lead was securely attached to the patient's chest. The corresponding sinogram is uniform, without evidence of data rejection and the cinematic display of the planar projections no longer shows "flashing".

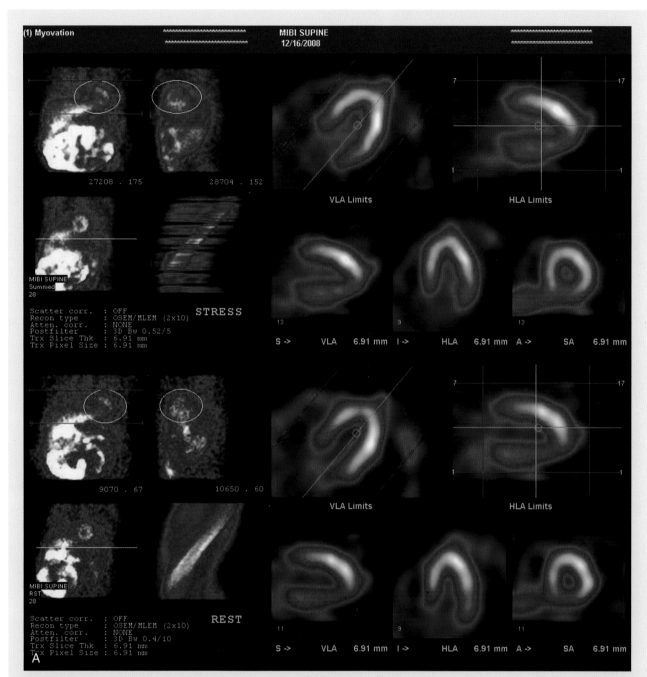

■ **Figure 3-13 A,** The poststress sinogram (vertically "stacked" sequential planar projection images that have been compressed in the *y*-axis) demonstrates rejection of data during many of the 64 planar projection images.* Cardiac cycles with an R-R interval falling outside of the predetermined ECG gating interval (usually the mean R-R interval ±50%) are rejected, thereby decreasing count density of that particular projection.

---

*With a dual-head detector, 32 frames acquired with one detector comprise the upper half of the sinogram, and the 32 frames simultaneously acquired with the other head comprise the lower half of the sinogram. Likewise, the first and second halves of the gated imaging quality control (QC) curve are derived from data from each of the two camera detectors, respectively.

(Continued)

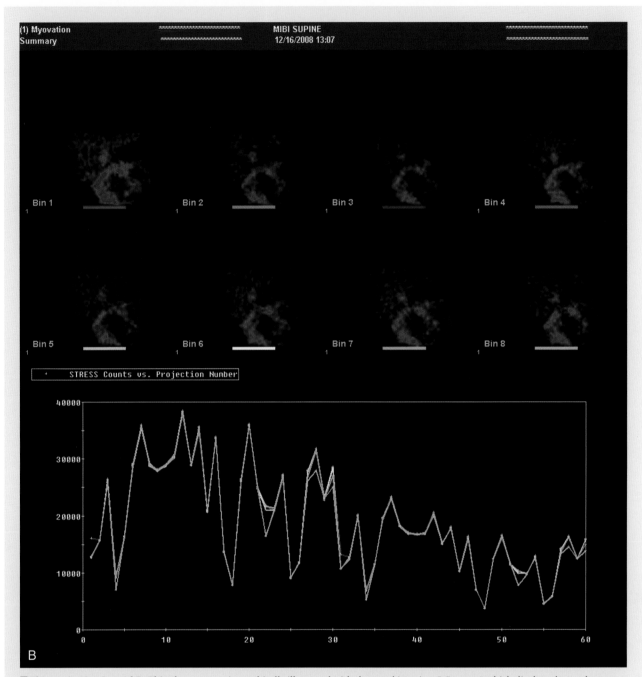

■Figure 3-13—Cont'd B, This phenomenon is graphically illustrated with the gated imaging QC curve,* which displays the total count density of each of the eight cardiac cycles (*y*-axis), each displayed in a different color, for the 64 projection images (*x*-axis). Compared to a normal curve (see **E**), the count density of many of the 64 frames is decreased, giving the QC curve a "jagged" appearance.

*See footnote on previous page.

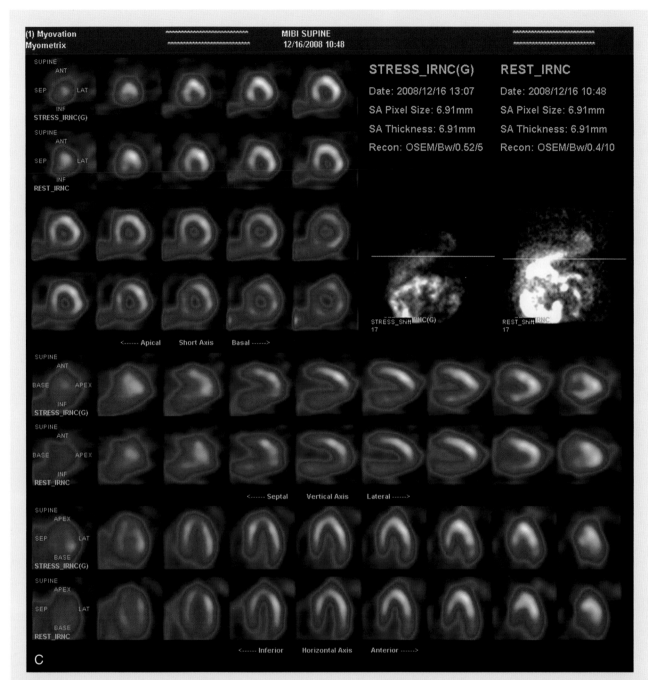

Figure 3-13—Cont'd C, In the reconstructed tomograms the count density of the poststress images is decreased due to data rejection, rendering these images somewhat compromised. The stress and rest tomograms are otherwise unremarkable except for a mild fixed defect in the inferior wall, very likely attributable to diaphragmatic attenuation.

(Continued)

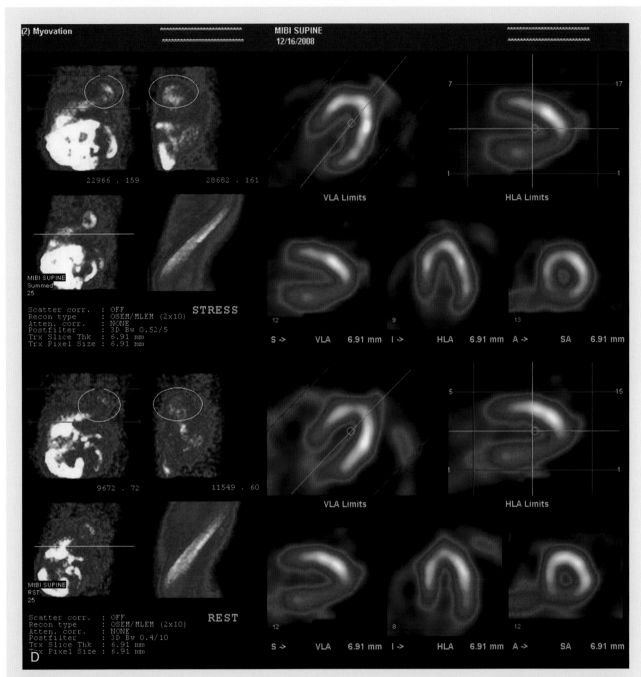

■ **Figure 3-13—Cont'd D,** The poststress images were reacquired after the ECG lead was securely attached to the patient's chest. Count density of the sinogram is uniform, without evidence of data rejection. Planar projection images no longer demonstrate "flashing" due to beat rejection.

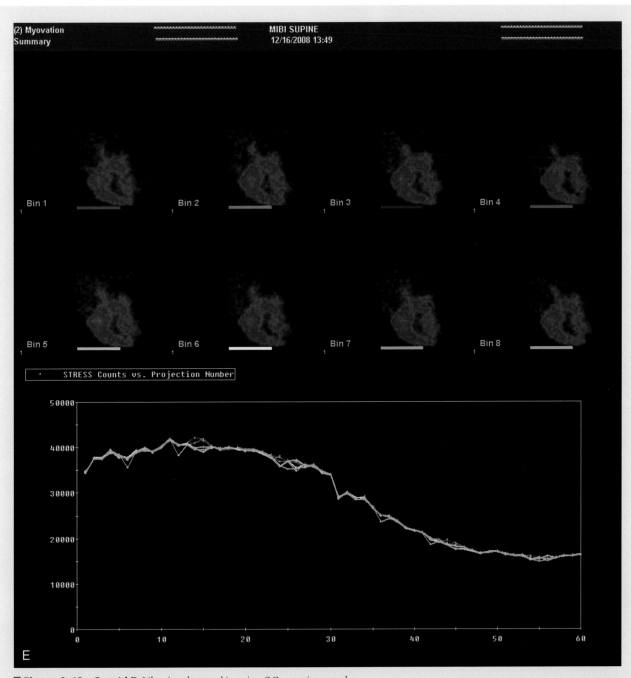

■ **Figure 3-13—Cont'd E,** Likewise, the gated imaging QC curve is normal.

(Continued)

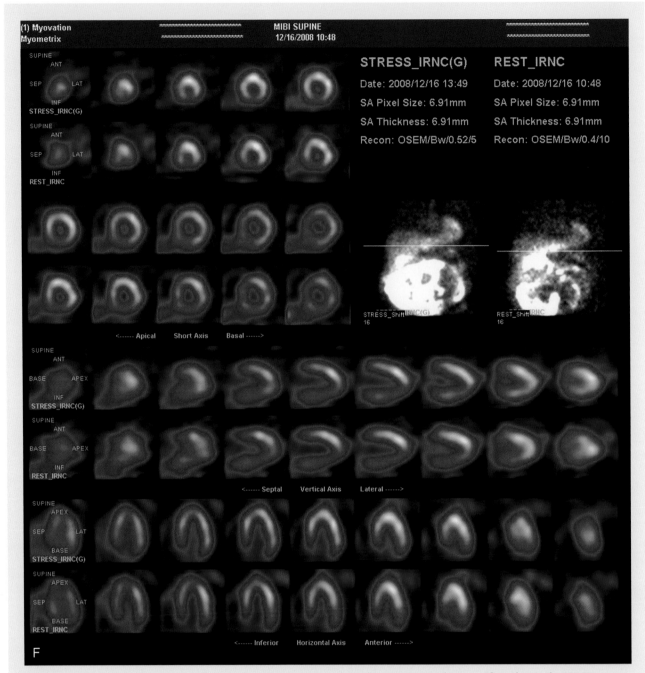

■ **Figure 3-13—Cont'd F,** Count density of the poststress tomograms shown here is greater and more uniform than in the SPECT acquisition for which beats were rejected. **A** and **D** are accompanied by dynamic displays (Video 3-10).

COMMENTS

Scan findings when the ECG leads were securely attached demonstrate normal myocardial perfusion and normal systolic LV function. Identical findings may be noted in patients with arrhythmias, where long and short cardiac cycles are rejected because they fall outside of the predetermined ECG gating interval. If the consequent decrease in count density of the summed tomographic images is too low for reliable interpretation, a nongated acquisition is recommended. Many commercially available scintillation cameras simultaneously acquire gated and nongated SPECT. If such a feature is not available, a repeat nongated acquisition is required.

Case 3-14   Effect of R-R Variability on ECG Gating (Figure 3-14)

A 76-year-old woman presented with multiple risk factors for CAD and nonanginal chest pains, usually occurring after meals. The resting ECG demonstrated nonspecific ST-T wave abnormalities. The patient underwent a single-day, low-dose (9 mCi)/high-dose (32 mCi) technetium-99m sestamibi scan. During dipyridamole pharmacologic vasodilatation, the patient experienced no chest pain and there were no ECG abnormalities.

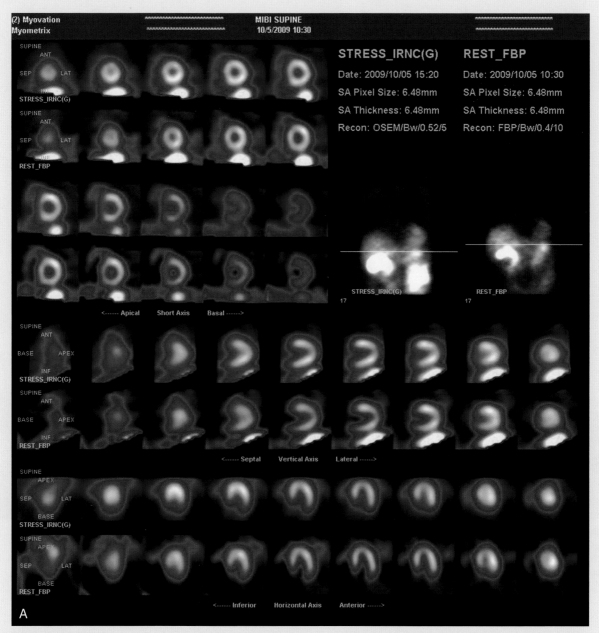

■ **Figure 3-14 A,** Planar projection images are unremarkable with the exception of marked radiotracer concentration in the stomach, consistent with duodenogastric reflux of radiotracer, excreted by the liver into the biliary tract and the duodenum. The patient's nonanginal chest pain could possibly be explained by this finding. Reconstructed tomograms demonstrate normal, physiologic tracer concentration throughout the LV myocardium in both the stress and rest images. Of note, the inferior wall of the left ventricle appears normal, affected by neither Compton scatter nor the Ramp filter artifact from the intense radiotracer concentration in the adjacent fundus of the stomach. Gated tomographic images viewed in eight frames per cardiac cycle, endless-loop cinematic format demonstrate normal LV wall motion and wall. LV ejection fraction is >70%. However, there is data dropout in the last two frames of the gated cine (i.e., a decrease in intensity of the entire image during the 7th and 8th gated frames). **A** is accompanied by a dynamic display (Video 3-11).

(Continued)

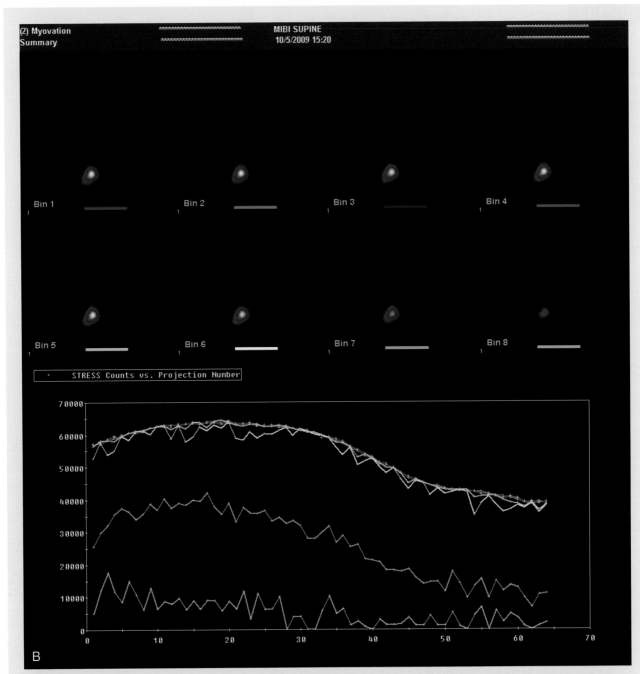

Figure 3-14—Cont'd B, Data drop-out in the last frame(s) of the gated cine is due to variation of the R-R interval of cardiac cycles *accepted* by electrocardiographic gating (usually beats within the mean R-R interval ±50% are electronically predetermined to be accepted). This phenomenon is graphically illustrated with the gated imaging quality control curve, which displays the total count density of each of the eight cardiac cycles (*y*-axis) (each displayed in a different color) for the 64 projection images (*x*-axis). Compared to a normal curve (see Figure 3-13, *E*), the count density of the seventh frame (*blue*) is moderately decreased, and that of the eighth frame (*gray*) is markedly decreased.

COMMENTS

Scan findings shown in Figure 3-14 demonstrate normal myocardial perfusion and normal systolic LV function in this patient with R-R interval variation. In general, such R-R interval variation does not affect quantification of LV volumes or ejection fraction, which are determined from the first frame (or frame with largest LV volume) of the cardiac cycle and the end-systolic frame (usually the third, fourth, or fifth frame). In this case example, the systolic portion of the LV volume curve is well defined.

SELECTED READINGS

DePuey EG: A stepwise approach to myocardial perfusion SPECT interpretation. In Gerson MC, editor: *Cardiac Nuclear Medicine*, ed 3, New York, 1987, McGraw-Hill, pp 81–142.

DePuey EG: Artifacts clarified by and caused by gated myocardial perfusion SPECT. In Germano G, Berman D, editors: *Clinical Gated Cardiac SPECT*, Armonk, NY, 1999, Futura, pp 183–238.

DePuey EG: Artifacts in SPECT myocardial perfusion imaging. In DePuey EG, Garcia EV, Berman DS, et al, editors: *Cardiac SPECT*, Philadelphia, 2001, Lippincott Williams and Wilkins, pp 231–262.

DePuey EG: Image artifacts. In Iskandrian AE, Garcia EV, editors: *Nuclear Cardiac Imaging*, ed 4, New York, 2008, Oxford University Press, pp 117–146.

DePuey EG: Single-photon emission computed tomography artifacts. In Zaret B, Beller G, editors: *Nuclear Cardiology: State of the Art and Future Directions*, ed 4, Philadelphia, 2010, Elsevier, pp 72–95.

Chapter 4

Radionuclide Angiography

Jaekyeong Heo and Ami E. Iskandrian

KEY POINTS

- RNA is a time-honored method for assessment of LVEF and RVEF.

- RNA-derived EF is based on count changes and not on geometric assumptions.

- RNA can be performed with first-pass and gated equilibrium methods.

- Gated RNA can be performed with either a planar technique or tomography.

- RNA can be performed at rest, with exercise, and many other interventions.

- RNA can be performed in patients with sinus rhythm, as well as those with atrial fibrillation.

- Planar RNA can be done in any projection, but gated planar RNA uses the septal LAO projection for EF measurements.

- RNA can provide information on wall motion, LV/RV size, pulmonary transit time, diastolic function, pulmonary blood volume, intracardiac shunts, and regurgitant volume.

- Gated RNA can be used to assess dyssynchrony.

- Alternative RNA methods using different hardware and tracers as well as non-imaging devices have been tested in research applications.

BACKGROUND

The use of RNA has declined considerably with the proliferation and advancements in echocardiography. In fact, most of the exercise RNA literature is more than 2 decades old. At the time, interest in RNA produced fascinating data in the study of cardiac adaptation to exercise, the diagnosis and risk assessment of patients with CAD, the evaluation of patients with valvular and congenital heart diseases, the assessment of diastolic LV function in many patient populations, including those with hypertrophic cardiomyopathy, and the assessment of activation sequences via evaluation of phase and amplitude images using Fourier analysis of the time-activity curve (TAC) in each pixel within the ROI. One RNA study that remains popular is the serial assessment of LVEF in patients with several solid tumors who are undergoing chemotherapy with drugs that are associated with cardiotoxicity. In our daily practice, we continue to use RNA in patients in whom the 2DE is of poor quality or has results that are not consistent with clinical judgment, especially in potential candidates for device treatment (intracardiac defibrillators or biventricular pacing).

An additional factor that has contributed to the decline of RNA use is the ability to measure LVEF by gated SPECT myocardial perfusion imaging; this technique can also be used to assess dyssynchrony. These new developments happened at a time when tomographic gated RNA had reached a stage at which it could be implemented for routine clinical use. Along the way, other methods have come and gone, one of them being the nonimaging probe known as the VEST, a nuclear counterpart to the ambulatory Holter monitor, capable of measuring LVEF on a beat-to-beat basis. Other devices included the multiwire gamma camera and a short-lived, generator-produced tracer (tantalum-178).

The most frequently used variant of RNA is gated RNA, also known as a MUGA (multiple gated acquisition), performed in multiple planar projections. This method is popular because it can readily be done with a standard gamma camera. A MUGA can also be acquired in tomographic fashion (SPECT MUGA), which is superior to the planar method in delineating LV, and especially RV, topography, and volume measurements. The SPECT MUGA is now more widely used than traditional MUGA. We almost always perform both, as the tomographic method can be completed in a shorter period of time.

An alternative method is the first-pass RNA, with which we have had extensive experience. Unlike MUGA, it requires a dedicated gamma camera with a high counting efficiency for best results. Further, the first-pass method also inherently requires more skill and a larger vein for the bolus injection of the tracer. These issues, combined with the others discussed here, have limited its use.

In this chapter, we shall revisit some of these uses and developments in the following images and legends.

| Case 4-1 | **Rest MUGA (Figure 4-1)** |

A 64-year-old woman is undergoing chemotherapy for breast cancer. She has a MUGA study. The images are shown in the LAO projection at end-diastole and end-systole (Figure 4-1, *A*). The LV function is normal.

In Figure 4-1, *B*, a 59-year-old man has severe LV dysfunction and is being considered for ICD therapy. The images in the anterior, shallow, and steep LAO projections are shown at end-diastole (top row) and end-systole (middle row) together with the time activity curve and its first derivative (bottom row). The LAO is used to derive the EF, as it allows for better separation of the LV and RV. A slight caudal angulation allows separation of the LV from the left atrium.

The dynamic images from a patient with heart failure symptoms are shown in Video 4-1.

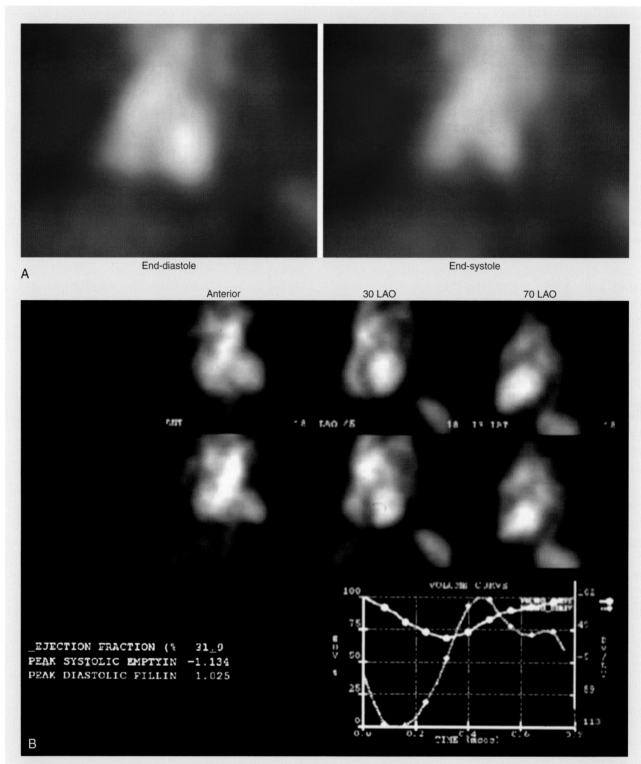

■ **Figure 4-1** Gated equilibrium radionuclide angiogram in a modified LAO projection is shown in a normal subject **(A)** and in a patient with severe LV dysfunction **(B)**. Dynamic images are shown in Video 4-1.

COMMENTS

The main indications for rest MUGA at our institution are serial studies in patients receiving chemotherapy for solid tumors and candidates for CRT/ICD therapy in whom the 2DE studies are, or are expected to be, of suboptimal quality.

Case 4-2   **Rest First-Pass RNA (Figure 4-2)**

This 43-year-old woman has a history of heart murmur and syncope. The images showed bolus transit through the central circulation and the LV silhouettes at end-diastole and end-systole with derived measurements. The EF is normal.

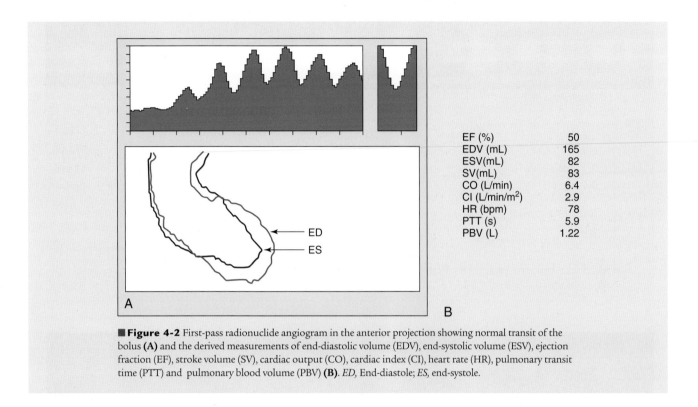

EF (%)	50
EDV (mL)	165
ESV(mL)	82
SV(mL)	83
CO (L/min)	6.4
CI (L/min/m²)	2.9
HR (bpm)	78
PTT (s)	5.9
PBV (L)	1.22

■ **Figure 4-2** First-pass radionuclide angiogram in the anterior projection showing normal transit of the bolus **(A)** and the derived measurements of end-diastolic volume (EDV), end-systolic volume (ESV), ejection fraction (EF), stroke volume (SV), cardiac output (CO), cardiac index (CI), heart rate (HR), pulmonary transit time (PTT) and pulmonary blood volume (PBV) **(B)**. *ED,* End-diastole; *ES,* end-systole.

COMMENTS

As mentioned, the 2DE in this patient was of suboptimal quality. This patient had aortic regurgitation; precise assessment of EF is critical in the timing of surgery to correct this problem.

Case 4-3   **SPECT MUGA (Figure 4-3)**

A 66-year-old woman was treated with chemotherapy for an ovarian tumor. The SPECT MUGA shows normal LV/RV function. In Figure 4-3, *A*, end-diastole frames in the short-axis projection, along with the volume-time curve and LV volumes, are shown.

In Figure 4-3, *B*, the SPECT MUGA of a 36-year-old man with dilated cardiomyopathy is shown in the same format. The 3D images at end-diastole and end–systole for both patients are shown in Figure 4-3, *C*, and the dynamic images are shown in Video 4-2, *A, B*.

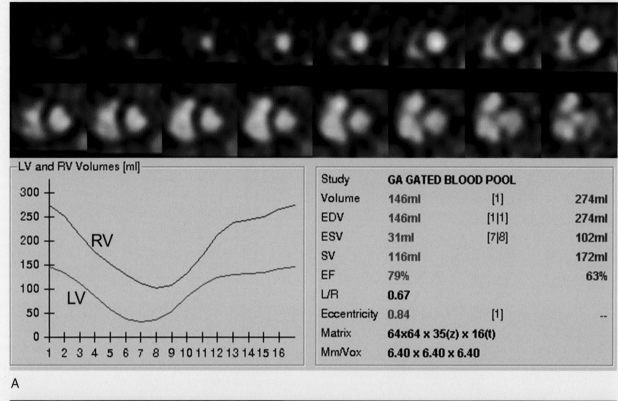

A

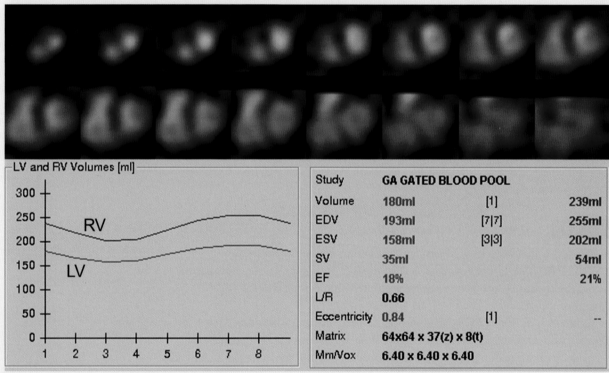

B

■ **Figure 4-3** Gated SPECT equilibrium RNA in the short-axis planes in a normal subject with time-activity curve and LV volumes (**A**) and in a patient with heart failure and abnormal function (**B**).

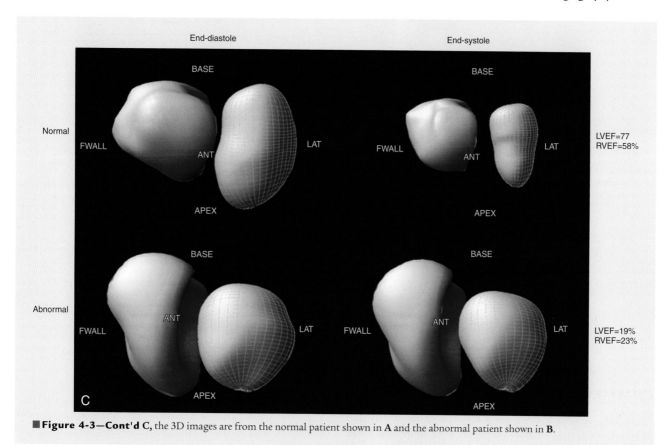

■**Figure 4-3—Cont'd C,** the 3D images are from the normal patient shown in **A** and the abnormal patient shown in **B**.

COMMENTS

The tomographic MUGA is superior to planar MUGA in assessment of LV topography and volumes and RV function.

Case 4-4   Rest and Exercise First-Pass RNA in a Normal Subject (Figure 4-4)

A 52-year-old man with atypical angina underwent rest and exercise first-pass RNA. The rest and peak exercise images are shown in a modified anterior projection (superimposed end-diastolic and end-systolic silhouettes). There is an increase in EF, EDV, SV, CO, and HR and a decrease in ESV. The wall motion becomes hyperdynamic during exercise.

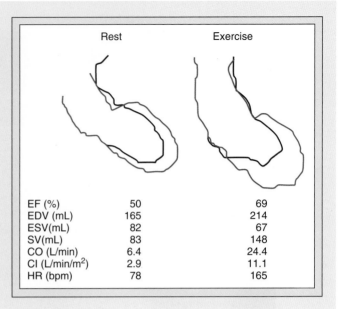

■ **Figure 4-4** Rest and exercise first-pass RNA in a normal subject is shown with superimposed end-diastolic and end-systolic silhouettes. There is an increase in EF, EDV, SV, and CO and a decrease in ESV.

	Rest	Exercise
EF (%)	50	69
EDV (mL)	165	214
ESV(mL)	82	67
SV(mL)	83	148
CO (L/min)	6.4	24.4
CI (L/min/m²)	2.9	11.1
HR (bpm)	78	165

COMMENTS

First-pass RNA captures data at peak exercise (unlike MUGA, which provides averaged data acquired over 2 minutes) and has been very helpful in the understanding of cardiac adaptation to exercise and the roles of the Starling mechanism and increased contractility in the augmentation of LV function during exercise.

Normal subjects increase the stroke volume by increasing the EDV and decreasing the ESV during peak exercise. The relative changes in these two parameters depend on age, intensity of exercise, gender, and body position, among other factors. The increase in cardiac output is due to increases in both stroke volume and heart rate.

Case 4-5   **Rest and Exercise First-Pass RNA in a Patient With CAD (Figure 4-5)**

A 72-year-old man with coronary risk factors underwent rest and exercise RNA. He developed angina during bike exercise and had 2-mm ST-segment depression in leads V₄ to V₆. The images are in the same format is as in Figure 4-4, *A*. Unlike a normal subject, there is a decrease in EF, an increase in ESV, and marked LV dilatation with new severe wall motion abnormality.

First-pass RNA can be combined with SPECT perfusion images (usually using two different gamma cameras). An example of combined perfusion and RNA is shown in Figure 4-5, *B*, from a patient with known CAD. Slices at stress (top) and rest (bottom) with the RNA images are shown. Images from before and after CABG in a patient with CAD are shown in Figure 4-5, *C*. There is marked improvement in response to exercise after surgery.

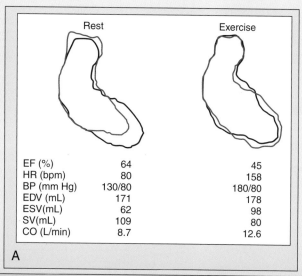

	Rest	Exercise
EF (%)	64	45
HR (bpm)	80	158
BP (mm Hg)	130/80	180/80
EDV (mL)	171	178
ESV(mL)	62	98
SV(mL)	109	80
CO (L/min)	8.7	12.6

A

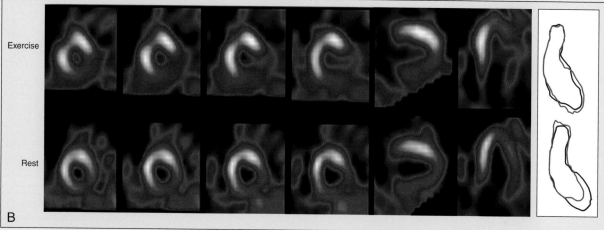

Exercise

Rest

B

	PreOp		PostOp	
	Rest	Exercise	Rest	Exercise
HR (bpm)	62	104	66	164
BP (mm Hg)	135/80	155/85	130/80	180/85
Ex duration (min)	—	5.2	—	11.0
Ex work (kpm)	—	400	—	800
LVEF (%)	50	42	57	64
LVEDVI (ml/m²)	92	101	95	110
LVESVI (ml/m²)	46	59	41	40
CI (L/min/m²)	2.9	4.4	3.6	11.5

C

■ **Figure 4-5** Rest and exercise first-pass RNAs in a patient with CAD are shown (format same as in Figure 4-4). **A,** There is a decrease in EF and an increase in ESV, with a new wall motion abnormality. In **B,** first-pass RNA at rest and exercise with a multicrystal gamma camera is combined with SPECT perfusion imaging using a dual head Anger gamma camera. In **C,** the improvement in exercise LV function is clearly seen after CABG (postoperative versus preoperative).

COMMENTS

The responses to exercise in patients with CAD are effectively captured by first-pass RNA. Unlike with gated SPECT perfusion imaging, they are true peak exercise data rather than postexercise data. In patients with CAD, there is an increase in ESV, a decrease in EF, and new wall motion abnormalities.

Case 4-6   **The Role of RNA-Derived Exercise LVEF in Predicting Outcome in CAD (Figure 4-6)**

The Kaplan-Meier survival curves (free of death and nonfatal myocardial infarction) for exercise EF are shown. Patients with higher exercise EFs have a much better event-free survival. This observation has been well documented in many studies.

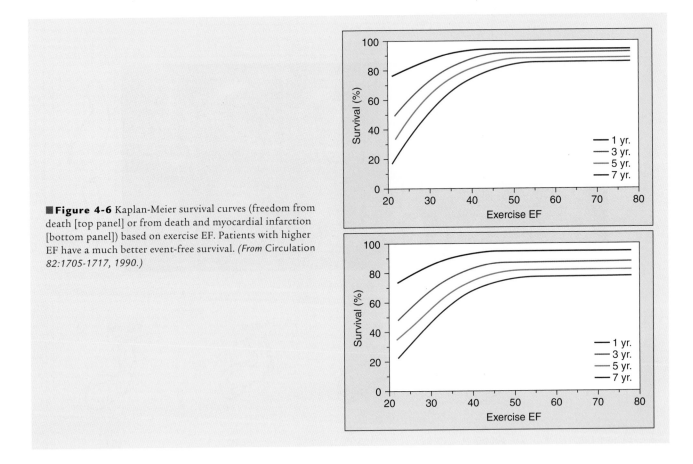

■**Figure 4-6** Kaplan-Meier survival curves (freedom from death [top panel] or from death and myocardial infarction [bottom panel]) based on exercise EF. Patients with higher EF have a much better event-free survival. *(From* Circulation *82:1705-1717, 1990.)*

COMMENTS

The exercise EF (which reflects the rest EF and the change from rest to exercise) has been a powerful predictor of outcomes; for each 1% decrease in exercise EF, there is a concomitant 2% increase in risk. The exercise EF is comparable to the summed stress score by perfusion imaging, which also incorporates rest data and the changes from rest to stress.

Case 4-7	**Rest and Exercise First-Pass RNA in a Patient**
	With Aortic Regurgitation (Figure 4-7)

A 45-year-old man with severe aortic regurgitation and atypical symptoms underwent rest and exercise (bicycle) first-pass RNA. The format of the images is the same as in Figures 4-4 and 4-5. Unlike patients with CAD, there is a decrease in EDV with exercise in the upright position because of a decrease in diastolic filling time and a decrease in regurgitant volume per beat.

The change in EF from rest to exercise has proved to be useful in the follow-up of asymptomatic patients in regard to the timing of surgery in some studies. However, resting EF remains the most widely used measurement.

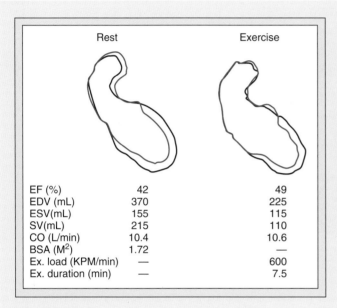

	Rest	Exercise
EF (%)	42	49
EDV (mL)	370	225
ESV(mL)	155	115
SV(mL)	215	110
CO (L/min)	10.4	10.6
BSA (M²)	1.72	—
Ex. load (KPM/min)	—	600
Ex. duration (min)	—	7.5

■**Figure 4-7** Rest and exercise first-pass RNA in a patient with aortic regurgitation (format same as in Figure 4-4). Unlike patients with CAD, there is a decrease in EDV with exercise in the upright position because of a decrease in the diastolic filling time and a decrease in regurgitant volume per beat.

COMMENTS

Rest and exercise RNA is seldom used in assessing patients with aortic regurgitation but has clearly provided useful data on cardiac adaptation with changes in regurgitant volume per beat, total and net cardiac output, and EF. The EF, being a load-dependent measurement, is nicely illustrated in patients in whom there are changes in both the blood pressure and EDV during exercise. Although the exercise EF and the change in EF from rest to exercise have been examined in relation to timing of surgery in asymptomatic patients, the results have not been more predictive than the rest EF alone, which is the standard of care found in the ACC/AHA guidelines.

Case 4-8	**Rest and Atrial Pacing First-Pass RNA (Figure 4-8)**

The 42-year-old man whose images are shown in Figure 4-8, *A*, had atypical symptoms and underwent cardiac catheterization to exclude CAD. The coronary angiogram was normal. He subsequently had pacing studies with hemodynamic assessment and RNA. With rapid atrial pacing, there is a decrease in EDV but no change in EF.

In Figure 4-8, *B*, the images from a 66-year-old woman with CAD by angiography are shown. There was deterioration in wall motion and step-wise decrease in EF with more rapid pacing. She developed ST depression (Figure 4-8, *C*) and had angina, both relieved promptly with discontinuation of pacing. As with exercise, pacing results in deterioration of LV function and ST depression. Unlike exercise, there is a decrease in EDV because of shortening of RR intervals.

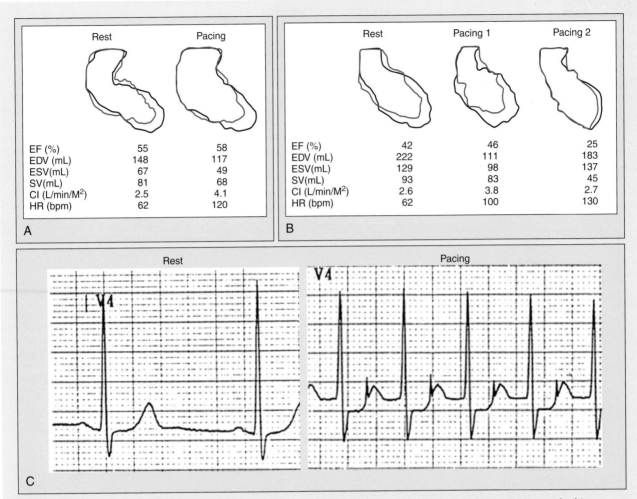

Figure 4-8 Rest first-pass RNA is shown (same format as in Figure 4-4) at baseline and during fast atrial pacing in a normal subject **(A)** and in a patient with CAD **(B)**. With pacing, there is a decrease in EF, ST depression **(C)**, and elevation of LV filling pressure (not shown). Unlike exercise, there is a decrease in EDV because of a shortening of the RR interval.

COMMENTS

Pacing represented an attractive stress alternative prior to the advent of pharmacologic stress testing, at a time when right heart catheterization was frequently performed in patients undergoing coronary angiography for chest pain syndromes. It may still have some value in patients with exercise limitations and contraindications to adenosine and dobutamine. It can be combined with RNA or perfusion imaging. Our center often leaves pacing catheters in place and moves patients from the catheterization lab to the nuclear lab, where the pacing studies are performed. Previously, mobile gamma cameras allowed such studies to be done in the catheterization lab.

Case 4-9   Phase Analysis of MUGA (Figure 4-9)

The planar MUGA and the phase and amplitude images of a normal subject (top) and those from a patient with an LV aneurysm (bottom). In the normal subject, there is a uniform histogram while in the patient with the aneurysm there is a wide histogram, and the phase at the apex is at a 180-degree phase differential from the base, indicating paradoxical motion (it is actually in phase with the atrium).

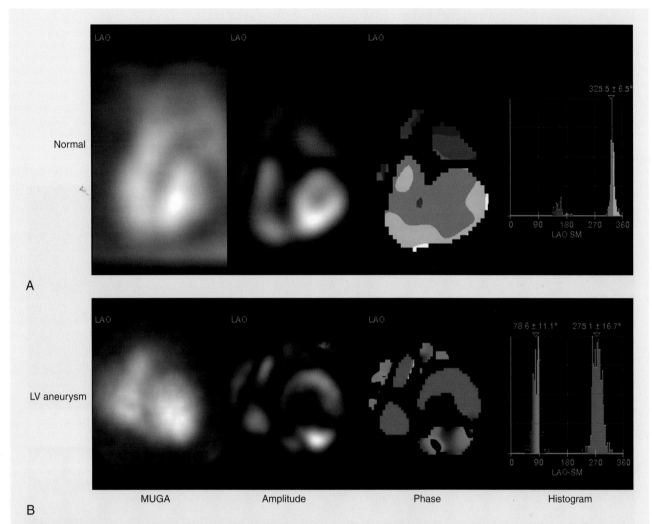

■ **Figure 4-9** Phase and amplitude images of planar MUGA are shown in a normal subject **(A)** and in a patient with LV aneurysm **(B)**. In the normal subject, there is a synchronous contraction (similar phase), while in the patient with aneurysm there is 180° phase difference in the apex, indicating paradoxical motion. Dynamic images are shown in Videos 4-3, A, B.

COMMENTS

Early interest in phase analysis of MUGA studies was directed toward identification of accessory pathways, such as in WPW syndrome, long before the advent of CRT. At present, phase analysis of gated SPECT perfusion images in patients undergoing CRT is more widely used than phase analysis of MUGA, as discussed elsewhere.

Case 4-10   **First-Pass RNA With a Multiwire Gamma Camera (Figure 4-10)**

A 55-year-old woman underwent cardiac catheterization for atypical angina and shortness of breath on exertion. She underwent the following study as a part of a research protocol. Tantalum-178 is injected as a bolus and the transit through the central circulation is recorded. The pulmonary artery pressure is simultaneously measured by thermodilution catheter (Figure 4-10, *A*). The RV ROI and the LV

ROI from two sequential studies before and after nitroglycerin administration are shown in Figure 4-10, *B*. The LV and RV silhouettes are shown in Figure 4-10, *C*. The RV pressure-volume loops are shown in Figure 4-10, *D*. Such studies were done in the cardiac catheterization lab because the camera was small enough and portable to bedside measurements. The pressure volume loop is seen at baseline and in response to nitroglycerin administration, where a leftward shift can be seen.

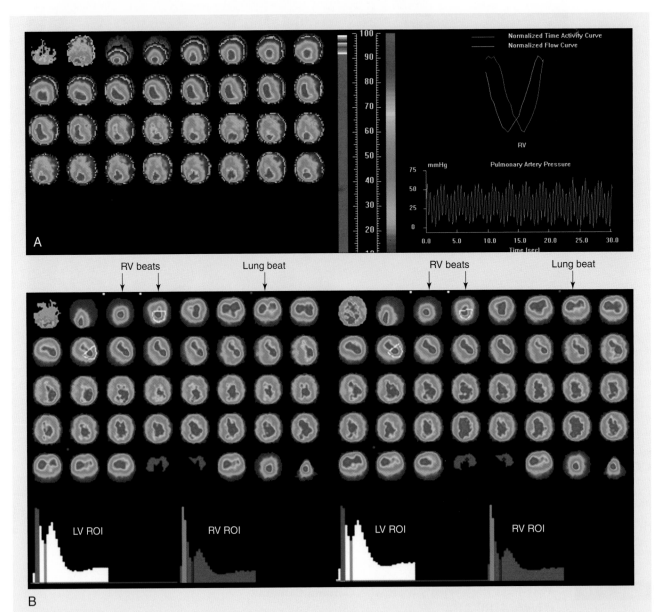

■ **Figure 4-10 A,** First-pass RNA with Ta-178 is shown as a bolus transit; the pulmonary artery pressure measured by a thermodilution catheter and the RV time activity curves are also shown. **B,** The RV ROI and the LV ROI from two sequential studies before and after nitroglycerin administration.

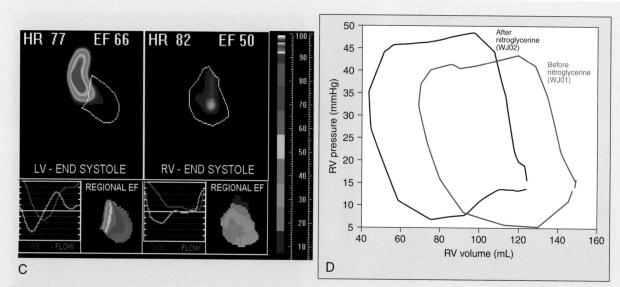

■ **Figure 4-10—Cont'd** The silhouettes of LV and RV **(C)**, and the RV pressure-volume loops (generated from simultaneous RNA and thermodilution measurements before and after nitroglycerin administration) **(D)**.

COMMENTS

The camera/tracer discussed above is not currently available for clinical use but it provided an extremely useful opportunity to study a myriad of variables. The high counting efficiency, high resolution, ability to correct for motion artifacts, and short-lived generator-produced tracers are distinct advantages of the procedure.

Case 4-11   Ambulatory Nuclear Monitor (VEST) (Figure 4-11)

A 69-year-old man underwent VEST study as part of a research protocol. The VEST position over the LV apex is shown in Figure 4-11, *A*, with the patient on a treadmill. The beat-to-beat histogram of HR, EF, EDV, ESV, and CO at baseline and during exercise and recovery are shown in Figure 4-11, *B*, together with the ECG.

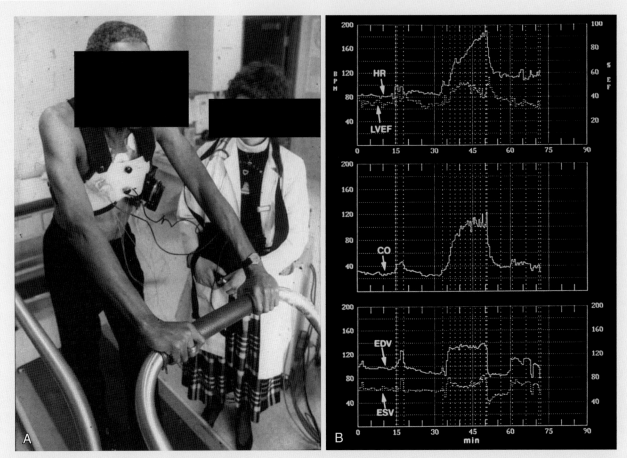

■ **Figure 4-11 A,** The VEST nuclear probe position over the LV is shown while the study is done during exercise. **B,** The beat-to-beat time-activity curve along with ECG. *HR,* Heart rate (bpm); *LVEF,* left ventricular ejection fraction (%); *CO,* cardiac output (as % change); *EDV,* end-diastolic volume; *ESV,* end-systolic volume (both as % changes from baseline).

COMMENTS

The VEST is, again, not currently in use but provided an opportunity to monitor LV function for hours and study the effect of various interventions. The VEST is the nuclear counterpart to the Holter monitor.

Case 4-12   **Dobutamine MUGA (Figure 4-12)**

A 44-year-old man with recent-onset heart failure and chest pain underwent left heart catheterization, which demonstrated an isolated 50% stenosis of the left main artery. The 2DE showed global LV dysfunction with an LVEF of 22%. Catheter-based measurements across the left main stenosis did not suggest a hemodynamically severe stenosis.

He underwent MUGA with dobutamine. Serial EF measurements were done in a modified LAO projection throughout the pharmacologic stress (during the last 2 minutes of each 3-minute stage) up to a peak heart rate of 150 bpm. The rest ECG was normal. There were no ischemic changes. The baseline EF was normal, increasing with stress (see Figure 4-12). The improvement of EF was accompanied by an improvement in wall motion.

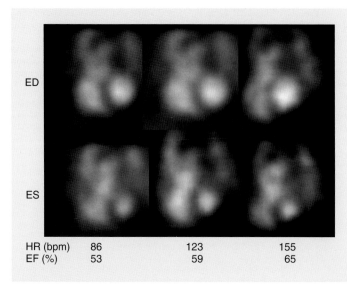

■**Figure 4-12** Serial MUGA studies in LAO projections; baseline, intermediate, and peak doses of dobutamine. The heart rates and LVEF are shown. Note the improvement in EF with stress.

| HR (bpm) | 86 | 123 | 155 |
| EF (%) | 53 | 59 | 65 |

COMMENTS

Dobutamine MUGA was attempted because there was only isolated left main stenosis by angiography. Stress myocardial perfusion imaging would likely not show perfusion defects even if the lesion were severe. This pattern of isolated left main disease is very unusual. The reason for the stress test was to determine whether the LV dysfunction was caused by left main disease and whether CABG was warranted. The MUGA results showed normal baseline EF. The response during dobutamine infusion was also normal. The response indicated that the left main lesion was not hemodynamically significant.

SELECTED READINGS

ASNC: Updated imaging guidelines for nuclear cardiology procedures, part 1, *J Nucl Cardiol* 8:G5–G58, 2001.

Botvinick E, Dunn R, Frais M, et al: The phase image: its relationship to patterns of contraction and conduction, *Circulation* 65:551–560, 1982.

Brindis RG, Douglas PS, Hendel RC, et al: ACCF/ASNC Appropriateness Criteria for Single-Photon Emission Computed Tomography Myocardial Perfusion Imaging (SPECT MPI) A Report of the American College of Cardiology Foundation Quality Strategic Directions Committee Appropriateness Criteria Working Group and the American Society of Nuclear Cardiology Endorsed by the American Heart Association, *J Am Coll Cardiol* 46:1587–1605, 2005.

Chen J, Garcia EV, Folks RD, et al: Onset of left ventricular mechanical contraction as determined by phase analysis of ECG-gated myocardial perfusion SPECT imaging: Development of a diagnostic tool for assessment of cardiac mechanical dyssynchrony, *J Nucl Cardiol* 12:687–695, 2005.

Daou D, Harel F, Helal BO, et al: Electrocardiographically gated blood-pool SPECT and left ventricular function: comparative value of 3 methods for ejection fraction and volume estimation, *J Nucl Med* 42:1043–1049, 2001.

De Bondt P, Nichols KJ, De Winter O, et al: Comparison among tomographic radionuclide ventriculography algorithms for computing left and right ventricular normal limits, *J Nucl Cardiol* 13:675–684, 2006.

Folse R, Braunwald E: Determination of fraction of left ventricular volume ejected per beat and of ventricular end-diastolic and residual volumes: experimental and clinical observations with a precordial dilution technic, *Circulation* 25:674–685, 1962.

Ferraresi V, Milella M, Vaccaro A, et al: Toxicity and activity of docetaxel in anthracycline-pretreated breast cancer patients: a phase II study, *Am J Clin Oncol* 23:132–139, 2000.

Freeman ML, Palac R, Mason J, et al: A comparison of dobutamine infusion and supine bicycle exercise for radionuclide cardiac stress testing, *Clin Nucl Med* 9:251–258, 1984.

Hendel RC, Berman DS, Di Carli MF, et al: ACCF/ASNC/ACR/AHA/ASE/SCCT/SCMR/SNM 2009 Appropriate Use Criteria for Cardiac Radionuclide Imaging: A Report of the American College of Cardiology Foundation Appropriate Use Criteria Task Force, the American Society of Nuclear Cardiology, the American College of Radiology, the American Heart Association, the American Society of Echocardiography, the Society of Cardiovascular Computed Tomography, the Society for Cardiovascular Magnetic Resonance, and the Society of Nuclear Medicine, *J Am Coll Cardiol* 53:2201–2229, 2009.

Heo J, Htay T, Mehta D, et al: Assessment of left ventricular function during upright treadmill exercise with tantalum-178 and multiwire gamma camera, *J Nucl Cardiol* 12:560–566, 2005.

Htay T, Mehta D, Sun L, et al: Right ventricular pressure-volume loops using simultaneous radionuclide angiography with a multiwire gamma camera and right heart catheterization, *J Nucl Cardiol* 12:435–440, 2005.

Hurwitz RA, Treves S, Freed M, et al: Quantitation of aortic and mitral regurgitation in the pediatric population: evaluation by radionuclide angiocardiography, *Am J Cardiol* 51:252–255, 1983.

Iskandrian AE, Garcia EV: *Nuclear Cardiac Imaging: Principles and Applications*, Ed 4, New York, 2008, Oxford University Press.

Iskandrian AS, Bemis CE, Hakki AH, et al: Ventricular systolic and diastolic impairment during pacing-induced myocardial ischemia in coronary artery disease: simultaneous hemodynamic, electrocardiographic, and radionuclide angiographic evaluation, *Am Heart J* 112:382–391, 1986.

Jones RH, Johnson SH, Bigelow C, et al: Exercise radionuclide angiocardiography predicts cardiac death in patients with coronary artery disease, *Circulation* 84:I52–I58, 1991.

Lee KL, Pryor DB, Pieper KS, et al: Prognostic value of radionuclide angiography in medically treated patients with coronary artery disease. A comparison with clinical and catheterization variables, *Circulation* 82:1705–1717, 1990.

Mitani I, Jain D, Joska TM, et al: Doxorubicin cardiotoxicity: prevention of congestive heart failure with serial cardiac function monitoring with equilibrium radionuclide angiocardiography in the current era, *J Nucl Cardiol* 10:132–139, 2003.

Nallamouthu N, Araujo L, Russell J, et al: Prognostic value of simultaneous perfusion and function assessment using technetium-99m sestamibi, *Am J Cardiol* 78:562–564, 1996.

Panjrath GS, Jain D: Monitoring chemotherapy-induced cardiotoxicity: role of cardiac nuclear imaging, *J Nucl Cardiol* 13:415–426, 2006.

Patrick ST, Glowniak JV, Turner FE, et al: Comparison of in vitro RBC labeling with the UltraTag RBC kit versus in vivo labeling, *J Nucl Med* 32:242–244, 1991.

Strauss HW, Zaret BL, Hurley PJ, et al: A scintiphotographic method for measuring left ventricular ejection fraction in man without cardiac catheterization, *Am J Cardiol* 28:575–580, 1971.

Tamas E, Broqvist M, Olsson E, et al: Exercise radionuclide ventriculography for predicting post-operative left ventricular function in chronic aortic regurgitation, *JACC Cardiovasc Imaging* 2:48–55, 2009.

Wolz DE, Flores AR, Grandis DJ, et al: Abnormal left ventricular ejection fraction response to mental stress and exercise in cardiomyopathy, *J Nucl Cardiol* 2:144–150, 1995.

Wright GA, Thackray S, Howey S, et al: Left ventricular ejection fraction and volumes from gated blood-pool SPECT: comparison with planar gated blood-pool imaging and assessment of repeatability in patients with heart failure, *J Nucl Med* 44:494–498, 2003.

Chapter 5

Choice of Stress Test

Gilbert J. Zoghbi, Fahad M. Iqbal, and Ami E. Iskandrian

KEY POINTS

- Exercise (treadmill or bicycle) is the preferred stress modality in patients who can exercise and achieve adequate exercise endpoints.

- Vasodilator stress is reserved for patients who have exercise limitations, left bundle branch block, or electronically paced rhythms.

- Dobutamine stress is reserved for patients who have exercise limitations and who have contraindications to vasodilator stress.

- The non-ST changes during exercise stress testing provide useful prognostic information.

- The site of ST depression during stress testing does not predict the site of coronary stenosis/ischemia location.

- The site of ST elevations during stress testing in leads without Q waves often is accurate in localizing the site of coronary stenosis/ischemia.

- Hybrid protocols are available, such as combination of dobutamine and atropine and exercise with vasodilators.

- The ST responses are characterized as positive, negative, or nondiagnostic for ischemia.

- There is increasing use of vasodilator stress testing; it may be as high as 50% of all stress tests.

- The dosages and mode of administration of the three current vasodilators in clinical use (dipyridamole, adenosine, and regadenoson) are different. Regadenoson is given as a bolus and is not weight-adjusted.

BACKGROUND

Exercise stress in conjunction with MPI is more commonly used in clinical practice in lieu of TET alone, due to the limitations of TET, such as its low sensitivity, specificity, and accuracy in diagnosing and localizing the extent and severity of ischemia and its inability to provide information on LV function and viability. Half of the patients referred for stress MPI undergo exercise MPI. Exercise is the preferred stress modality in patients who can achieve exercise endpoints such as ≥85% of peak age-adjusted HR and >5 METs. Around 50% of outpatients and 75% of inpatients who undergo exercise stress testing fail to achieve adequate exercise endpoints. Vasodilator stress is reserved for patients who cannot achieve adequate exercise endpoints or who have exercise limitations, LBBB, or pacemakers (Table 5-1). Dobutamine stress is reserved for those who have exercise limitations and contraindications to vasodilator stress.

Exercise or pharmacological stress augment MBF; the MBF in coronary beds without significant stenoses increases ~3-fold with exercise, 2.5-fold with dobutamine, and 3- to 5-fold with vasodilator stressors.

The ECG response to stress testing is classified as negative, positive, or nondiagnostic. A positive ECG response is defined by ≥1-mm flat or downsloping ST depression 60 to 80 milliseconds from the J point, ≥1.5-mm upsloping ST depression 80 ms from the J point, or ≥1-mm ST elevation. These changes should be present in three consecutive beats. A nondiagnostic ECG response is seen in the presence of baseline ECG abnormalities that preclude interpretation of ECG changes, such as in the presence of LV hypertrophy, LBBB, WPW syndrome, paced rhythm, digitalis therapy, or ST depression at rest. Failure to achieve a target age-predicted HR in the

TABLE 5-1 Choice of Stress Test

Factors That Favor Vasodilator Stress MPI

- Peripheral vascular disease
- Muscular disorders
- Skeletal disorders
- Neurologic disorders
- Left bundle branch block
- Electronically paced rhythm
- Chronotropic incompetence
- Inability to achieve exercise endpoints
    - Limited exercise capacity
    - Morbid obesity
    - Poor motivation
    - Poor physical conditioning
    - Pulmonary disease
    - Diabetes mellitus
- Presence of large abdominal aortic aneurysm
- Acute myocardial infarction (within 72 hours)
- Percutaneous coronary intervention (within 48 to 72 hours)

Factors That Favor Dobutamine Stress MPI When Exercise Is Not Indicated

- Bronchospasm
- Second- or third-degree heart block without a functioning pacemaker
- Use of dipyridamole, aspirin/dipyridamole (Aggrenox), or aminophylline within the past 24 hours
- Sick sinus syndrome
- Systolic blood pressure <90 mm Hg

absence of positive ECG changes is considered a nondiagnostic response during exercise testing. The site of ST depression is not predictive of the location of the coronary stenosis. The severity and extent of ST depressions have a low correlation with the extent of ischemia seen on MPI.

Case 5-1 Normal Exercise ECG, Abnormal Perfusion (Figure 5-1)

A 71-year-old white man with HTN, dyslipidemia, remote tobacco abuse, COPD, and erectile dysfunction presented to his primary care physician with a 2-week history of exertional chest pain. He was referred for exercise MPI. The baseline BP was 162/96 mm Hg and HR was 103 bpm. He exercised on the treadmill for 6 minutes 31 seconds according to the Bruce protocol and stopped due to fatigue. He achieved a peak HR of 150 bpm (111% of age-predicted HR) and 7.7 METs (100% of predicted). The exercise ECG was negative for ischemia (Figure 5-1, *A, B*). The SPECT images showed a large area of ischemia in the LAD territory with TID and poststress stunning (Figure 5-1, *C, D*). The rest LVEF was 47%. He had distal anterior and apical wall akinesis after stress. Coronary angiography showed 80% proximal LAD stenosis and 90% mid LAD stenosis. The LCX had minimal disease and the RCA had a 70% proximal stenosis and a 60% mid stenosis (Figure 5-1, *E*). He underwent CABG to the LAD, diagonal, and RCA.

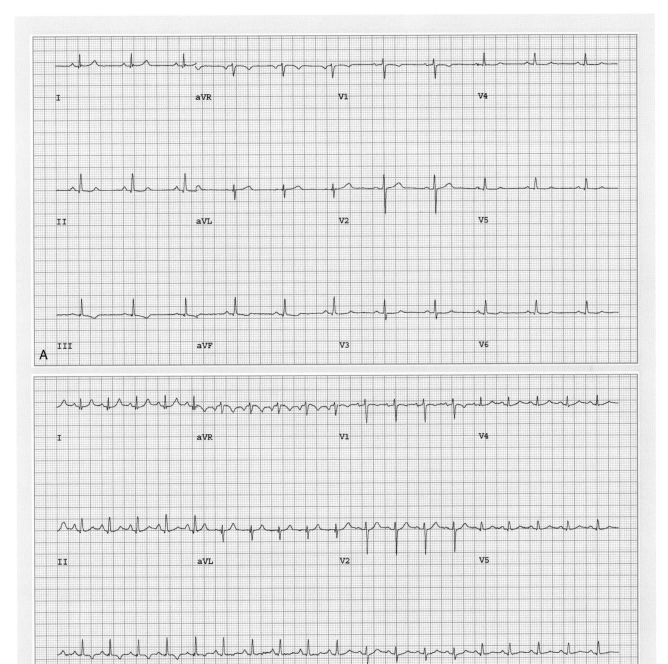

■ **Figure 5-1** The ECG at rest (**A**) and peak exercise (**B**) showing a normal response with no ST changes.

(Continued)

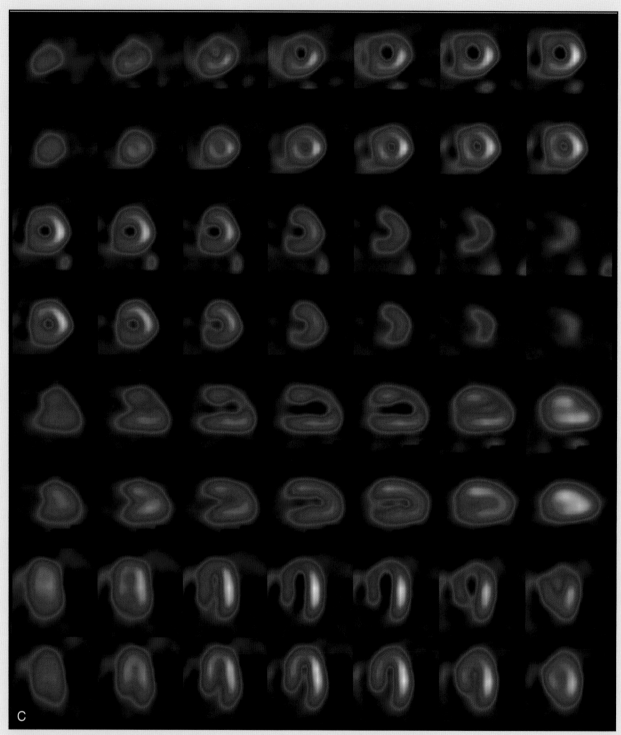

■**Figure 5-1—Cont'd** The SPECT images show a reversible LAD perfusion abnormality with TID **(C)**.

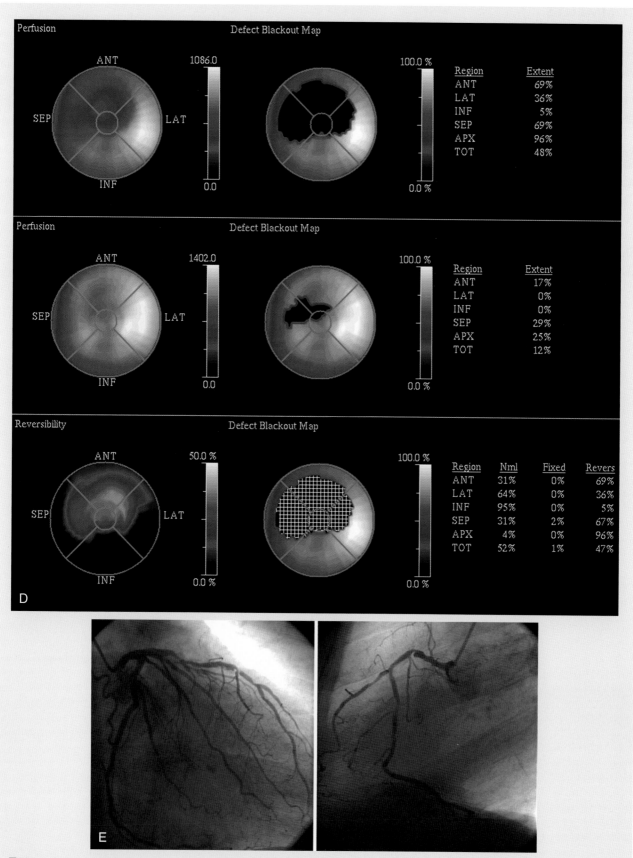

■ Figure 5-1—Cont'd The LVEF was normal. The polar maps show a large abnormality **(D)**. Coronary angiography showing severe proximal and mid LAD stenoses, mild LCX disease, and severe proximal RCA stenosis **(E)**.

COMMENTS

The exercise ECG showed no ischemia, although the perfusion images showed high-risk features (large perfusion defect, TID, and postexercise stunning).

In a meta-analysis of 147 studies involving around 24,000 patients, the sensitivity and specificity of exercise testing for detection of CAD were 68% and 77%, respectively, with a positive predictive value of 73%. In a meta-analysis of 27 studies involving about 3200 patients, the sensitivity and specificity of exercise MPI were 87% and 64% compared to 54% and 71% with exercise alone, respectively. The yearly rate of major adverse cardiac events in the setting of high-risk perfusion abnormalities is 5.9% (25th percentile 4.6%, 75th percentile 8.5%).

| Case 5-2 | Abnormal Exercise ECG, Normal Perfusion (Figure 5-2) |

A 63-year-old African American woman with GERD, osteoporosis, and hypothyroidism was referred for exercise MPI for evaluation of atypical chest pain. Her baseline BP was 131/65 mm Hg and HR was 55 bpm. She exercised on the treadmill for 7 minutes according to the Bruce protocol. She stopped due to fatigue. She achieved a peak HR of 151 bpm (107% of age-predicted HR) and 8.5 METs (127% of predicted). The exercise ECG was positive for ischemia (Figure 5-2, *A*, *B*). The SPECT images showed normal perfusion (Figure 5-2, *C*, *D*) and normal LVEF and wall motion/thickening.

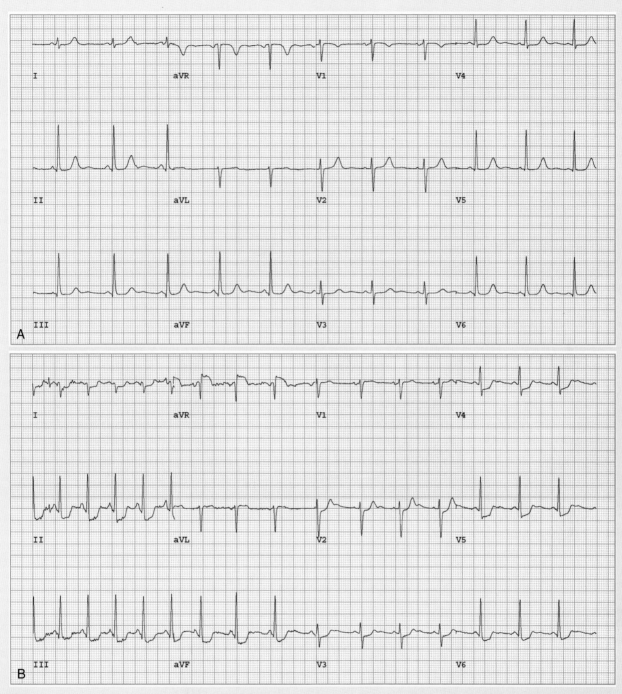

■ **Figure 5-2** The ECG at rest (**A**) and peak exercise (**B**) showing ST depressions indicative of an ischemic response.

(Continued)

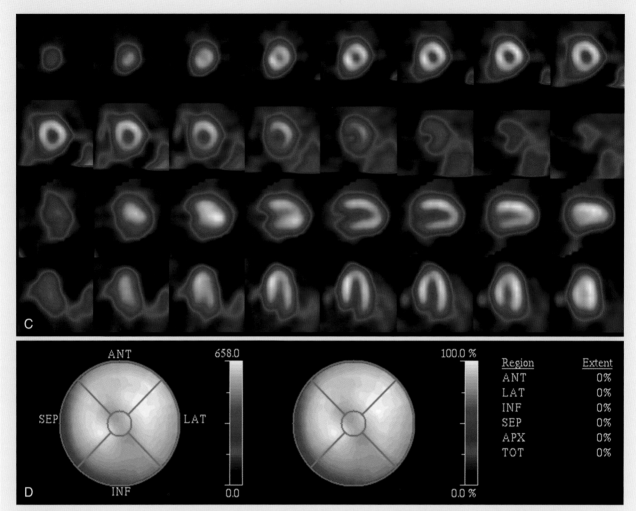

■**Figure 5-2—Cont'd** The stress-only SPECT images are normal **(C)**. The LVEF was normal. The polar maps show uniform tracer distribution **(D)**.

Case 5-3   Abnormal Exercise ECG, Abnormal Perfusion (Figure 5-3)

A 61-year-old white man with diabetes mellitus, idiopathic ventricular tachycardia (post RV outflow ablation), and dyslipidemia presented with a 1-month history of new-onset exertional chest pain on mild-to-moderate exertion. He was referred for further evaluation with exercise MPI. The baseline BP was 113/79 mm Hg and HR was 69 bpm. He exercised on the treadmill for 7 minutes 15 seconds according to the Bruce protocol. He stopped due to fatigue and chest pain. He achieved a peak HR of 159 bpm (113% of age-predicted HR) and 8.9 METs (91% of predicted). He had a hypotensive BP response. The exercise ECG was positive for ischemia (Figure 5-3, *A, B*). The SPECT images showed a large area of ischemia in the LAD, RCA, and LCX territories with TID and poststress stunning (Figure 5-3, *C, D*). The rest LVEF was 71% and the poststress LVEF was 58%. Coronary angiography showed 90% proximal to mid LAD stenosis, 90% stenosis of the proximal LCX artery, and 90% stenosis of the proximal RCA with left-to-right collaterals. He underwent CABG.

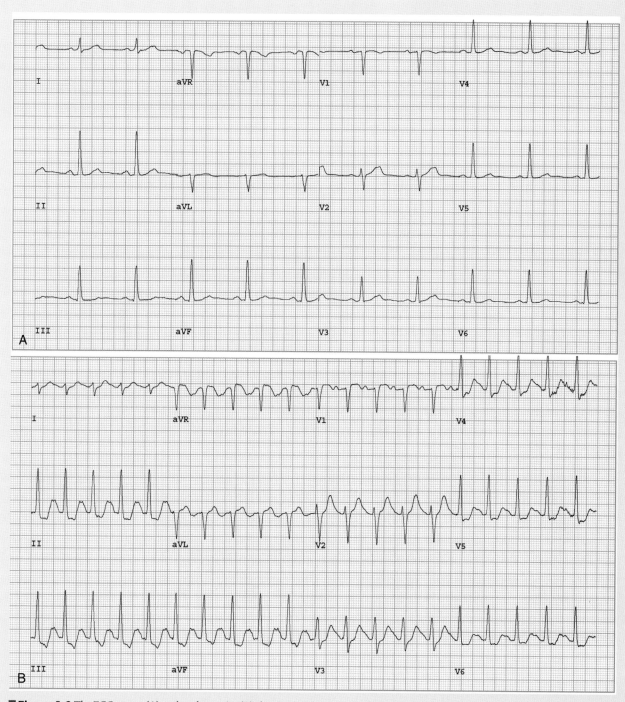

■ **Figure 5-3** The ECG at rest **(A)** and peak exercise **(B)** showing ST depressions indicative of an ischemic response.

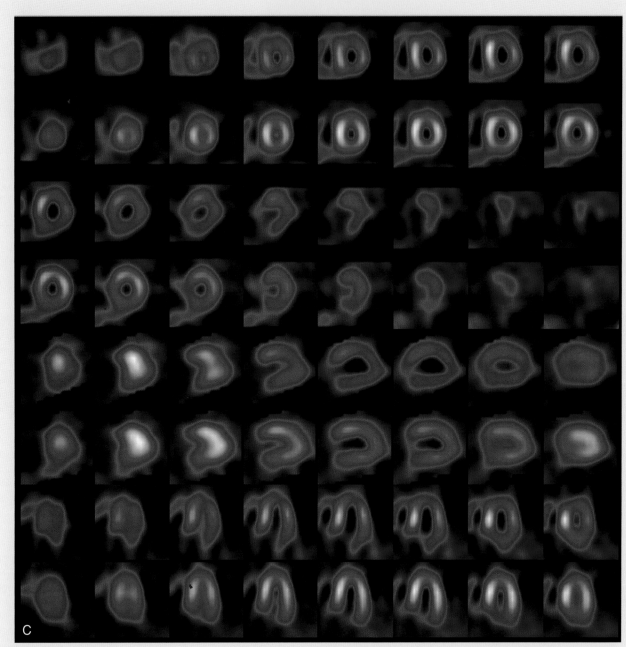

■ **Figure 5-3—Cont'd** The SPECT images show reversible perfusion abnormality in the three vascular territories **(C)**.

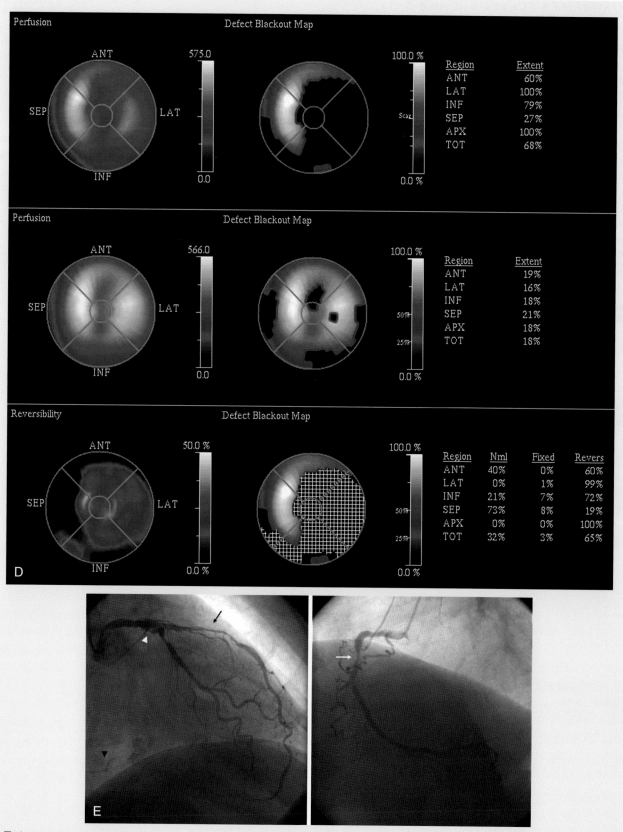

■ **Figure 5-3—Cont'd** The LVEF was normal. The polar maps show a large abnormality **(D)**. Coronary angiography showed severe LAD *(black arrow)*, LCX *(white arrowhead)*, and RCA stenoses *(white arrow)*. Note the presence of left-to-right collaterals *(black arrowhead)* **(E)**.

COMMENTS (Cases 5-2 and 5-3)

Case 5-2 demonstrates a false-positive ECG response. The exercise ECG shows >1-mm flat ST depressions in the inferior and lateral leads. The perfusion images were normal. The patient had a low pretest probability for CAD. The accuracy of TET in women is lower than in men, with a higher rate of false-positive results. In a meta-analysis of 19 studies of exercise testing in women, the respective weighted sensitivity, specificity, and likelihood ratio for CAD detection were 61%, 70%, and 2.25, respectively.

In a study that compared the performance of exercise ECG to MPI in men and women, the false-positive ECG results were 14% in women and 10% in men. The respective sensitivity and positive predictive value of a positive ECG were 30% and 34% in women compared to 42% and 70% in men.

Case 5-3 demonstrates a true-positive ECG response with flat to downsloping ST depressions in the inferior and lateral leads. Factors that increase the sensitivity of the exercise ECG for detection of CAD include older patients, presence of multivessel disease, severe CAD, typical angina, multiple CAD risk factors, and resting ECG changes. A hypotensive BP response is a predictor of the presence of severe and extensive CAD and portends a poor prognosis. Other exercise ECG predictors of severe and extensive CAD include ≥2-mm downsloping ST depressions, ST depressions occurring in stage 1 or 2 of the Bruce protocol or at low double product, persistent ST depressions (>6 minutes into recovery), ST depressions in ≥-5 leads, exercise-induced typical angina at low level of exercise, poor exercise capacity (<5 METs), ventricular ectopy, abnormal HR recovery, high-risk Duke treadmill score, and exercise-induced LBBB at HR <125 bpm.

| **Case 5-4** | **ST Elevation During Exercise, Abnormal Perfusion (Figure 5-4)** |

A 65-year-old white man with history of dyslipidemia and family history of CAD presented with a 2-week history of vague left precordial chest discomfort and was referred for exercise MPI. His baseline BP was 144/94 mm Hg and HR was 95 bpm. He exercised on the treadmill for 8 minutes 30 seconds according to the Bruce protocol. He stopped due to ST elevation at peak exercise. He achieved a peak HR of 139 bpm (90% of age-predicted HR) and 10.1 METs (105% of predicted). The rest ECG is normal (Figure 5-4, *A*). The exercise ECG showed ST elevation in leads II, III, and aVF (Figure 5-4, *B*). The SPECT images showed a large and severe reversible inferior abnormality (Figure 5-4, *C*). The rest LVEF was 57%. Coronary angiography showed mild proximal LAD and LCX disease but the RCA was occluded at its mid portion and received mature collaterals from the left coronary system (Figure 5-4, *D*). He underwent emergent PCI of the RCA.

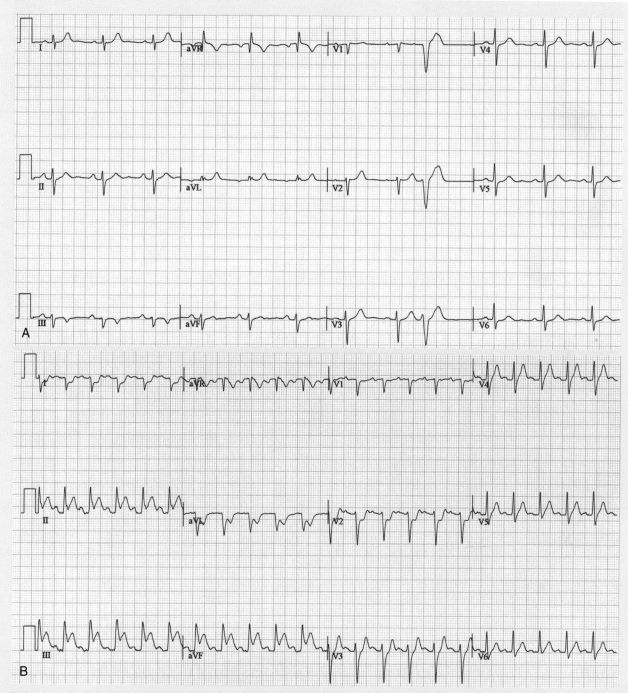

■ **Figure 5-4** The ECG at rest **(A)** and peak exercise **(B)** showing ST elevation.

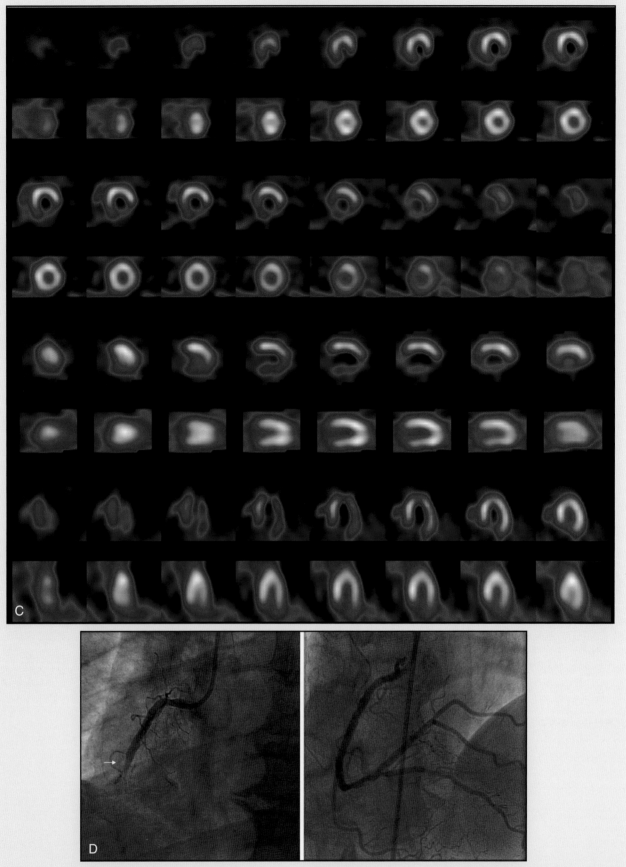

■ **Figure 5-4—Cont'd** The SPECT images show a reversible severe perfusion defect in the RCA territory **(C)**. Coronary angiography showed mild LAD and LCX disease (not shown) and an occluded mid RCA *(white arrow)* **(D)**. The angiogram after PCI is also shown.

COMMENTS

ST elevation during exercise in leads with Q waves is due to wall motion abnormality from scar or aneurysms and, as such, is not due to ischemia. ST elevations during exercise occurs in 30% of patients with anterior MI and 15% of patients with inferior MI. ST elevations occur more commonly in patients with larger infarcts and lower LVEF. ST elevation during exercise in leads without Q waves indicates transmural ischemia that could be due to coronary spasm, high-grade stenosis, or both. The incidence of ST elevation during exercise was 0.5% in healthy men, 3% to 6.5% in symptomatic patients, and 10% to 30% in patients with variant angina. The leads with ST elevations accurately predict the stenotic coronary artery or the respective area of ischemia on MPI.

| Case 5-5 | Normal Adenosine ECG, Normal Perfusion (Figure 5-5) |

A 54-year-old white man with HTN, dyslipidemia, and a history of stroke, scoliosis, depression, DM, peripheral vascular disease, and CAD with prior CABG and PCI presented with atypical angina. He underwent adenosine MPI. His baseline BP was 114/70 mm Hg and HR was 60 bpm. The peak HR was 83 bpm and the peak BP was 122/76 mm Hg. The adenosine ECG was negative for ischemia (Figure 5-5, *A, B*). The SPECT images showed a normal perfusion pattern (Figure 5-5, *C*) with normal LVEF. He had septal hypokinesis secondary to prior CABG.

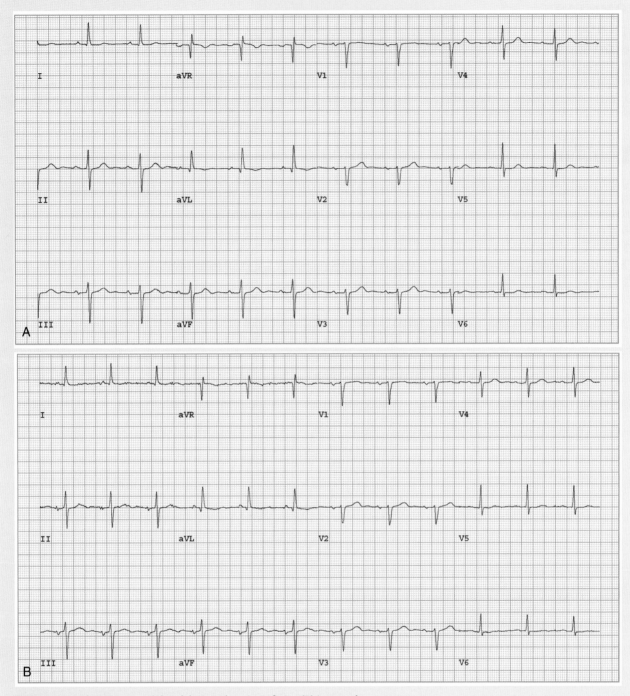

■ **Figure 5-5** The ECG at rest (**A**) and during adenosine infusion (**B**) is normal.

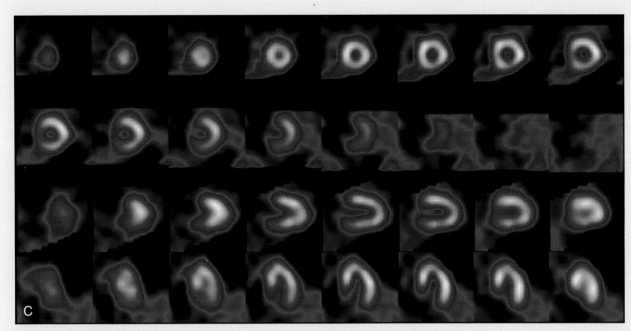

■ **Figure 5-5—Cont'd** The stress-only SPECT images show normal perfusion **(C)**. The LVEF was normal.

COMMENTS

Pharmacologic stress is reserved for patients who cannot exercise (see Table 5-1). ST depression during adenosine occurs less commonly than with exercise (<20% of patients), although it is more specific (90%). A meta-analysis of 9 adenosine SPECT MPI studies involving ~1200 patients showed weighted mean sensitivities and specificities of 90% and 75%, respectively, for CAD detection (>50% stenosis) and 92% weighted mean sensitivity for multivessel CAD detection. The sensitivity of adenosine MPI to detect one-vessel, two-vessel, and three-vessel CAD was 83%, 91%, and 97%, respectively.

The presence of normal perfusion in Case 5-6 confers a low annual rate of events, whereas the annual event rate for Case 5-7 is high given the pattern of multivessel ischemia. Features that are indicative of high risk include moderately to severely abnormal perfusion abnormalities, multivessel perfusion abnormalities, poststress LVEF <45%, TID, and increased lung thallium uptake. The annual risk of cardiac death or MI is higher in patients referred to pharmacologic MPI than those referred to exercise MPI. The annual event rate in low-risk and high-risk patients undergoing pharmacologic MPI is 1.2% and 8.3%, respectively, compared with 0.7% and 5.6% in low- and high-risk patients undergoing exercise MPI.

Case 5-6   Positive Adenosine ECG, Abnormal Perfusion (Figure 5-6)

A 78-year-old white man with obstructive sleep apnea, depression, dyslipidemia, erectile dysfunction, ankle and knee arthritis, and CAD with CABG twice and multiple PCIs was referred for adenosine MPI because of recurrent chest pain. His baseline BP was 102/60 mm Hg and HR was 52 bpm. The peak HR was 58 bpm and his peak BP was 126/68 mm Hg. The adenosine ECG was positive for ischemia (Figure 5-6, *A, B*). The SPECT images showed LCX and RCA ischemia (Figure 5-6, *C, D*) with normal LVEF. He had septal hypokinesis secondary to prior CABG. Coronary angiography showed severe in-stent stenosis of distal LCX and occlusion of RCA (Figure 5-6, *E*). LIMA graft to the LAD was patent. He underwent PCI to distal LCX (Figure 5-6, *E*).

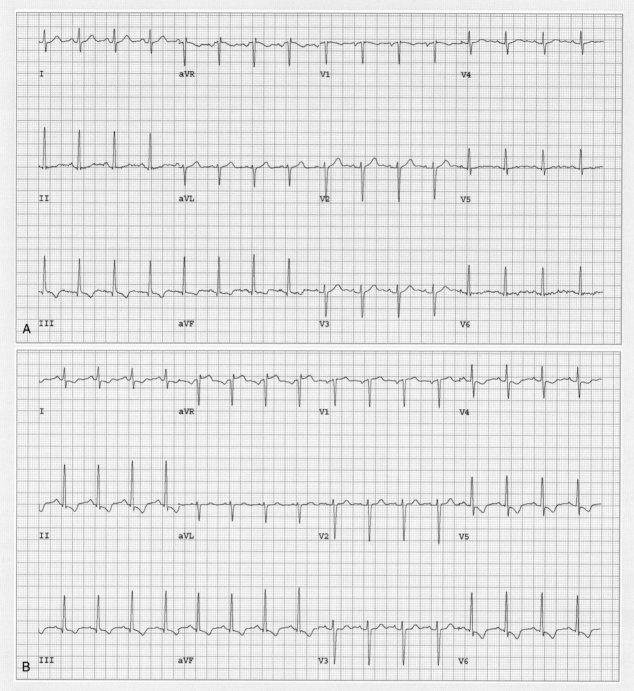

■ **Figure 5-6** The ECG at rest (**A**) and during adenosine infusion (**B**) showing ischemic changes.

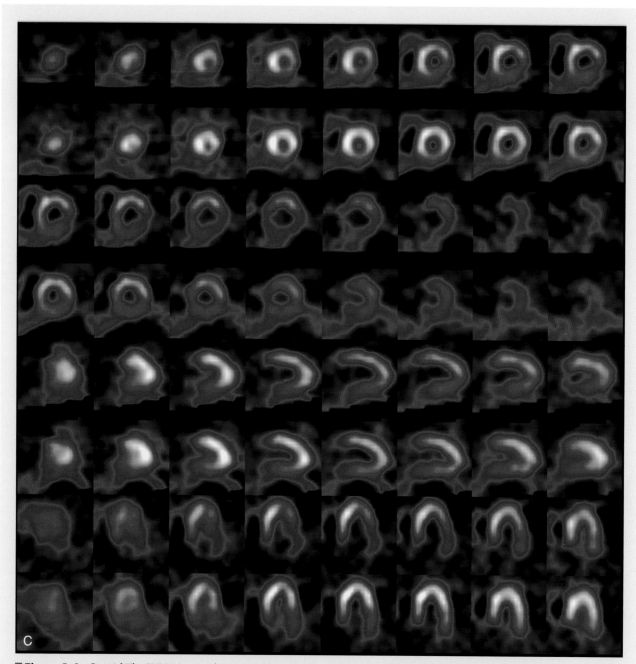

■ **Figure 5-6—Cont'd** The SPECT images show reversible perfusion abnormality in the LCX and RCA territories **(C).**

(Continued)

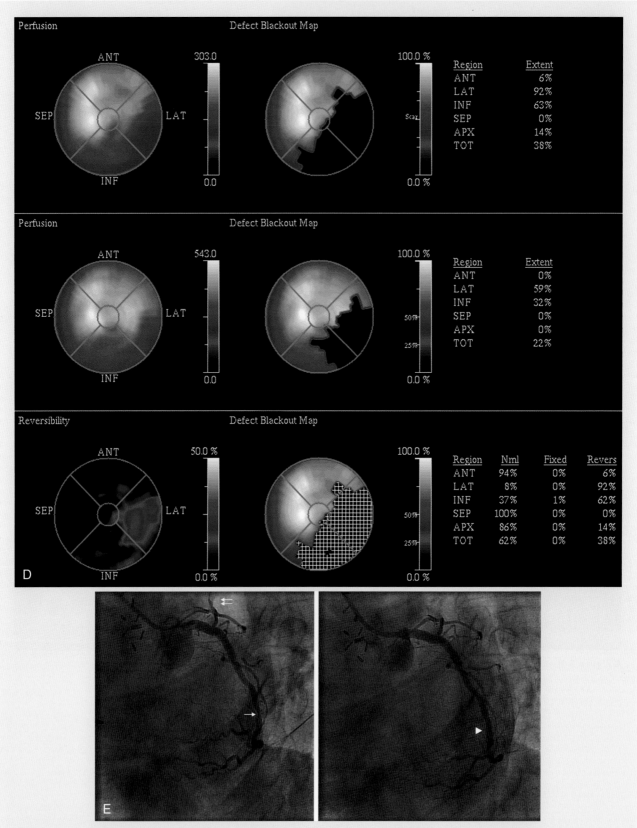

■ Figure 5-6—Cont'd The polar maps show a large abnormality **(D)**. Coronary angiography showed severe LCX in-stent restenosis *(white arrow)* **(E)**. The distal LCX after PCI *(white arrowhead)* is shown **(E)**. The LAD is occluded *(double white arrows)* but the LIMA is patent (not shown).

COMMENTS

Adenosine-induced ischemic ECG changes with normal perfusion occur in 1% to 2% of patients undergoing adenosine MPI. The majority of such patients are elderly women (80% to 90%), and in our experience, these patients have a benign prognosis and certainly not consistent with balanced ischemia due to multivessel disease. Ischemia during vasodilator stress can occur due to increased myocardial oxygen demand, decreased distal coronary perfusion, collapse at the stenosis, and coronary steal, either collateral dependant or, less likely, collateral independent.

Case 5-7   **Negative Regadenoson ECG Response, Abnormal Perfusion (Figure 5-7)**

A 60-year-old African American woman with HTN, end-stage renal disease, GERD, and CAD with prior PCI underwent regadenoson MPI for renal transplant evaluation. The baseline BP was 142/85 mm Hg and HR was 70 beats/min. The peak HR was 100 bpm and her nadir BP was 116/71 mm Hg. The regadenoson ECG was negative for ischemia (Figure 5-7, *A, B*). The SPECT images showed a large area of ischemia in the LCX distribution with TID (Figure 5-7, *C*) with normal LVEF and wall motion. Coronary angiography showed mild-to-moderate LAD stenosis, 90% stenosis of a marginal branch, and occluded distal posterior descending artery (Figure 5-7, *D*). She underwent PCI of the second marginal branch (Figure 5-7, *D*).

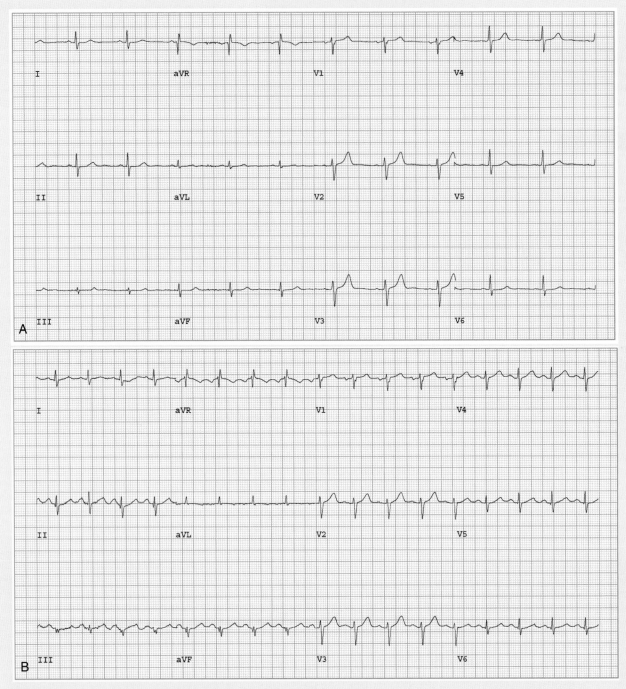

■**Figure 5-7** The ECG at rest (**A**) and in response to regadenoson (**B**) is normal.

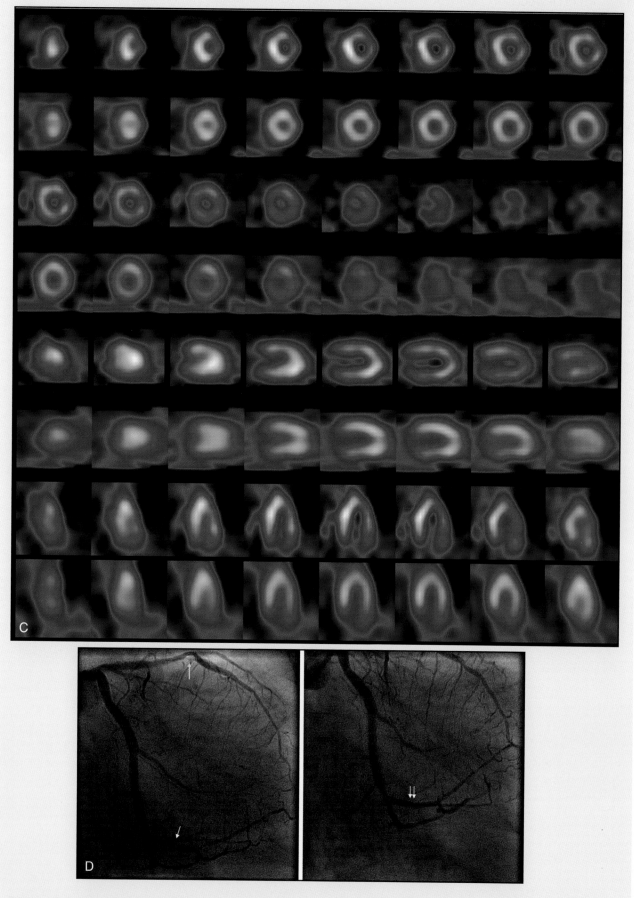

■**Figure 5-7—Cont'd** The SPECT images show a large area of reversible perfusion abnormality in the LCX distribution, with TID **(C)**. Coronary angiogram showed mild-to-moderate LAD disease *(yellow arrow)*, and severe marginal branch of LCX disease *(white arrow)*. The stenosis was corrected with a drug–eluting stent *(double white arrows)* **(D)**.

COMMENTS

Regadenoson is a new selective A_{2a} receptor agonist that is given as a single intravenous bolus. In the phase 3 multicenter trial that compared regadenoson to adenosine, ischemic ECG changes occurred in 17% of regadenoson and 17% of adenosine stress tests. Regadenoson was better tolerated than adenosine. Regadenoson provided diagnostic information comparable to adenosine. The average agreement rate was 0.63 ± 0.03 for regadenoson-adenosine and 0.64 ± 0.04 for adenosine-adenosine SPECT. There were no significant differences in total or ischemic perfusion defect sizes between regadenoson and adenosine. Linear regression showed a close correlation between adenosine and regadenoson for total ($r = 0.97$, $p < .001$) and ischemic ($r = 0.95$, $p < .001$) perfusion defect sizes. Regadenoson has been shown to be well tolerated in patients with mild-to-moderate asthma and in patients with moderate and severe COPD.

| Case 5-8 | Normal Dobutamine ECG, Abnormal Perfusion (Figure 5-8) |

An 80-year-old white man with HTN, GERD, DM, low back pain, cerebrovascular disease, asthma, dyslipidemia, and CAD with prior PCI underwent dobutamine MPI for evaluation of exertional angina. The baseline BP was 100/70 mm Hg and HR was 60 bpm. He received intravenous dobutamine at a maximal dose of 40 µg/kg/min. He achieved a peak HR of 117 bpm (83% of age predicted) and a peak BP of 170/90 mm Hg. The dobutamine ECG was negative for ischemia (Figure 5-8, *A*, *B*). The SPECT images showed a moderate-sized defect in the LCX territory (Figure 5-8, *C*). The LVEF was 68%. Coronary angiography showed minimal LAD and RCA disease but severe LCX disease (yellow arrow) (Figure 5-8, *D*). The coronary angiogram after PCI is also shown.

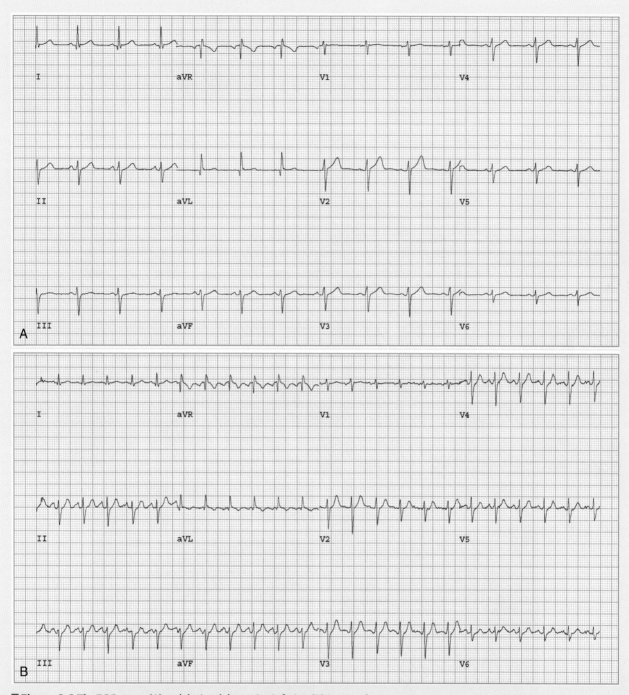

■ **Figure 5-8** The ECG at rest **(A)** and during dobutamine infusion **(B)** is normal.

(Continued)

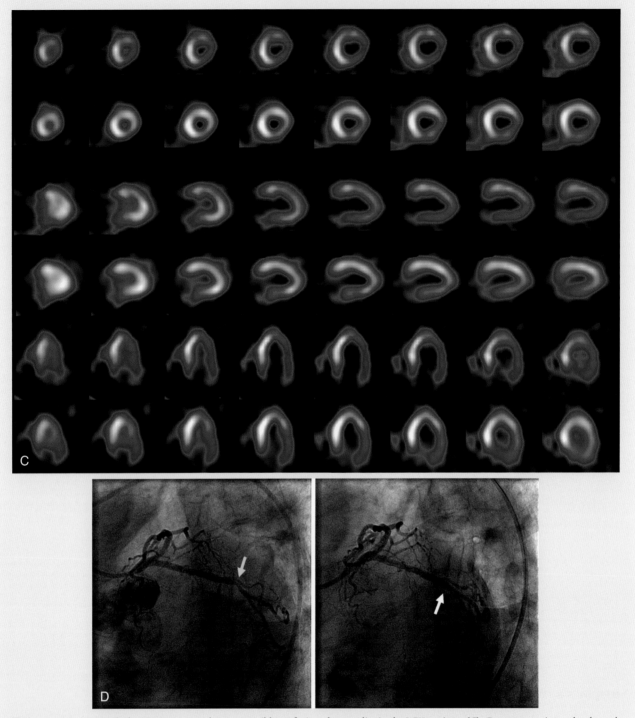

■**Figure 5-8—Cont'd** The SPECT images show a reversible perfusion abnormality in the LCX territory **(C)**. Coronary angiography showed mild LAD and RCA disease and severe mid LCX stenosis *(yellow arrow)* **(D)**. The LCX is also shown post PCI *(white arrow)*.

COMMENTS

Dobutamine stress is reserved for patients who are not a candidate for exercise and vasodilator stress (see Table 5-1). As such, patients undergoing dobutamine stress tend to be sicker patients. ST depressions occur in 30% to 50% of such patients. In a meta-analysis of 20 studies involving around 1000 patients who underwent dobutamine SPECT, weighted sensitivity, specificity, and accuracy for CAD detection were 88%, 74%, and 84%, respectively. The sensitivity increased from 82% to 90% with the use of atropine in addition to maximal dobutamine dose. The respective sensitivities of dobutamine MPI to detect one-vessel, two-vessel, and three-vessel CAD were 84%, 95%, and 100%, respectively. In patients with chest pain who underwent dobutamine MPI, the annual cardiac event rate was 0.8% in those with normal perfusion. Patients with increasing reversible defect scores had increasing annual event rates of 2.1%, 5.0%, 5.5%, 13.0%, and 14.6%, respectively. In a study of patients with known or suspected CAD who underwent dobutamine MPI, the cardiac death rate was 1% per year in patients with a normal MPI compared to 5.1% per year in patients with an abnormal MPI. The presence of perfusion abnormalities provided incremental prognostic information to clinical, electrocardiographic, and hemodynamic data.

SELECTED READINGS

Abbott BG, Afshar M, Berger AK, Wackers FJ: Prognostic significance of ischemic electrocardiographic changes during adenosine infusion in patients with normal myocardial perfusion imaging, *J Nucl Cardiol* 10:9–16, 2003.

Amanullah AM, Aasa M: Significance of ST-segment depression during adenosine-induced coronary hyperemia in angina pectoris and correlation with angiographic, scintigraphic, hemodynamic, and echocardiographic variables, *Int J Cardiol* 48:167–176, 1995.

Dunn RF, Freedman B, Kelly DT, et al: Exercise-induced ST-segment elevation in leads V1 or aVL. A predictor of anterior myocardial ischemia and left anterior descending coronary artery disease, *Circulation* 63:1357–1363, 1981.

Fleischmann KE, Hunink MG, Kuntz KM, et al: Exercise echocardiography or exercise SPECT imaging? A meta-analysis of diagnostic test performance, *JAMA* 280:913–920, 1998.

Geleijnse ML, Elhendy A, Fioretti PM, et al: Dobutamine stress myocardial perfusion imaging, *J Am Coll Cardiol* 36:2017–2027, 2000.

Geleijnse ML, Elhendy A, van Domburg RT, et al: Prognostic value of dobutamine-atropine stress technetium-99m sestamibi perfusion scintigraphy in patients with chest pain, *J Am Coll Cardiol* 28:447–454, 1996.

Gibbons RJ, Balady GJ, Bricker JT, et al: ACC/AHA 2002 Guideline Update for Exercise Testing: Summary Article. A report of the American College of Cardiology/American Heart Association Task Force on Practice Guidelines (Committee to Update the 1997 Exercise Testing Guidelines), *J Am Coll Cardiol* 40:1531–1540, 2002.

Gulati M, Pratap P, Kansal P, et al: Gender differences in the value of ST-segment depression during adenosine stress testing, *Am J Cardiol* 94:997–1002, 2004.

Hage FG, Dubovsky EV, Heo J, et al: Outcome of patients with adenosine-induced ST-segment depression but with normal perfusion on tomographic imaging, *Am J Cardiol* 98:1009–1011, 2006.

Henzlova MJ, Cerqueira MD, Mahmarian JJ, Yao S: Stress protocols and tracers, *J Nucl Cardiol* 13:e80–90, 2006.

Hung M, Hung M, Cheng C, et al: Clinical characteristics of patients with exercise-induced ST-segment elevation without prior myocardial infarction, *Circ J* 70:254–261, 2006.

Iskandrian A, Garcia E, editors: *Nuclear Cardiac Imaging: Principles and Applications*, ed 4, New York, 2008, Oxford University Press.

Iskandrian AE, Bateman TM, Belardinelli L, et al: Adenosine versus regadenoson comparative evaluation in myocardial perfusion imaging: results of the ADVANCE phase 3 multicenter international trial, *J Nucl Cardiol* 14:645–658, 2007.

Iskandrian AS, Chae SC, Heo J, et al: Independent and incremental prognostic value of exercise single-photon emission computed tomography (SPECT) thallium imaging in coronary artery disease, *J Am Coll Cardiol* 22:665–670, 1993.

Kim C, Kwok YS, Heagerty P, et al: Pharmacologic stress testing for coronary disease diagnosis: a meta-analysis, *Am Heart J* 142:934–944, 2001.

Klocke FJ, Baird MG, Lorell BH, et al: ACC/AHA/ASNC Guidelines for the Clinical Use of Cardiac Radionuclide Imaging—Executive Summary: A Report of the American College of Cardiology/American Heart Association Task Force on Practice Guidelines (ACC/AHA/ASNC Committee to Revise the 1995 Guidelines for the Clinical Use of Cardiac Radionuclide Imaging), *J Am Coll Cardiol* 42:1318–1333, 2003.

Klodas E, Miller TD, Christian TF, et al: Prognostic significance of ischemic electrocardiographic changes during vasodilator stress testing in patients with normal SPECT images, *J Nucl Cardiol* 10:4–8, 2003.

Kwok Y, Kim C, Grady D, et al: Meta-analysis of exercise testing to detect coronary artery disease in women, *Am J Cardiol* 83:660–666, 1999.

Leaker BR, O'Connor B, Hansel TT, et al: Safety of regadenoson, an adenosine A2A receptor agonist for myocardial perfusion imaging, in mild asthma and moderate asthma patients: a randomized, double-blind, placebo-controlled trial, *J Nucl Cardiol* 15:329–336, 2008.

Mahmarian JJ, Cerqueira MD, Iskandrian AE, et al: Regadenoson induces comparable left ventricular perfusion defects as adenosine: a quantitative analysis from the ADVANCE MPI 2 trial, *JACC Cardiovasc Imaging* 2:959–968, 2009.

Mahmarian JJ, Verani MS: Myocardial perfusion imaging during pharmacologic stress testing, *Cardiol Clin* 12:223–245, 1994.

Marshall ES, Raichlen JS, Kim SM, et al: Prognostic significance of ST-segment depression during adenosine perfusion imaging, *Am Heart J* 130:58–66, 1995.

Miller TD, Roger VL, Milavetz JJ, et al: Assessment of the exercise electrocardiogram in women versus men using tomographic myocardial perfusion imaging as the reference standard, *Am J Cardiol* 87:868–873, 2001.

Schinkel AFL, Elhendy A, van Domburg RT, et al: Prognostic value of dobutamine-atropine stress (99m)Tc-tetrofosmin myocardial perfusion SPECT in patients with known or suspected coronary artery disease, *J Nucl Med* 43:767–772, 2002.

Shaw LJ, Iskandrian AE: Prognostic value of gated myocardial perfusion SPECT, *J Nucl Cardiol* 11:171–185, 2004.

Thomas GS, Tammelin BR, Schiffman GL, et al: Safety of regadenoson, a selective adenosine A2A agonist, in patients with chronic obstructive pulmonary disease: a randomized, double-blind, placebo-controlled trial (RegCOPD trial), *J Nucl Cardiol* 15:319–328, 2008.

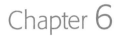

Chapter 6

Use in Stable Patients With Known or Suspected Coronary Artery Disease

Gilbert J. Zoghbi, Eva V. Dubovsky, and Ami E. Iskandrian

KEY POINTS

- Stress MPI remains the most common imaging modality used in patients with known or suspected CAD.

- The improvement in hardware and software and the availability of multiple stress modalities and imaging protocols have contributed to the continued growth and success of stress MPI.

- There is an increasing awareness of the radiation risk and the means to minimize it.

- There are appropriateness criteria and guidelines that define the proper indications for stress MPI.

- Stress MPI provides comprehensive information on myocardial perfusion and regional and global LV function that have incremental diagnostic and prognostic information.

- The results of stress MPI have had a major impact on the role of coronary angiography as the "gold standard" for sensitivity and specificity reporting.

- The terms "false negative" and "false positive" in regard to MPI results should be reconsidered in lieu of the serious limitations of coronary angiography in predicting myocardial blood flow.

- The size of the perfusion defect has stood the test of time in predicting patient outcome and the presence of either fixed defects (scar) or reversible defects (ischemia) are important.

- The presence of additional non-perfusion data may be helpful in managing patients with conditions such as stunning, transient dilatation, and RV dysfunction.

- Not all patients with multivessel disease will have perfusion defects in all diseased territories—not unlike the results of functional assessment of coronary stenoses by flow or pressure wire. which showed not all diseased vessels are physiologically important.

BACKGROUND

CAD represents a major worldwide health problem. It is estimated that in the United States, 17.6 million individuals have CAD. Around 8.5 million individuals have a history of MI, and 10.2 million individuals have angina pectoris. The lifetime risk of developing CAD is 49% for males and 32% for females aged >40 years. Although the CAD mortality has been declining, it is anticipated that the prevalence of CAD will continue to increase. Stress testing with MPI is one of the most commonly used noninvasive modalities for evaluation of individuals who have or are suspected of having CAD. Stress MPI is generally indicated for diagnosing CAD, risk-stratifying patients with known CAD, assessing therapeutic interventions and progression/regression of CAD, and assessing the physiological significance of an intermediate coronary stenosis. Appropriateness criteria and national guidelines have been published to assist in the proper use of stress MPI (Table 6-1).

Exercise and pharmacologic stress agents increase MBF, although via different mechanisms. The peak, or hyperemic, MBF is inversely related to the degree of coronary stenosis but the relationship is not linear. Several studies have shown considerable discordance between the percent diameter stenosis, a measure of anatomic significance of coronary stenosis, and FFR, a measure of the physiologic significance of coronary stenosis in patients with one-, two-, and three-vessel disease. This crucial observation casts doubt on prior studies that used coronary angiography as the "gold standard" to assess the performance of stress MPI (sensitivity and specificity). There is one more overlooked fact—that FFR does not provide data on the extent of a perfusion abnormality or on the nature of the abnormality (scar, ischemia, or mixed). These latter data combined with LVEF and volume have been proven to be powerful predictors of outcome in patients with known or suspected CAD.

TABLE 6-1 Appropriateness Criteria for Stress MPI in Patients With Known or Suspected CAD

	SCORE
1. Detection of CAD	
• Symptomatic patients	
• Low CAD pretest probability + uninterpretable ECG or cannot exercise	7
• Intermediate CAD pretest probability + uninterpretable ECG and can exercise	7
• Intermediate CAD pretest probability + ECG or cannot exercise	9
• High CAD pretest probability regardless of ECG or ability to exercise	8
2. Detection of CAD/Risk Assessment	
• Asymptomatic patients	
• High ATP III CHD risk	7
• Miscellaneous cardiac conditions	
• New CHF with LV dysfunction + no prior CAD evaluation and nor planned coronary angiography (without ischemia equivalent symptoms)	8
• Ventricular tachycardia + low ATP III CHD risk	7
• Ventricular tachycardia + intermediate or high ATP III CHF risk	8
• Syncope + intermediate or high ATP III CHF risk	7
3. Risk Assessment in Asymptomatic or Stable Symptoms	
• Equivocal, discordant, or borderline stress testing results with concern for presence of obstructive CAD	8
• New or worsening symptoms + abnormal coronary angiography or abnormal prior stress test	9
• Coronary stenosis or abnormality of indeterminate significance	9
• Asymptomatic patient + high CHD risk with Agatston score 100-400	7
• Asymptomatic patient + Agatston score >400	7
• Intermediate risk Duke treadmill score	7
• High risk Duke treadmill score	8

Appropriateness scores are based on a score from 1 to 9 based on the consensus of experts. Scores of 7 to 9 are considered appropriate indications, scores of 4 to 6 are considered uncertain indications, and scores of <4 are considered inappropriate indications.

The accuracy of stress MPI (or any testing modality) for the diagnosis of CAD depends on the disease severity and the test's characteristics. Despite the limitations of coronary angiography, in a meta-analysis of 27 studies involving around 3200 patients who underwent exercise MPI, the weighted respective sensitivities and specificities of exercise SPECT for CAD detection were 87% and 64%. The normalcy rate of exercise SPECT MPI for detecting CAD in patients with low likelihood of CAD was 90% in 10 pooled studies involving 628 patients. The mean sensitivities and specificities of vasodilator SPECT MPI for detection of CAD were 86% and 73%, respectively, from pooled studies of about 2500 patients. In a meta-analysis of nine adenosine SPECT MPI studies involving about 1200 patients, the respective mean sensitivity and specificity for CAD detection were 90% and 75%, respectively, with a normalcy rate of 90% in patients with low likelihood of disease. In a meta-analysis of 24 studies involving about 1200 patients, the respective sensitivity, specificity, and accuracy of dobutamine SPECT MPI for CAD detection were 85%, 72%, and 77%, respectively. The use of gating and attenuation correction in one study of adenosine SPECT imaging significantly improved the sensitivity and normalcy rates to >90%.

Case 6-1   Stress Testing After MI (Figure 6-1)

An 81-year-old African American woman with history of HTN, dyslipidemia, end-stage renal disease status post renal transplantation, osteoporosis, and GERD had a non–ST-elevation MI 6 months ago at an outside facility. She did not undergo coronary angiography because of concerns about her renal function. She underwent regadenoson MPI for evaluation of dyspnea on exertion 6 months after her MI. The stress MPI showed normal perfusion (Figure 6-1, *A, B*), LVEF, and wall motion/thickening (Figure 6-1, *C*).

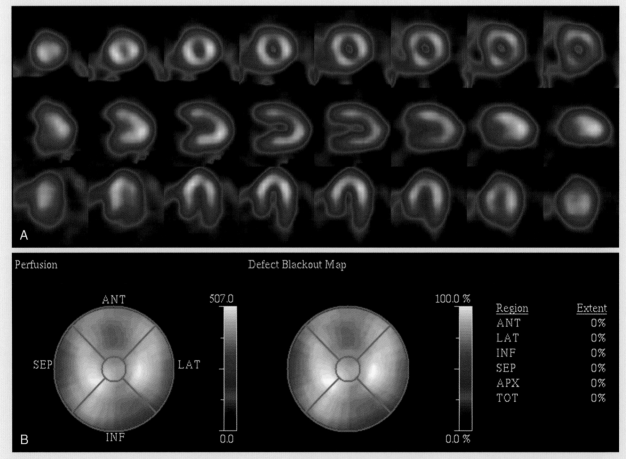

■ **Figure 6-1** Stress-only regadenoson SPECT sestamibi images showing a normal perfusion pattern **(A)**. The polar maps are normal **(B)**.

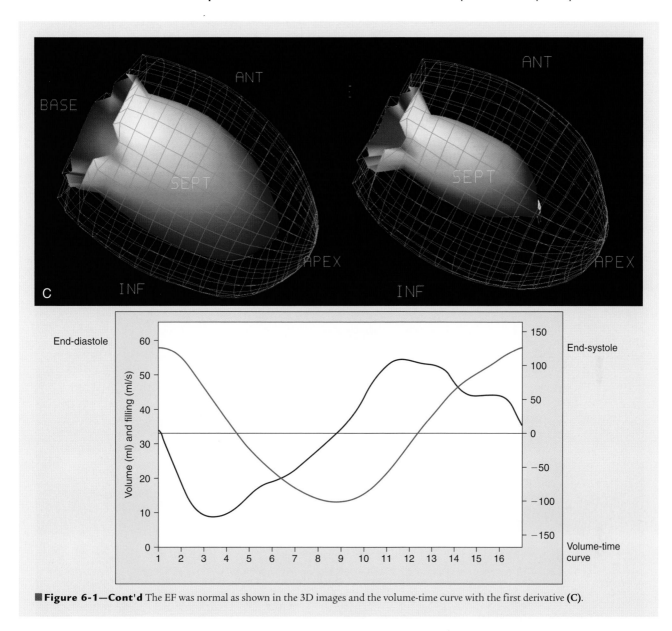

■ **Figure 6-1—Cont'd** The EF was normal as shown in the 3D images and the volume-time curve with the first derivative **(C)**.

COMMENTS

The normal stress MPI in this patient predicts good prognosis. The diagnosis of non–ST elevation MI is not easy in patients with severe renal disease as the chest pain, troponin elevation, and ECG changes could be due to severe LV hypertrophy. The normal MPI in this patient spared her from contrast nephrotoxicity. The shortness of breath is likely due to diastolic LV dysfunction.

Case 6-2 **Stress Testing in a Patient With Known CAD (Figure 6-2)**

An 80-year-old white man with HTN, cerebrovascular disease with history of bilateral carotid endarterectomy, chronic renal insufficiency, mild-to-moderate CAD, and dyslipidemia was referred for exercise MPI for evaluation of a 3-month history of exertional angina. He exercised for 4 minutes 49 seconds according to the Bruce protocol. He attained a peak HR of 142 bpm and a peak BP of 160/100 mm Hg. The ECG did not show ischemic changes. The SPECT images showed a large area of ischemia in the LAD distribution with normal LVEF (Figure 6-2, *A*, *B*). Coronary angiography showed 50% distal left main stenosis and 95% proximal LAD stenosis involving the major diagonal (Figure 6-2, *C*).

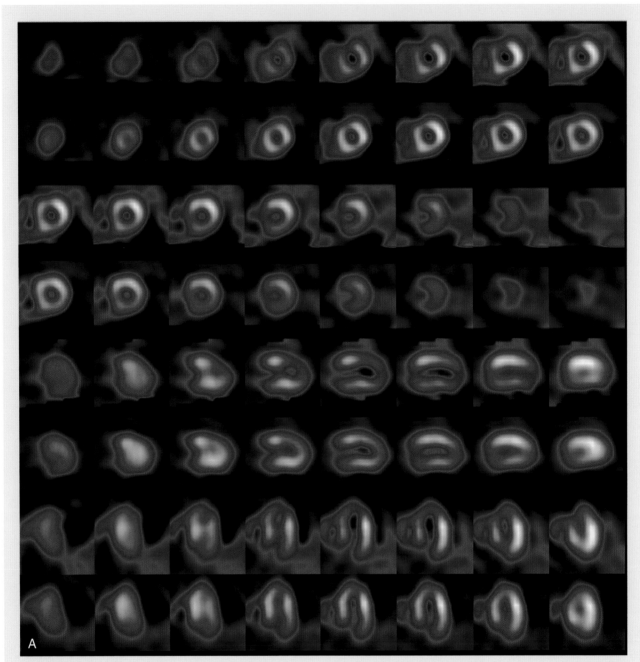

■ **Figure 6-2** Exercise/rest SPECT sestamibi images showing a reversible perfusion abnormality in the LAD territory **(A)**.

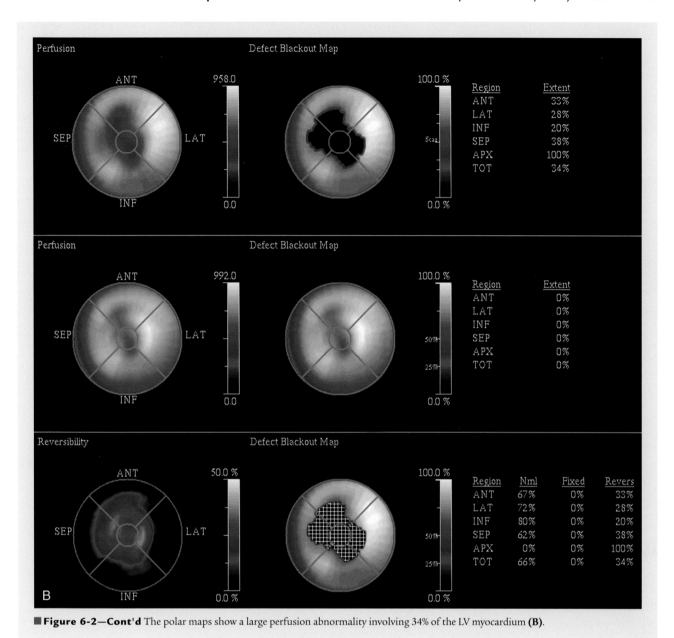

Region	Extent
ANT	33%
LAT	28%
INF	20%
SEP	38%
APX	100%
TOT	34%

Region	Extent
ANT	0%
LAT	0%
INF	0%
SEP	0%
APX	0%
TOT	0%

Region	Nml	Fixed	Revers
ANT	67%	0%	33%
LAT	72%	0%	28%
INF	80%	0%	20%
SEP	62%	0%	38%
APX	0%	0%	100%
TOT	66%	0%	34%

■ **Figure 6-2—Cont'd** The polar maps show a large perfusion abnormality involving 34% of the LV myocardium **(B)**.

(Continued)

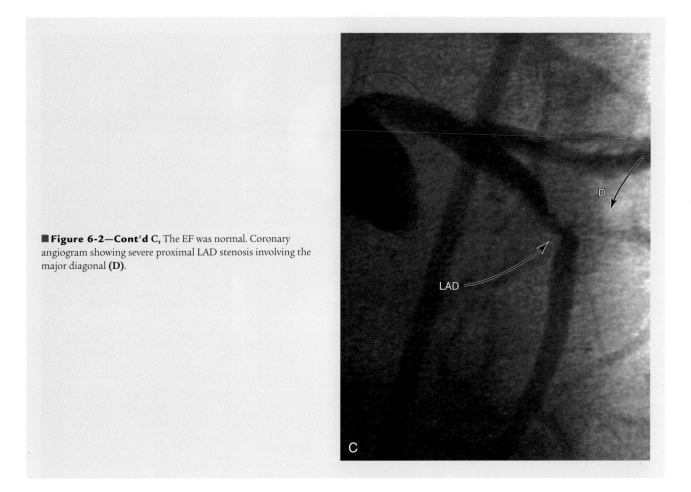

■ **Figure 6-2—Cont'd C,** The EF was normal. Coronary angiogram showing severe proximal LAD stenosis involving the major diagonal **(D)**.

Case 6-3   Stress Testing in a Patient With Shortness of Breath (Figure 6-3)

A 39-year-old African American woman with type 1 DM and dyslipidemia underwent exercise MPI for evaluation of dyspnea on exertion. She exercised for 8 minutes according to the Bruce protocol. She attained a peak HR of 184 bpm and a peak systolic BP of 118/70 mm Hg. She stopped exercise due to shortness of breath. The ECG showed ST depression at peak exercise. The SPECT images showed a large area of ischemia in the LCX distribution with normal LVEF (Figure 6-3, *A, B*). Coronary angiography showed severe LCX disease. She underwent PCI of the LCX with a drug-eluting stent.

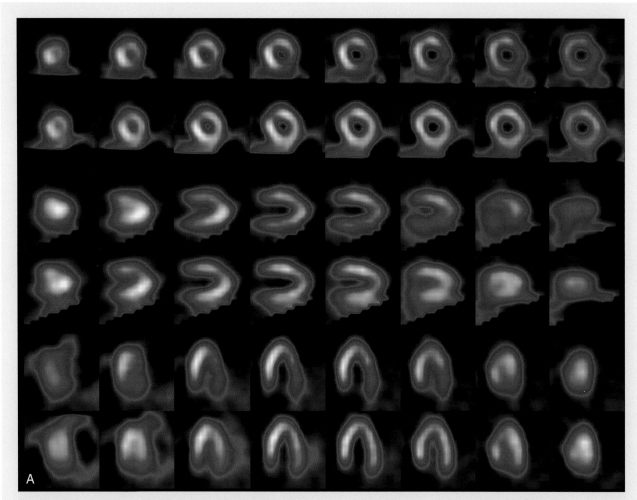

■ **Figure 6-3** Exercise/rest SPECT sestamibi images showing a reversible perfusion abnormality in the LCX territory **(A)**.

(Continued)

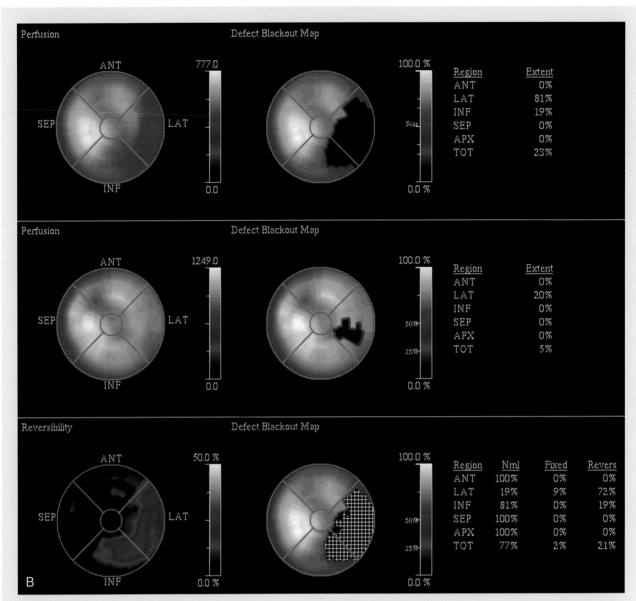

■**Figure 6-3—Cont'd** The polar maps show a large abnormality involving 23% of the LV myocardium **(B)**. The EF was normal. Coronary angiography showed severe LCX disease.

Case 6-4 **Stress Testing in a Patient With an Intermediate Pretest Likelihood of CAD (Figure 6-4)**

A 54-year-old white woman with systemic lupus erythematosus and hypothyroidism underwent exercise MPI for evaluation of fatigue and shortness of breath. She exercised for 7 minutes 16 seconds according to the Bruce protocol. She stopped due to fatigue. The peak HR was 153 bpm and her peak systolic BP was 140/74 mm Hg. The exercise ECG was negative for ischemia. The SPECT images showed ischemia in the RCA and LCX territories with normal LVEF (Figure 6-4, *A–C*). Coronary angiography showed 80% mid RCA stenosis and 95% mid LCX stenosis (Figure 6-4, *D*). She underwent staged stenting of the RCA and LCX stenoses.

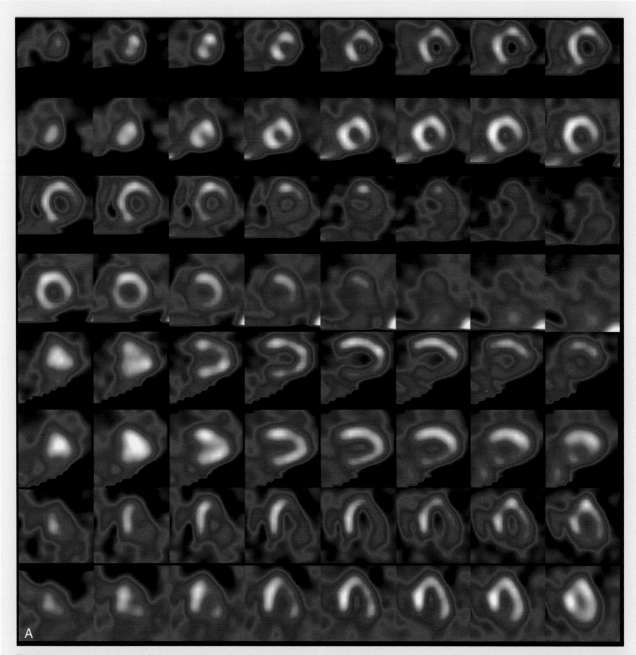

■ **Figure 6-4** Stress/rest regadenoson SPECT sestamibi images showing a reversible perfusion abnormality in the RCA and LCX territories **(A)**.

(Continued)

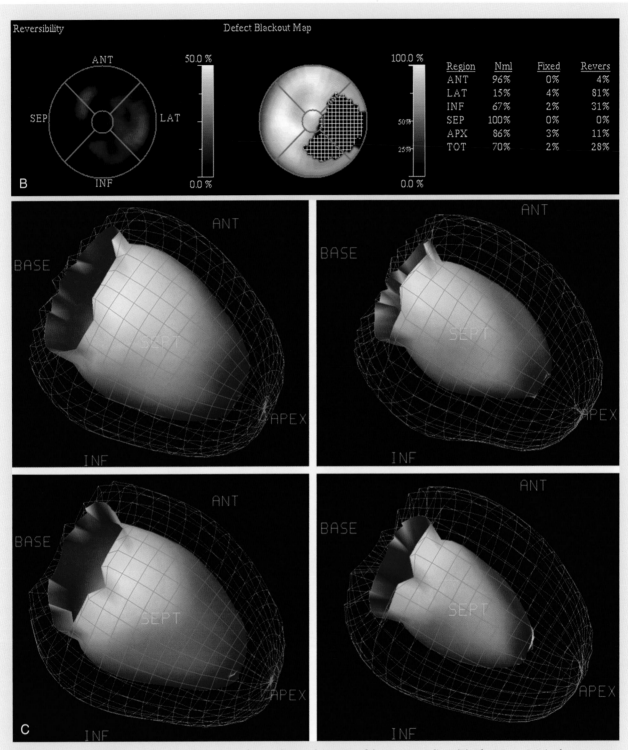

■Figure 6-4—Cont'd The polar maps show a large abnormality involving 28% of the LV myocardium **(B)**. The EF was 54% in the post-stress images and 68% in the rest images, suggesting poststress stunning **(C)**.

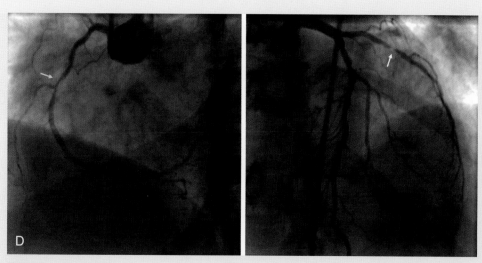

■**Figure 6-4—Cont'd** Coronary angiogram showing severe mid RCA *(yellow arrow)* and mid LCX *(white arrow)* stenoses **(D)**.

| Case 6-5 | Stress Testing in a Patient With a High Pretest Likelihood of CAD (Figure 6-5) |

A 64-year-old white man with DM, tobacco abuse, peripheral vascular disease, and dyslipidemia underwent regadenoson MPI for evaluation of exertional chest pain of 8 months duration. His HR increased from 58 at baseline to 92 bpm after regadenoson. The SPECT images showed a multivessel reversible perfusion abnormality in the RCA and LAD territories (Figure 6-5, *A, B*). The LVEF was normal. Coronary angiography showed severe LCX, RCA, and LAD disease (Figure 6-5, *C*). He had a remarkable symptomatic improvement after CABG.

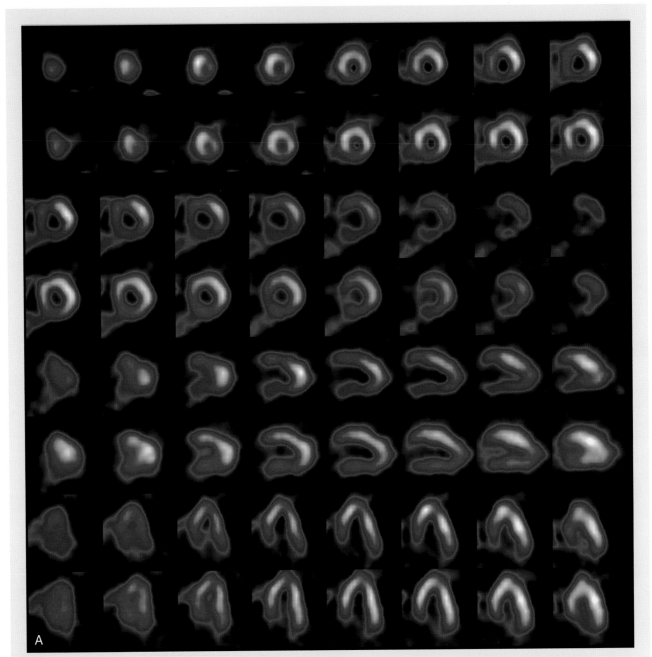

■ **Figure 6-5** Stress/rest regadenoson SPECT sestamibi images showing a reversible perfusion abnormality in the RCA and LAD territories **(A)**.

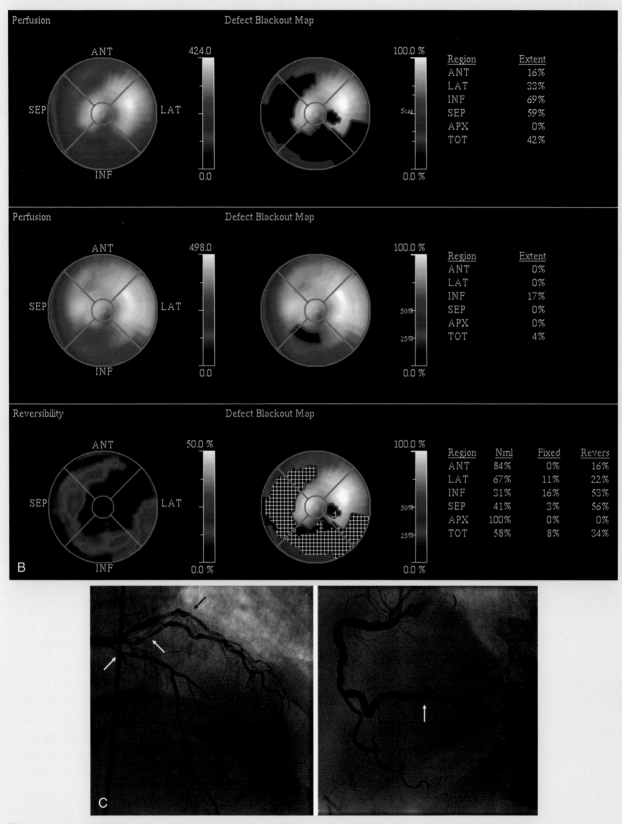

■ **Figure 6-5—Cont'd** The polar maps show a large abnormality involving 42% of the LV myocardium **(B)**. The EF was normal. Coronary angiogram showing severe LAD, LCX, and RCA disease (**C,** *arrows* show stenotic sites).

COMMENTS ON CASES 6-2 TO 6-5

These cases demonstrate a spectrum of perfusion abnormalities in patients with an intermediate to high pretest probability of CAD. Perfusion abnormalities can be quantified using one of several methods as discussed in Chapter 2. The automated analysis is a distinct advantage of MPI. The respective sensitivity and specificity of exercise MPI for the detection of significant LAD disease are 83% and 88%; for significant RCA disease, 89% and 93%; and for significant LCX disease, 77% and 90%. The respective sensitivity and specificity of adenosine MPI for the detection of significant LAD disease are 75% and 97%; for significant RCA disease, 75% and 96%; and for significant LCX disease, 60% and 90%. The respective accuracy for LAD, RCA, and LCX disease is 85%, 86%, and 75%. The respective mean sensitivity and specificity of dobutamine MPI for the detection of significant LAD disease are 68% and 90%; for significant RCA disease, 88% and 81%; and for significant LCX disease, 50% and 94%. These results must be considered cautiously as the comparison is made to coronary angiography.

| Case 6-6 | Stress Testing in a Patient With Recurrent Symptoms After Coronary Revascularization (Figure 6-6) |

An 81-year-old white man with HTN, DM, sick sinus syndrome (status post permanent pacemaker implantation), dyslipidemia, arthritis, and CAD with prior CABG and PCI underwent regadenoson MPI for evaluation of recurrent exertional angina and dyspnea on exertion. The ECG response was nondiagnostic for ischemia due to underlying paced rhythm. The HR increased from 71 at baseline to 83 bpm after regadenoson. The SPECT images showed a large area of ischemia in all three vascular territories, severely depressed LVEF, TID, and poststress stunning (Figure 6-6, *A–C*). The EF on rest imaging was 24% (not shown). Coronary angiography showed occlusion of the grafts but reasonable distal runoffs. He underwent repeat CABG.

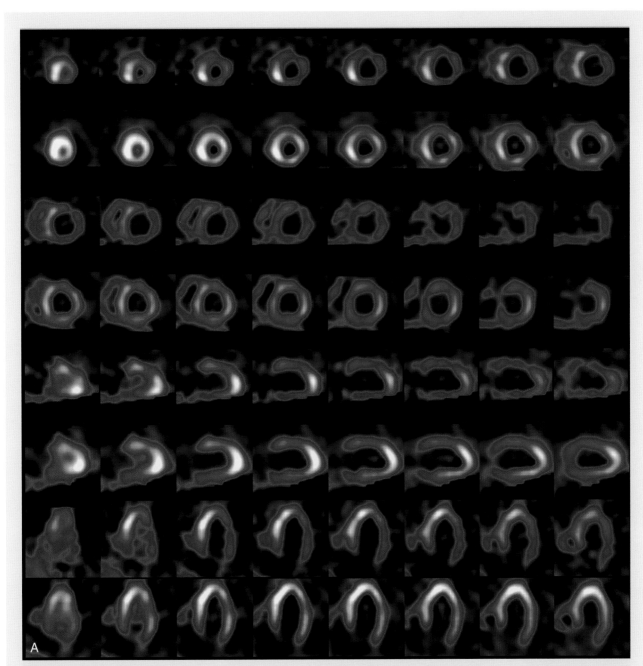

■**Figure 6-6** Stress/rest regadenoson SPECT sestamibi images showing reversible and partially reversible perfusion abnormalities in all three vascular territories **(A)**.

(Continued)

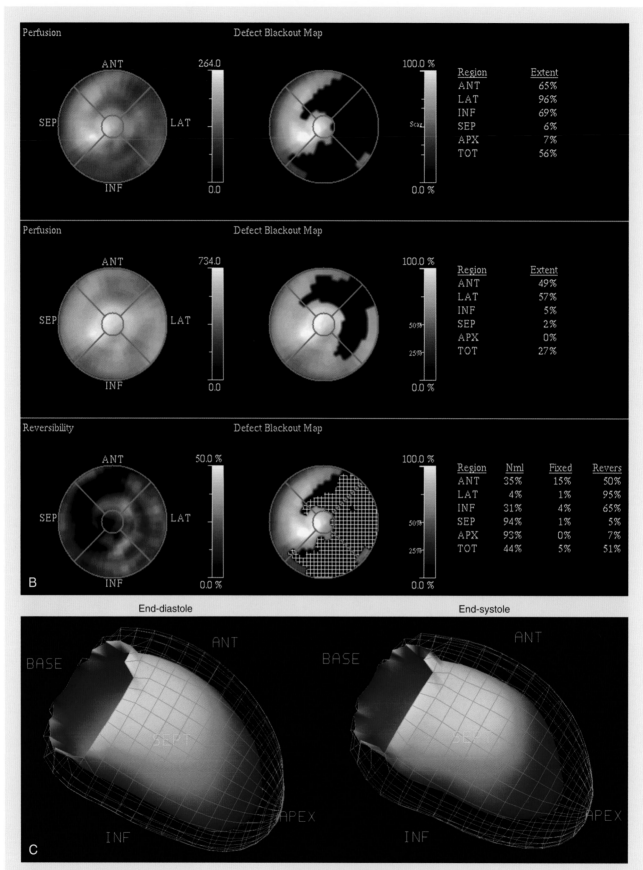

Figure 6-6—Cont'd The polar maps show a large abnormality involving 56% of the LV myocardium **(B)**. The poststress EF was markedly reduced, suggesting stunning and hibernation **(C)**.

COMMENTS

This case illustrates a frequent chapter in the lives of patients with CAD; recurrence of symptoms and the need for additional interventions. The symptoms and scan findings suggested a high-risk profile and a repeat CABG was considered the best option as the patient was already on maximum medical therapy.

SELECTED READINGS

Abreu A, Mahmarian JJ, Nishimura S, et al: Tolerance and safety of pharmacologic coronary vasodilation with adenosine in association with thallium-201 scintigraphy in patients with suspected coronary artery disease, *J Am Coll Cardiol* 18:730–735, 1991.

Amanullah AM, Kiat H, Friedman JD, Berman DS: Adenosine technetium-99m sestamibi myocardial perfusion SPECT in women: diagnostic efficacy in detection of coronary artery disease, *J Am Coll Cardiol* 27:803–809, 1996.

Berman DS, Kang X, Hayes SW, et al: Adenosine myocardial perfusion single-photon emission computed tomography in women compared with men. Impact of diabetes mellitus on incremental prognostic value and effect on patient management, *J Am Coll Cardiol* 41: 1125–1133, 2003.

Fleischmann KE, Hunink MG, Kuntz KM, Douglas PS: Exercise echocardiography or exercise SPECT imaging? A meta-analysis of diagnostic test performance, *JAMA* 280:913–920, 1998.

Geleijnse ML, Elhendy A, Fioretti PM, et al: Dobutamine stress myocardial perfusion imaging, *J Am Coll Cardiol* 36:2017–2027, 2000.

Hendel RC, Berman DS, Di Carli MF, et al: ACCF/ASNC/ACR/AHA/ASE/SCCT/SCMR/SNM 2009 Appropriate Use Criteria for Cardiac Radionuclide Imaging: A Report of the American College of Cardiology Foundation Appropriate Use Criteria Task Force, the American Society of Nuclear Cardiology, the American College of Radiology, the American Heart Association, the American Society of Echocardiography, the Society of Cardiovascular Computed Tomography, the Society for Cardiovascular Magnetic Resonance, and the Society of Nuclear Medicine, *J Am Coll Cardiol* 53:2201–2229, 2009.

Iskandrian A, Garcia E, editors: *Nuclear Cardiac Imaging: Principles and Applications*, ed 4, New York, 2008, Oxford University Press.

Kim C, Kwok YS, Heagerty P, et al: Pharmacologic stress testing for coronary disease diagnosis: a meta-analysis, *Am Heart J* 142(6):934–944, 2001.

Klocke FJ, Baird MG, Lorell BH, et al: ACC/AHA/ASNC guidelines for the clinical use of cardiac radionuclide imaging—executive summary: a report of the American College of Cardiology/American Heart Association Task Force on Practice Guidelines (ACC/AHA/ASNC Committee to Revise the 1995 Guidelines for the Clinical Use of Cardiac Radionuclide Imaging), *J Am Coll Cardiol* 42:1318–1333, 2003.

Lloyd-Jones D, Adams RJ, Brown TM, et al: Executive summary: heart disease and stroke statistics–2010 update: a report from the American Heart Association, *Circulation* 121:948–954, 2010.

Mahmarian JJ, Boyce TM, Goldberg RK, et al: Quantitative exercise thallium-201 single photon emission computed tomography for the enhanced diagnosis of ischemic heart disease, *J Am Coll Cardiol* 15:318–329, 1990.

Pereztol-Valdés O, Candell-Riera J, Santana-Boado C, et al: Correspondence between left ventricular 17 myocardial segments and coronary arteries, *Eur Heart J* 26:2637–2643, 2005.

Shaw LJ, Iskandrian AE: Prognostic value of gated myocardial perfusion SPECT, *J Nucl Cardiol* 11:171–185, 2004.

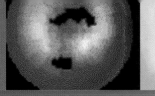

Chapter 7

Serial Testing

Fadi G. Hage, Fahad M. Iqbal, and Ami E. Iskandrian

KEY POINTS

- MPI has been extensively studied to examine the effects of interventions or changes using well-validated techniques.

- Variations in imaging protocol, tracer dose, processing, and quality could contribute to variability in the presence, type, and severity of perfusion abnormalities.

- Side-by-side visual comparison and the use of supervised automated methods are helpful in serial testing to study improvement/worsening in regional and global indices of MPI.

- Serial MPI can be helpful in determining the success and or complications of PCI and CABG and in the evaluation of patients with recurrent or new symptoms.

- Serial MPI can be used to compare the effects of a treatment or intervention versus an alternative or placebo.

- Serial MPI can be used to assess the effect of a new treatment in patients with conditions other than CAD, such as alcohol septal ablation in patients with hypertrophic cardiomyopathy.

- Serial MPI studies can be used to evaluate the effectiveness of optimum medical therapy in suppressing ischemia.

- Serial MPI can be used to determine the effectiveness of newer forms of treatment for angina pectoris, such as angiogenesis or stem cell therapy.

- Serial MPI studies can be used to compare an already approved tracer or stress agent with a new and, as yet, unapproved tracer or stress agent.

- Serial gated blood pool imaging for the evaluation of LVEF has been extensively used to monitor patients receiving chemotherapy

BACKGROUND

Gated SPECT MPI is an established method for the assessment of myocardial perfusion and LVEF. In patient care and research, there is a need for serial testing either because of a change in the clinical presentation, because of a desire to examine the effects of a variety of treatments or interventions, or the introduction of newer imaging tracers or stress agents. The comparison of two or more serial studies is anything but straightforward. The reader needs to decide whether there is an improvement or worsening in extent, severity, location, and type (reversible or fixed) of perfusion abnormality. For example, there could be an improvement in one region and a worsening in another region and yet the global score remains unchanged.

Guidelines by the American Society of Nuclear Cardiology endorse the adoption of a model in which the LV is represented by 17 segments to localize the perfusion defect and define its extent as the number of myocardial segments involved. This is usually combined with the use of a scoring system to assess the activity level in each segment (e.g., 0 = normal and 4 = absent). The summed scores (summed rest score, summed stress score, and summed difference score) therefore represent extent and severity (but not location). Alternatively, polar maps can define the extent, severity, and reversibility of the perfusion abnormality (expressed as percent of LV myocardium or as a percent of the vascular territory). As mentioned in Chapter 2, these scores could be obtained by visual interpretation or by automated programs. It should be noted that any differences between the two sets of images could be real, due to technical problems, or because of variability (intraindividual and interindividual) in the interpretation of serial images. Therefore, all acquisition and processing parameters should be standardized, image artifacts minimized, and image quality enhanced as much as possible. Image quality is probably the single most important variable that impacts the precision of the comparison.

For clinical applications, serial studies should be compared side-by-side using both visual and automated analysis. For research purposes, side-by-side analysis is as important as long as the readers are blinded to the sequence of the images. Although most of the above discussion focused on the perfusion pattern, attention to gating is also very important to assess improvement or deterioration in LV function.

Here are a few of the many questions that should be answered in comparing two or more sets of images:

- Are the images normal or abnormal?
- Do the images show fixed or reversible defects (or both)?
- If present, what is the number of abnormal segments in each?
- If present, what is the number of reversible segments in each?
- What is the rate of agreement based on summed stress score or summed difference score?
- What is the rate of agreement based on polar maps for total abnormality or reversible abnormality?
- What are the rates of agreement in regional perfusion?

Generally, concordance is highest for simple comparisons (such as normal vs. abnormal) and concordance is highest when most images are normal.

The following cases will address some of the salient features of serial testing:

Case 7-1 Progression of Disease (Figure 7-1)

A 71-year-old woman with a history of DM, paroxysmal atrial fibrillation, HTN, and hyperlipidemia presented with atypical chest pains of several weeks' duration. Due to the presence of rate-dependent left bundle branch block (LBBB) (Figure 7-1, *A*) she underwent adenosine MPI, which showed a normal perfusion pattern and LVEF (Figure 7-1, *B*). She was managed medically with risk factor modification. Approximately 3.5 years later, she sustained a traumatic injury to the left knee and underwent regadenoson MPI before planned major surgery. The images showed a large area of ischemia with normal LVEF (Figure 7-1, *C*). On coronary angiography she had severe stenosis of the proximal LAD, which was treated with a bare metal stent. She underwent total knee replacement 3 months later without incident.

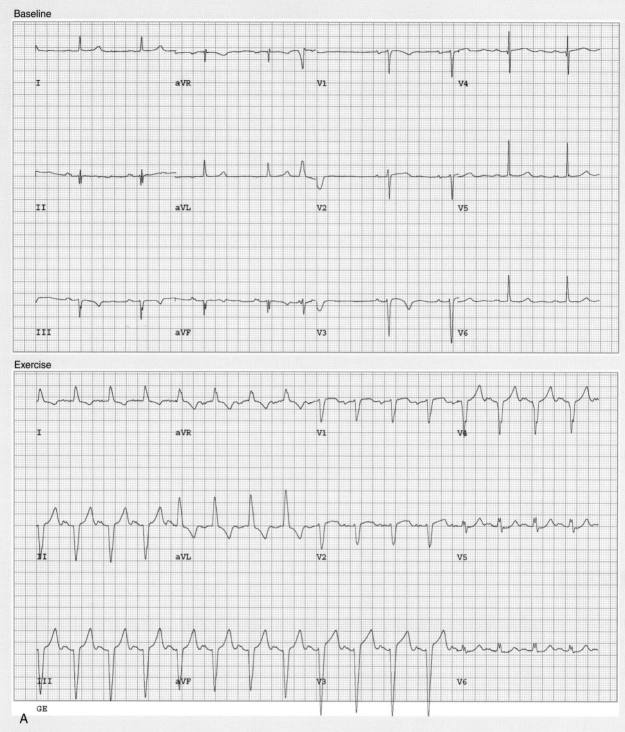

■ **Figure 7-1** The ECG shows normal QRS at rest, but rate-related LBBB during exercise **(A)**.

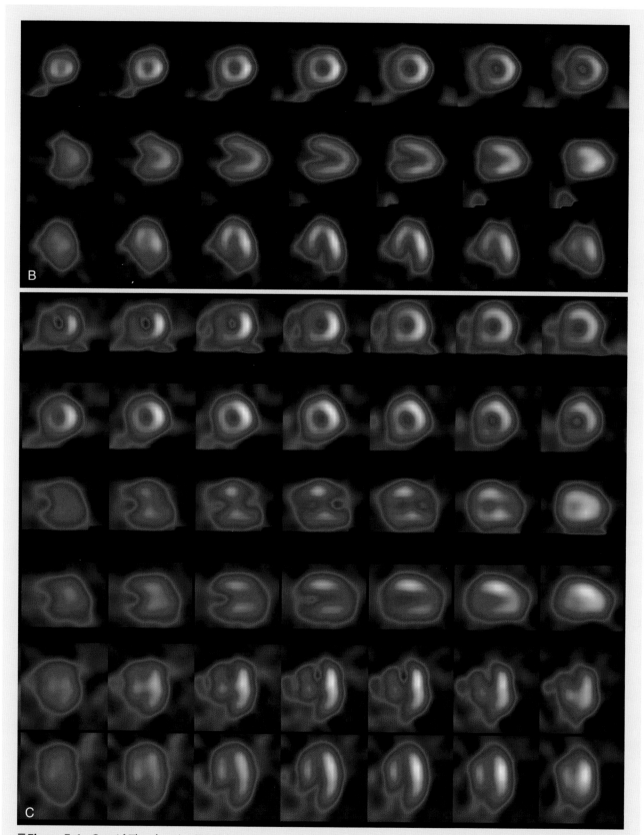

■**Figure 7-1—Cont'd** The adenosine SPECT MPI images are normal **(B)** despite the rate-related LBBB. The LVEF was normal. The regadenoson MPI 3 years later, however, revealed a reversible perfusion abnormality in the LAD territory **(C)**.

(Continued)

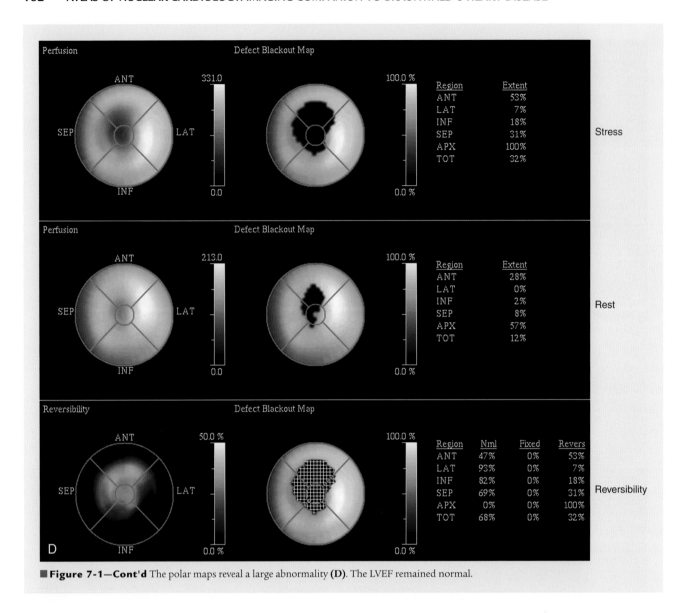

■ Figure 7-1—Cont'd The polar maps reveal a large abnormality (**D**). The LVEF remained normal.

COMMENTS

The comparison of the serial MPI images in this patient is arguably an easy task because the earlier images were normal. Nevertheless, the recent images should always be examined side-by-side with the earlier images and not be based on the report alone. This practice is important in maintaining quality and consistency in interpretation. The earlier study also serves the useful purpose of defining the normal variation in tracer concentration in different myocardial segments, which is very valuable in determining the degree of reversibility in the current study.

Case 7-2   Serial Testing for a Change in Symptoms (Figure 7-2)

A 56-year-old woman, known to have mitral valve prolapse, presented to her primary care physician with atypical chest pain of several months duration that are not associated with exertion. Her comorbidities include family history of premature CAD, HTN, and hyperlipidemia. The baseline ECG showed right bundle branch block. She ran on a treadmill for 7.5 minutes, reaching a heart rate of 150 bpm with no ischemic ST changes. The MPI showed normal perfusion and normal LVEF (Figure 7-2, *A*). Five years later, she presented with left-sided chest pain that woke her from sleep and was described as being different from her previous episodes.

She was seen in the emergency room 2 hours later but the pain had subsided by this time and biomarkers were normal. She underwent exercise MPI 2 days later and had no chest pain or ECG changes after 6.5 minutes of exercise achieving 80% of maximum predicted heart rate. The gated SPECT MPI again showed essentially normal perfusion (except for apical attenuation) and normal LVEF (Figure 7-2, *B*).

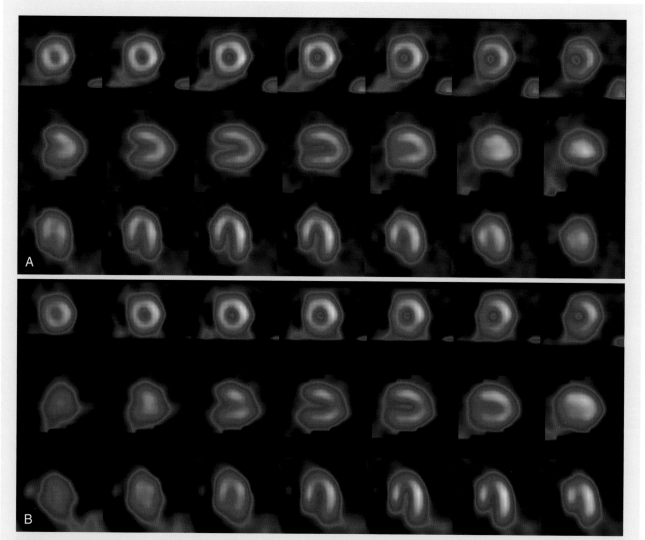

■**Figure 7-2** Normal exercise-only SPECT images **(A)**. Repeat imaging 5 years later reveals essentially normal images except for mild apical thinning **(B)**. The LVEF was normal at both times.

COMMENTS

The evaluation of atypical symptoms can be difficult, especially in women in whom typical angina occurs much less frequently than in men. Considering the change in symptoms, risk factors, and 5 years since the last stress test, a repeat stress MPI was appropriate for this patient. Again, the two sets of images needed to be evaluated side-by-side with special attention to breast location and body habitus. In lean tall women with mitral valve prolapse, attenuation artifacts could be due to the right ventricle (affecting the septum and inferior wall) as well as the breasts (affecting the anterior wall).

Case 7-3   Serial Testing in a Patient With Known CAD and New Symptoms (Figure 7-3)

A 48-year-old man with prior anterior myocardial infarction underwent an exercise MPI 3 weeks after failed thrombolysis. Coronary angiography showed occluded LAD, which was collateralized from the RCA. The LCX had 50% diameter stenosis. He had HTN, COPD, hyperlipidemia, and gastroesophageal reflux symptoms. He was an active smoker. He did well with medical therapy. Two years later, he had one episode of prolonged lower substernal pain, which abated after a sublingual nitroglycerin tablet and antacids. He had a repeat stress test. The images from both tests are shown in Figure 7-3, *A, B*.

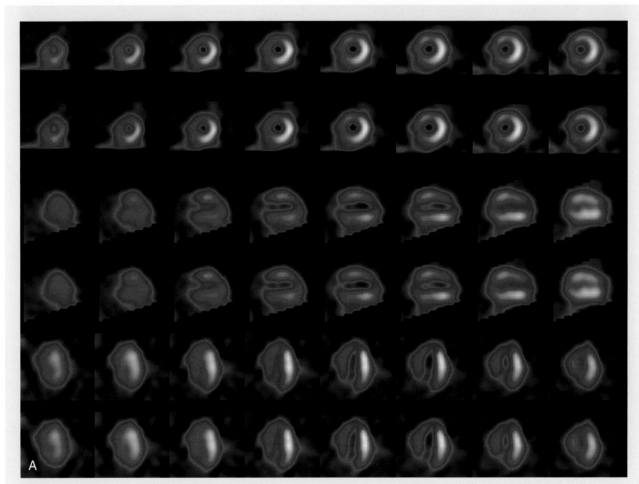

■ **Figure 7-3** Exercise/rest images showing a fixed perfusion abnormality in LAD territory **(A)**.

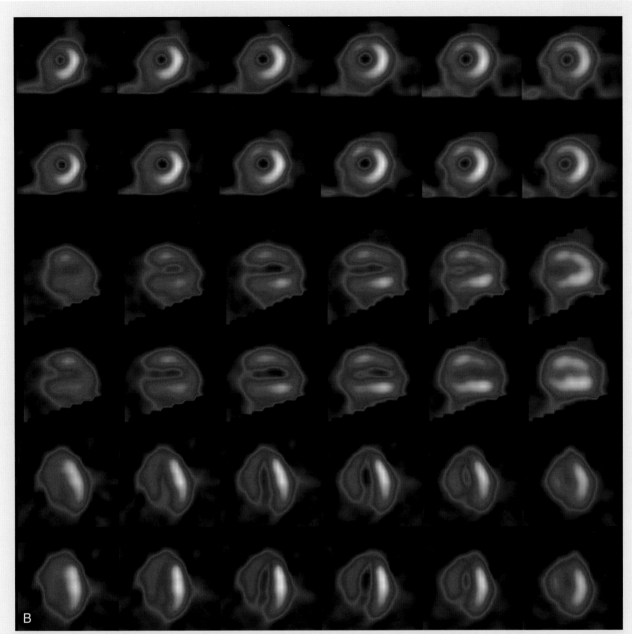

■ Figure 7-3—Cont'd The LVEF was normal. Repeat exercise/rest images 2 years later show no change and no evidence of ischemia in LCX territory **(B)**.

COMMENTS

Both sets of images reveal a large scar (fixed defect) in the distribution of the LAD. Myocardial infarct size can be quantified with MPI. The infarct size has prognostic implications since patients with larger infarcts have a high mortality and the size of the infarct is also associated with a lower LVEF and a larger LV end-systolic volume. There is no evidence of ischemia in either the LAD or the LCX, which had a moderate stenosis 2 years earlier. The LV function has remained unchanged.

In the early era of interventional therapy, assessment of infarct size, area at risk, and salvage area was popularized with injection of the tracer before the intervention (and imaging after the intervention such as fibrinolysis, angioplasty, or stenting) and then a repeat rest study before hospital discharge. The perfusion defect on the early image (before treatment when presumably the infarct-related artery is occluded) reflects the area at risk (the area that could potentially undergo necrosis without revascularization), while the perfusion defect on the predischarge study reflects necrosis area, and the difference between the two reflects the salvaged myocardium.

Case 7-4   **Serial Testing After Coronary Revascularization (Figure 7-4)**

A 62-year-old man presented with recurrent angina 2 years after he underwent CABG. After exercising for 10 minutes on a treadmill, he achieved a peak heart rate of 130 bpm (despite being on beta-blocker therapy); he developed chest pain and 1-mm ST depression in leads V_4-V_6. The MPI showed an abnormal perfusion pattern (Figure 7-4, *A*). Coronary angiography showed multivessel native CAD, patent LIMA graft to the LAD, and occluded vein graft to the OM1 branch of the LCX artery that was not amenable to percutaneous revascularization. His medical therapy was intensified and he was enrolled in a structured cardiac rehabilitation program. His symptoms improved and an exercise MPI confirmed improved perfusion (Figure 7-4, *B*). Repeat exercise MPI 2 years later showed a stable perfusion pattern.

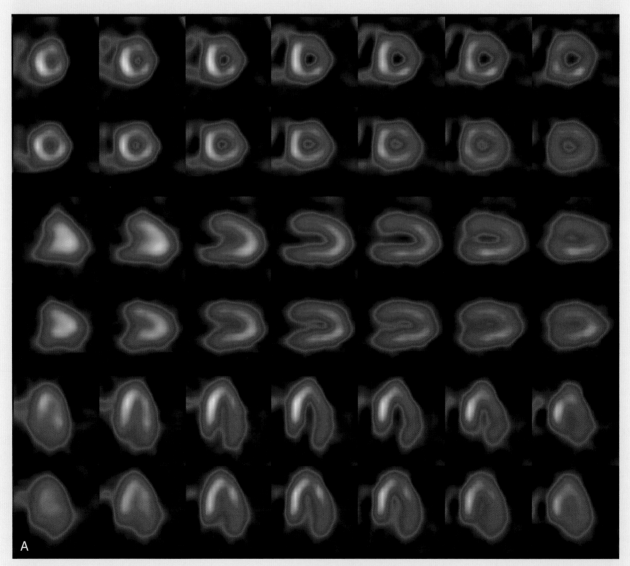

■**Figure 7-4** Exercise/rest images showing a reversible perfusion abnormality in LCX territory **(A)**.

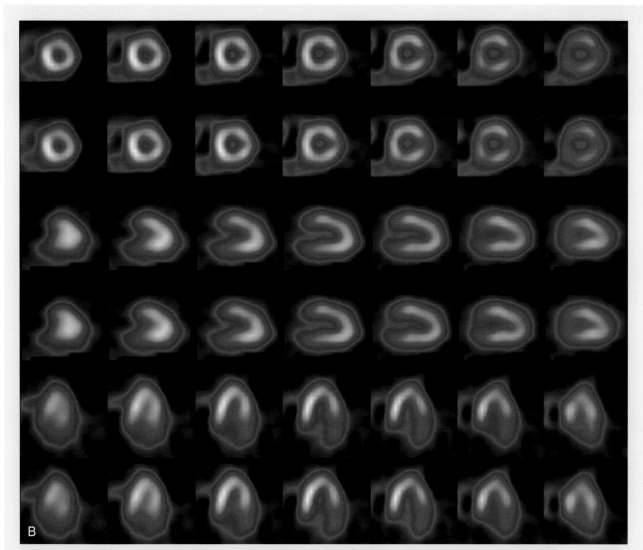

■**Figure 7-4—Cont'd** Repeat exercise/rest images after intensification of medical therapy and completion of an 8-week cardiopulmonary rehabilitation program showed marked improvement in the extent of ischemia **(B)**.

COMMENTS

Stress MPI is endorsed by current practice guidelines and appropriateness criteria as an accepted method for evaluating patients with symptoms after CABG. The main advantage of MPI over ECG is its ability to localize the area of perfusion abnormality and to quantify its extent. Perfusion abnormalities after CABG can be due to graft attrition, progression of disease in grafted vessels, incomplete revascularization, and, rarely, due to misplaced grafts. Our patient had multivessel CAD as well as disease in the bypass grafts that was not amenable to revascularization. Optimal medical therapy and regular exercise were effective in decreasing the ischemic burden. The lack of progression of ischemia over time indicated stability of the disease in response to therapy.

Case 7-5   **Serial Testing Long After PCI (Figure 7-5)**

A 62-year-old woman with DM, HTN, and hyperlipidemia presented with a
6-month history of exertional dyspnea. Exercise MPI showed a very large reversible
perfusion abnormality in the distribution of the LAD with marked transient ischemic
dilatation (Figure 7-5, *A*, *B*). Coronary angiography showed severe disease in the
proximal LAD with collaterals from the RCA. The patient was treated with a drug-
eluting stent and her symptoms resolved. Five years later, she underwent a repeat
exercise MPI before shoulder surgery. The perfusion pattern was normal and she had
an uneventful surgery.

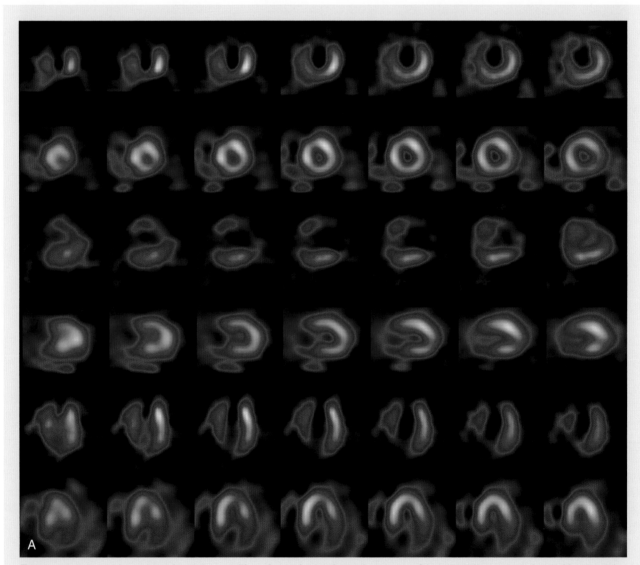

■ **Figure 7-5** Exercise/rest images showing a reversible perfusion abnormality in the territory of the LAD with transient ischemic dilatation **(A)**.

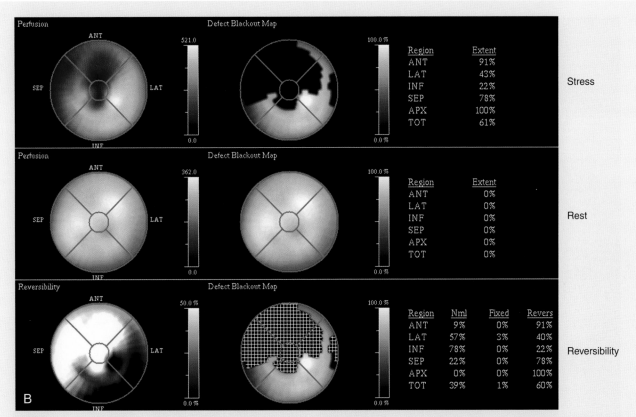

■**Figure 7-5—Cont'd** The polar maps show the extent of the abnormality (**B**). Repeat imaging 5 years later before noncardiac surgery had a normal myocardial perfusion pattern (not shown). The LVEF was normal.

COMMENTS

MPI can be used to select patients for coronary revascularization and to guide therapeutic decision making. A major role of MPI is to identify patients at high risk of cardiovascular events and thus serve as a gateway to coronary angiography. A large perfusion abnormality and transient LV dilatation are considered markers of high risk, as was the case in this patient. The need for repeat testing 5 years after coronary intervention, especially in a patient who did not have angina on initial presentation and who has DM, seems to be appropriate.

In the study by Johansen et al., of 384 patients with stable angina who were managed medically or with coronary revascularization, symptomatic improvement was more pronounced with coronary revascularization in those with reversible ischemia on baseline MPI. In an analysis of more than 10,000 patients, coronary revascularization was associated with a 50% risk-adjusted reduction in cardiac death in patients with myocardial ischemia involving > 10% of the LV. More recently, data from the Clinical Outcomes Utilizing Revascularization and Aggressive Drug Evaluation (COURAGE) study showed that PCI in addition to medical therapy resulted in a greater reduction in ischemia, as compared to medical therapy alone. Complete normalization of the MPI, as seen in our patient, was more common with PCI than medical therapy alone in the COURAGE trial, and this pattern is likely associated with a better outcome.

Case 7-6   Serial Testing After CABG for Atypical Angina (Figure 7-6)

A 59-year-old previously healthy woman presented to her primary physician with left-sided chest and shoulder pain of a few weeks duration. She underwent exercise MPI, which showed a reversible perfusion defect with a normal LVEF (Figure 7-6, *A*). Coronary angiography showed a severe ostial LAD stenosis. Single-vessel CABG was performed with LIMA graft to the LAD. Repeat exercise MPI done 1 year later (Figure 7-6, *B*), when she presented with atypical chest pain, showed normal perfusion and LVEF.

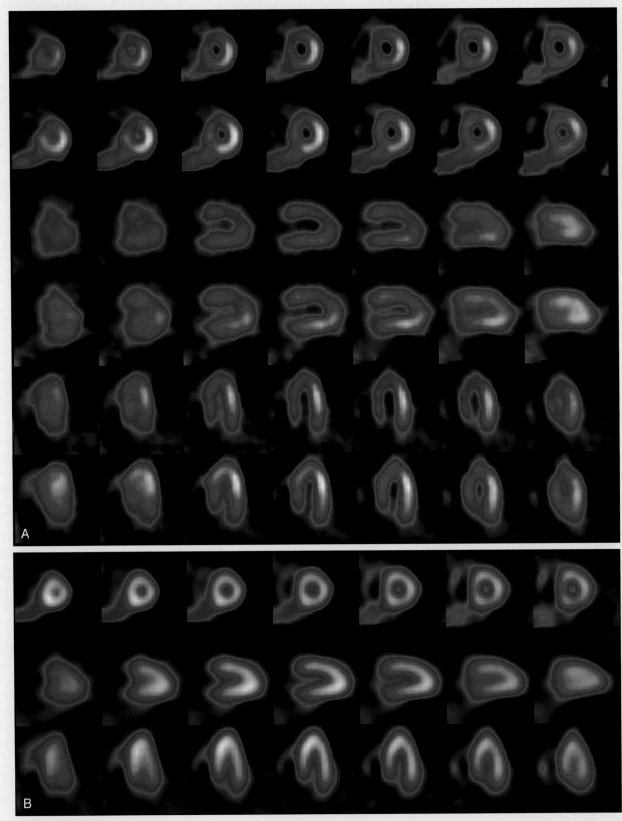

■**Figure 7-6** Exercise/rest images showing a reversible perfusion abnormality in LAD territory **(A).** Repeat imaging after CABG shows normal perfusion pattern **(B).**

COMMENTS

The American College of Cardiology Foundation Appropriateness Criteria state that the performance of routine MPI within the first 5 years after CABG is of uncertain indication except in those with incomplete revascularization or in those with recurrent symptoms. Residual ischemia can be present with patent grafts due to a number of reasons (see Chapter 8). In the study by Miller et al., of 411 patients from the Mayo Clinic who underwent MPI within 2 years of CABG, 12% of the patients had ischemia proximal to the bypass graft insertion, but this was not associated with worse outcomes. The timing of the MPI after CABG is also relevant since a considerable proportion of vein grafts will fail within the first 1 to 5 years. A remarkable improvement in perfusion pattern and LV function in many patients attests to the benefit of successful and complete revascularization and is a measure of why CABG has been shown to improve outcome in many patients, especially those with large ischemic areas, poor LVEF, or multivessel disease.

Case 7-7   **Serial Testing in a Patient With Known CAD and DM (Figure 7-7)**

A 59-year-old man with DM, multiple cardiac risk factors, and multiple prior PCIs (last one 8 years ago) has stable angina equivalent symptoms of fatigue and shortness of breath on exertion. Approximately 5 years ago, he had an exercise MPI. He exercised for 7.0 minutes and achieved a peak heart rate of 126 bpm. The test was terminated because of fatigue, with no chest pain or ECG changes. The MPI showed a normal perfusion pattern and normal LVEF.

On a repeat exercise testing, he exercised for 6.5 minutes, reaching a peak heart rate of 121 bpm. There were no ECG changes. The test was stopped because of fatigue and shortness of breath. The MPI showed a new large reversible perfusion abnormality (Figure 7-7, *A, B*). Coronary angiography showed severe three-vessel disease in the native vessels as well as an in-stent stenosis. He underwent revascularization and did well at last follow-up 3 years later.

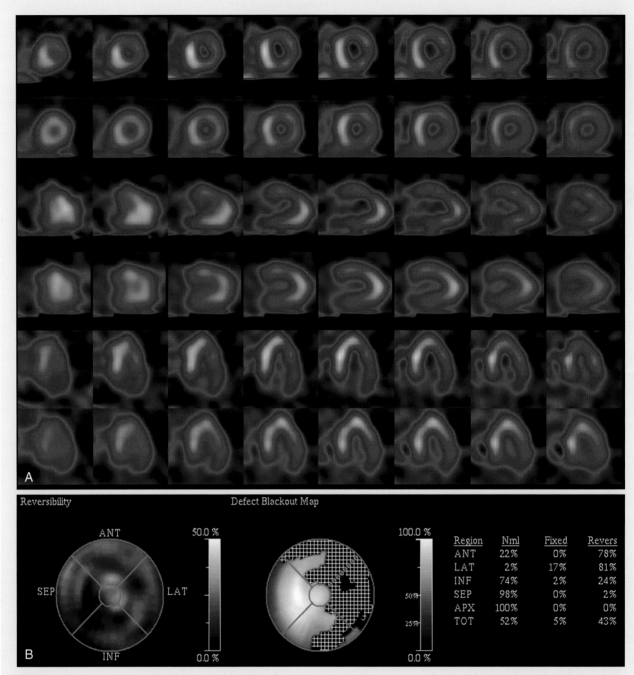

Region	Nml	Fixed	Revers
ANT	22%	0%	78%
LAT	2%	17%	81%
INF	74%	2%	24%
SEP	98%	0%	2%
APX	100%	0%	0%
TOT	52%	5%	43%

■ **Figure 7-7** Exercise/rest images showing multivessel perfusion abnormality (**A**); the stress polar maps shown in **B** reveal a large abnormality *(cross-hatched area)*. The LVEF was normal.

COMMENTS

The problem of in-stent stenosis is a very real concern, especially in patients with multiple stents. Part of the problem can be attributed to stents that are placed in less than ideal vessels. Further, ischemia could be silent in diabetic patients or may present with atypical features. Nevertheless, routine and frequent testing in entirely asymptomatic patients is not appropriate. Knowledge of coronary anatomy and comparison of serial images can help localize the problem and guide management.

Case 7-8   Serial Testing After Intensification of Medical Therapy (Figure 7-8)

A 71-year-old man with DM, HTN, hyperlipidemia, and known CAD with prior PCI presented with recurrence of a stable pattern of angina despite maximization of medical therapy with a statin, aspirin, clopidogrel, a beta-blocker, a calcium channel blocker, and a long-acting nitrate. After exercising for 6 minutes on the treadmill, he had 2- to 3-mm ST depression with chest pain at a peak heart rate of 125 bpm. The images were abnormal but the LVEF was normal. Ranolazine was added to his medical regimen at a dose of 1000 mg twice daily. His symptoms improved. A repeat MPI was performed 6 weeks later. He exercised for 7 minutes on the treadmill with no ST changes and stopped due to fatigue. The second MPI showed an improvement in the perfusion pattern (Figure 7-8).

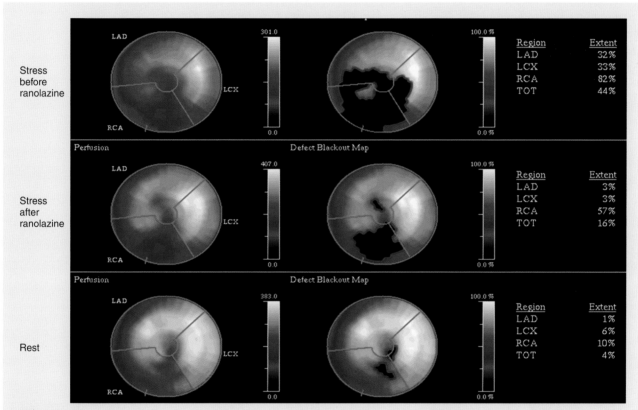

■ **Figure 7-8** Polar maps from exercise/rest studies before and after the addition of ranolazine to medical regimen. There is marked reduction in ischemic burden. Only the first rest study is shown because the repeat rest study was unchanged. The LVEF was normal on both studies.

COMMENTS

Anti-ischemic medications (nitrates, calcium channel–blocking agents, beta-blockers, statins, and ranolazine) can improve myocardial perfusion and decrease the size and/or severity of perfusion defects. There is considerable individual variability in the degree of improvement in response to any of these medications (or other interventions). Complete normalization of the perfusion pattern may contribute to lowering the sensitivity of stress MPI in detecting CAD. The improvement in perfusion is most marked with exercise MPI but has been reported with pharmacologic testing as well. In the COURAGE trial, medic therapy resulted in a reduction of > 5% of ischemic myocardium in 19% of patients (compared to 33% of patients treated with PCI plus medical therapy). In the Adenosine Sestamibi SPECT Post-Infarction Evaluation (INSPIRE) trial of myocardial infarction survivors, medical therapy produced a similar reduction, compared to coronary revascularization, in total perfusion defect size (–16.2 ± 10% vs. –17.8 ± 12%) and reversible perfusion defect size (–15 ± 9% vs.

−16.2 ± 9%). Suppression of ischemia was seen in ~ 80% of patients in either arm.

Ranolazine, which inhibits the late sodium current, relieves ischemia by reducing myocardial cellular sodium and calcium overload and, hence, extravascular compression of small vessels. Human studies have shown that ranolazine can increase exercise tolerance, and reduce angina episodes and the use of nitroglycerin without affecting heart rate and blood pressure. In the study by Venkataraman et al., a 4-week treatment course with ranolazine improved myocardial perfusion in 70% of patients who had ischemia on their baseline scan (ischemia improved from 16 ± 10% to 8 ± 6%, and the total perfusion defect decreased from 26 ± 17% to 19 ± 15%).

Case 7-9   Serial Assessment of LV Function After Chemotherapy (Figure 7-9)

A 33-year-old man presented with cervical adenopathy that, upon excisional biopsy, was consistent with a diffuse large B-cell lymphoma. Work-up revealed an 8-cm retroperitoneal lymph node and enlarged spleen. He received several cycles of chemotherapy that included doxorubicin but failed to achieve complete remission. A gated radionuclide angiogram (MUGA) showed normal LV function (Figure 7-9, *A*). He underwent allogenic bone marrow transplantation with a conditioning regimen of busulfan, cyclophosphamide, and antithymocyte globulin. A repeat MUGA showed a decrease in LVEF (Figure 7-9, *B*). The time activity curves are shown in (Figure 7-9, *C*). The videos are shown in Video 7-1, *A*, *B*. He was started on beta-blockers and an angiotensin-converting enzyme inhibitor, which he tolerated well. A transthoracic echocardiogram 12 weeks later showed a normal LVEF.

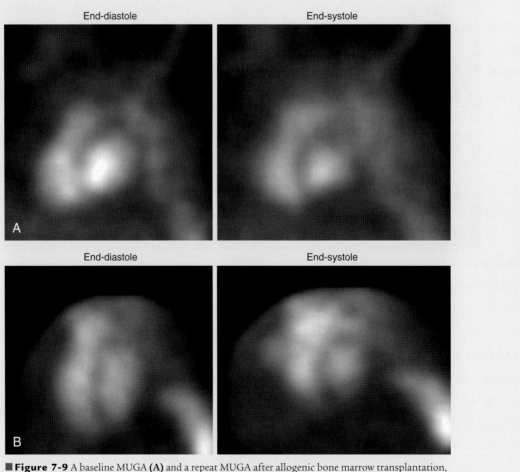

■ **Figure 7-9** A baseline MUGA (**A**) and a repeat MUGA after allogenic bone marrow transplantation, showing deterioration of LV function due to cardiotoxicity (**B**). The splenomegaly is better seen in **B** because the image angulation is different, which also explains why the LV looks more elongated.

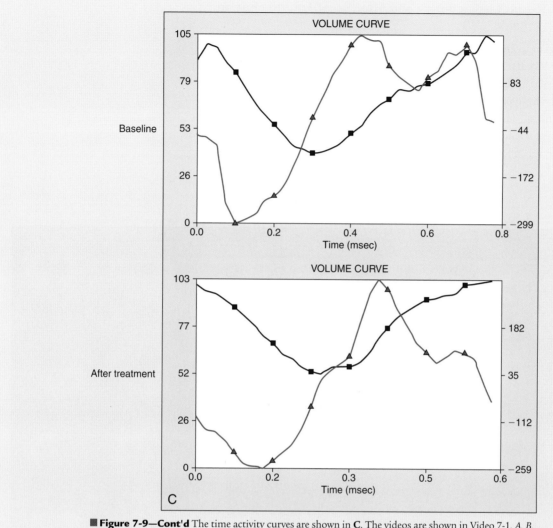

■ **Figure 7-9—Cont'd** The time activity curves are shown in **C**. The videos are shown in Video 7-1, *A, B.*

COMMENTS

MUGA remains the preferred method for serial testing at our institution in patients receiving chemotherapy that is potentially cardiotoxic. Monitoring of cardiac function has been shown to be an effective strategy for preventing progression to heart failure, especially with anthracycline-based regimens. The management of cardiotoxicity should include withdrawal of the offending agent(s), if possible, and standard medical therapy for heart failure with beta-blockers, angiotensin-converting enzyme inhibitors, or angiotensin receptor blockers. Regrettably, in some patients the deterioration in LV function continues despite discontinuation of chemotherapy.

Case 7-10   Serial Testing Before and After Renal Transplantation
(Figure 7-10)

A 62-year-old Asian woman with ESRD underwent renal transplantation after being on hemodialysis for 9 years. Pretransplant evaluation included an adenosine MPI, which revealed a depressed LVEF with a mild decrease in tracer activity in the lateral wall due to downscaling from hypertrophied septum (Figure 7-10, *A*). Coronary angiography showed nonsignificant obstructive CAD. Two months after the transplantation, she underwent a repeat adenosine MPI for nonspecific chest pains and ECG changes. The perfusion pattern was unchanged but the LVEF had improved (Figure 7-10, *B*).

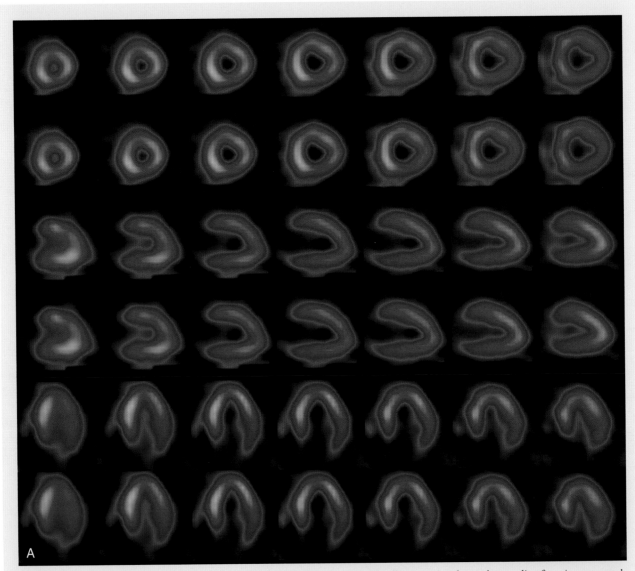

■ **Figure 7-10** Adenosine/rest images before renal transplantation showing lateral wall attenuation due to downscaling from intense septal activity **(A)**.

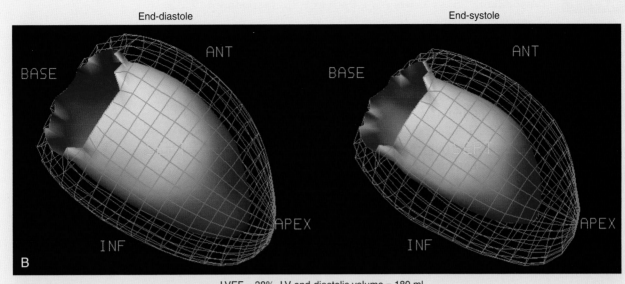

End-diastole   End-systole

LVEF = 38%, LV end-diastolic volume = 180 ml

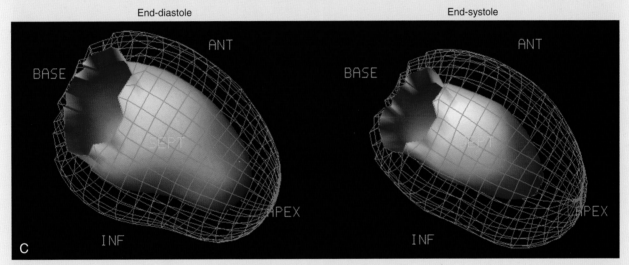

End-diastole   End-systole

LVEF = 53%, LV end-diastolic volume = 102 ml

■ **Figure 7-10—Cont'd** The LVEF was depressed (**B**). Repeat imaging 2 months after renal transplantation showed improvement in LVEF (**C**).

COMMENTS

Patients with ESRD constitute a special population that is at high risk for cardiac events. The evaluation of these patients prior to renal transplantation is addressed in Chapter 11. A depressed LVEF is a poor prognostic indicator prior to and after renal transplantation. Wali et al. evaluated 103 patients with depressed LVEF who underwent renal transplantation; they were able to show a dramatic improvement in LVEF from a mean of 30% to 52% with normalization of LV function in 70% of the patients, which was accompanied by improvements in functional status.

In patients with ESRD, the septum is often the brightest area of the myocardium, which results in down scaling of activity in the lateral wall. Attention to this pattern is important to avoid labeling many such patients as having prior MI. The reason for disproportional septal hypertrophy may be due to a combination of pressure and volume overload on both ventricles.

Case 7-11 Vasodilator Stress Testing in a Patient With Inadequate Exercise Performance (Figure 7-11)

A 63-year-old woman with no prior history of CAD, but who has DM, HTN, and hyperlipidemia was referred for an exercise MPI for evaluation of new onset atypical chest pain. Her medical regimen included aspirin, a beta-blocker, simvastatin, and metformin. She exercised on the treadmill for 4.5 minutes, reaching 65% of her maximum predicted heart rate, and stopped because of fatigue. She did not report having chest pain and the ECG did not show ischemic changes. The MPI revealed normal perfusion at rest and stress (Figure 7-10, *A*). Due to a high pretest likelihood of CAD and persistence of symptoms, she was referred back for adenosine MPI. The images show a large reversible abnormality in LCX territory (Figure 7-10, *B*).

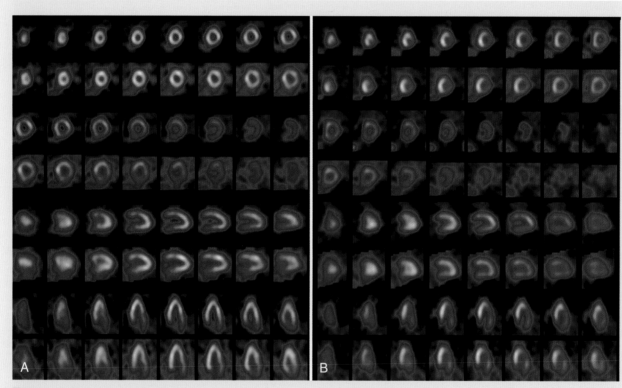

■ **Figure 7-11** Exercise/rest images showing a normal perfusion pattern at submaximal heart rate **(A)**. Repeat imaging with adenosine reveals a large reversible perfusion abnormality **(B)**.

COMMENTS

Although the diagnostic accuracy for CAD of pharmacologic and exercise MPI are generally comparable, exercise stress is generally preferred since it provides prognostic information is unavailable in patients who are stressed pharmacologically. The caveat is that a large proportion of patients who are referred for stress testing are unable to reach target heart rate on the treadmill because of exercise limitation or receiving a medication such as beta-blocker that attenuates the exercise-induced increase in heart rate, or a combination of both. Submaximal exercise decreases the diagnostic accuracy of MPI and underestimates the extent and severity of ischemia. In this patient, it is clear that submaximal exercise was misleading not only in missing the diagnosis of CAD, but also in that it missed an extensive area of ischemia.

Case 7-12   Serial Testing After Alcohol Septal Ablation (Figure 7-12)

A 37-year-old man with no prior medical history developed chest pain and episodes of syncope on exertion. Evaluation uncovered hypertrophic cardiomyopathy with dynamic outflow tract obstruction. He was placed on medical therapy, but his symptoms persisted. Coronary angiography did not show obstructive lesions in the coronary arteries. In the interventional laboratory, he had a resting gradient of 80 mm Hg across the LV outflow tract that increased to 200 mm Hg after a premature ventricular contraction on invasive hemodynamic monitoring. Absolute alcohol was then infused in the first septal artery, which resulted in resolution of the gradient. Resting MPI done 2 days afterward showed a small perfusion defect at the base of the septum with normal global LV function (Figure 7-12). The size of the perfusion abnormality was smaller on repeat MPI done 2 months later. The patient had a good response to the procedure, with resolution of symptoms and amelioration of the LV gradient.

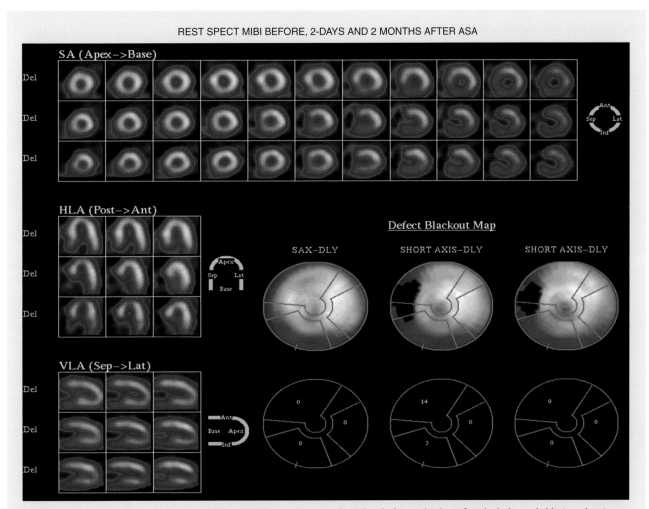

■ Figure 7-12 Rest images in a patient with hypertrophic cardiomyopathy 2 days before and 2 days after alcohol septal ablation, showing a small perfusion defect at the base of the septum *(middle)*. Repeat imaging 2 months later shows a decrease in the size of the defect *(lower)*.

COMMENTS

Although medical therapy is the first line of treatment in hypertrophic cardiomyopathy, surgical septal myectomy or, more recently, alcohol septal ablation is recommended for the small subgroup of patients (5%) who have a large outflow gradient (usually >50 mm Hg at rest or on provocation) and moderate to severe heart failure or angina symptoms unresponsive to maximal medical therapy. For alcohol ablation, a small amount of alcohol is injected into the septal branch of the LAD to induce a myocardial infarction at the base of the septum, as shown in immediate postprocedure images in our patient. Unexpectedly, a third scan done 2 months later, showed a reduction in the perfusion abnormality. The reasons are not clear but it might be due to resolution of edema or regeneration of myocytes. However, the outflow tract gradient continued to be small and the patient remained asymptomatic.

SELECTED READINGS

Aqel RA, Hage FG, Zohgbi GJ, et al: Serial evaluations of myocardial infarct size after alcohol septal ablation in hypertrophic cardiomyopathy and effects of the changes on clinical status and left ventricular outflow pressure gradients, *Am J Cardiol* 101:1328–1333, 2008.

Aqel R, Zoghbi GJ, Hage F, et al: Hemodynamic evaluation of coronary artery bypass graft lesions using fractional flow reserve, *Catheter Cardiovasc Interv* 72:479–485, 2008.

Berman DS, Kang X, Gransar H, et al: Quantitative assessment of myocardial perfusion abnormality on SPECT myocardial perfusion imaging is more reproducible than expert visual analysis, *J Nucl Cardiol* 16:45–53, 2009.

Dilsizian V, Narula J: Qualitative and quantitative scrutiny by regulatory process: is the truth subjective or objective? *JACC Cardiovasc Imaging* 2:1037–1038, 2009.

Elhendy A, Schinkel A, Bax JJ, et al: Long-term prognosis after a normal exercise stress Tc-99m sestamibi SPECT study, *J Nucl Cardiol* 10:261–266, 2003.

Gibbons RJ, Valeti US, Araoz PA, et al: The quantification of infarct size, *J Am Coll Cardiol* 44:1533–1542, 2004.

Hachamovitch R, Hayes S, Friedman JD, et al: Determinants of risk and its temporal variation in patients with normal stress myocardial perfusion scans: what is the warranty period of a normal scan? *J Am Coll Cardiol* 41:1329–1340, 2003.

Hachamovitch R, Hayes SW, Friedman JD, et al: Comparison of the short-term survival benefit associated with revascularization compared with medical therapy in patients with no prior coronary artery disease undergoing stress myocardial perfusion single photon emission computed tomography, *Circulation* 107:2900–2907, 2003.

Hage FG, Aqel R, Aljaroudi W, et al: Correlation between serum cardiac markers and myocardial infarct size quantified by myocardial perfusion imaging in patients with hypertrophic cardiomyopathy after alcohol septal ablation, *Am J Cardiol* 105:261–266.

Hage FG, Smalheiser S, Zoghbi GJ, et al: Predictors of survival in patients with end-stage renal disease evaluated for kidney transplantation, *Am J Cardiol* 100:1020–1025, 2007.

Hage FG, Venkataraman R, Zoghbi GJ, et al: The scope of coronary heart disease in patients with chronic kidney disease, *J Am Coll Cardiol* 53:2129–2140, 2009.

Hage FG, Venkataraman R, Aljaroudi W, et al: The impact of viability assessment using myocardial perfusion imaging on patient management and outcome, *J Nucl Cardiol* 7:378–389, 2010.

Hansen CL, Goldstein RA, Akinboboye OO, et al: Myocardial perfusion and function: single photon emission computed tomography, *J Nucl Cardiol* 14:e39–e60, 2007.

Hendel RC, Berman DS, Di Carli MF, et al: ACCF/ASNC/ACR/AHA/ASE/SCCT/SCMR/SNM 2009 appropriate use criteria for cardiac radionuclide imaging: a report of the American College of Cardiology Foundation Appropriate Use Criteria Task Force, the American Society of Nuclear Cardiology, the American College of Radiology, the American Heart Association, the American Society of Echocardiography, the Society of Cardiovascular Computed Tomography, the Society for Cardiovascular Magnetic Resonance, and the Society of Nuclear Medicine, *Circulation* 119:e561–e587, 2009.

Iskandrian AE, Garcia EV, Faber T, et al: Automated assessment of serial SPECT myocardial perfusion images, *J Nucl Cardiol* 16:6–9, 2009.

Johansen A, Hoilund-Carlsen PF, Christensen HW, et al: Use of myocardial perfusion imaging to predict the effectiveness of coronary revascularisation in patients with stable angina pectoris, *Eur J Nucl Med Mol Imaging* 32:1363–1370, 2005.

Mahmarian JJ, Moye LA, Verani MS, et al: High reproducibility of myocardial perfusion defects in patients undergoing serial exercise thallium-201 tomography, *Am J Cardiol* 75:1116–1119, 1995.

Mahmarian JJ, Dakik HA, Filipchuk NG, et al: An initial strategy of intensive medical therapy is comparable to that of coronary revascularization for suppression of scintigraphic ischemia in high-risk but stable survivors of acute myocardial infarction, *J Am Coll Cardiol* 48:2458–2467, 2006.

Miller TD, Christian TF, Hodge DO, et al: Prognostic value of exercise thallium-201 imaging performed within 2 years of coronary artery bypass graft surgery, *J Am Coll Cardiol* 31:848–854, 1998.

Shaw LJ, Iskandrian AE: Prognostic value of gated myocardial perfusion SPECT, *J Nucl Cardiol* 11:171–185, 2004.

Shaw LJ, Berman DS, Maron DJ, et al: Optimal medical therapy with or without percutaneous coronary intervention to reduce ischemic burden: results from the Clinical Outcomes Utilizing Revascularization and Aggressive Drug Evaluation (COURAGE) trial nuclear substudy, *Circulation* 117:1283–1291, 2008.

Siedlecki A, Foushee M, Curtis JJ, et al: The impact of left ventricular systolic dysfunction on survival after renal transplantation, *Transplantation* 84:1610–1617, 2007.

Venkataraman R, Hage FG, Dorfman T, et al: Role of myocardial perfusion imaging in patients with end-stage renal disease undergoing coronary angiography, *Am J Cardiol* 102:1451–1456, 2008.

Venkataraman R, Belardinelli L, Blackburn B, et al: A study of the effects of ranolazine using automated quantitative analysis of serial myocardial perfusion images, *JACC Cardiovasc Imaging* 2:1301–1309, 2009.

Wali RK, Wang GS, Gottlieb SS, et al: Effect of kidney transplantation on left ventricular systolic dysfunction and congestive heart failure in patients with end-stage renal disease, *J Am Coll Cardiol* 45:1051–1060, 2005.

Yeh ET, Tong AT, Lenihan DJ, et al: Cardiovascular complications of cancer therapy: diagnosis, pathogenesis, and management, *Circulation* 109:3122–3131, 2004.

Young LH, Wackers FJ, Chyun DA, et al: Cardiac outcomes after screening for asymptomatic coronary artery disease in patients with type 2 diabetes: the DIAD study: a randomized controlled trial, *JAMA* 301:1547–1555, 2009.

Zoghbi GJ, Dorfman TA, Iskandrian AE: The effects of medications on myocardial perfusion, *J Am Coll Cardiol* 52:401–416, 2008.

Chapter 8

Patients With PCI and CABG

Gilbert J. Zoghbi, Eva V. Dubovsky, and Ami E. Iskandrian

KEY POINTS

- PCI and CABG are commonly used modalities for revascularization in patients with stable and unstable CAD.

- Ideally, stress testing (in conjunction with imaging) should be used to guide the need for coronary angiography, PCI, or CABG in patients with stable symptoms.

- Stress MPI is helpful in patients with recurrent symptoms after PCI or CABG to assess for in-stent stenosis, bypass graft disease, progression of disease in native vessels, or incomplete revascularization.

- Stress MPI is helpful for risk stratification of patients after PCI or CABG.

- Stress MPI is acceptable for routine evaluation of high-risk asymptomatic patients who are more than 5 years post-CABG, especially those who had no angina before CABG.

- After successful PCI, new fixed perfusion defects might indicate periprocedural MI, while reversible defects might be due to jailed branches, such as diagonal or septal branches in the case of LAD stenting.

- After CABG, new fixed defects might be due to periprocedural MI, while reversible defects at the basal septum and anterior wall could be due to jeopardized branches prior to left internal mammary artery (LIMA) anastomosis. These abnormalities should not be confused with LIMA or downstream disease, where the reversible defects almost always involve the distal septum, anterior wall, and the apex.

- After CABG, septal wall motion, but not thickening, is abnormal despite a normal perfusion pattern and normal EF. The presence of a thickening abnormality suggests necrosis.

- Contrary to popular belief, normalization of the perfusion pattern in patients with stable angina after PCI is immediate and any residual abnormality should not be ascribed to the technique but to the results of the intervention.

- Unlike patients with stable CAD mentioned earlier, residual defects might persist immediately after PCI in patients with acute MI and resolve gradually after 1 to 2 weeks.

Coronary artery revascularization with either PCI or CABG is commonly performed in patients with stable angina and severe CAD for the alleviation of symptoms and for improved survival in a subset of patients with high-risk anatomy. PCI and CABG remain the mainstays of therapy in patients with unstable angina or MI. Stress testing is valuable before and after revascularization to evaluate recurrent symptoms or in asymptomatic high-risk patients. Stress MPI can identify restenosis after PCI, significant stenosis in bypass grafts, progression of native CAD, or assess the significance of disease in territories that were not completely revascularized.

Current guidelines recommend the use of imaging in conjunction with stress testing when evaluating patients with prior revascularization. Imaging can localize the site and extent of ischemia and improves the sensitivity of ischemia detection, compared to exercise testing alone. In a pooled analysis of studies that assessed restenosis after balloon angioplasty, the sensitivity of exercise ECG alone was 54% compared to 83% with stress MPI, with comparable specificities of 77% and 78%, respectively. Exercise is the preferred stress modality in patients who can exercise and achieve adequate exercise end points, while vasodilator stress is reserved for patients who cannot exercise or for those who have an underlying LBBB or a ventricular paced rhythm. Dobutamine stress is reserved for patients who have contraindications to vasodilator stress. Appropriateness guidelines have been published to assist in the proper selection of patients with prior revascularization who are referred for stress MPI (Table 8-1).

Earlier stress MPI studies that evaluated restenosis post-PCI were done in the era of balloon angioplasty and bare metal stenting, where the restenosis rates approached 30% to 50% and 20% to 30%, respectively. The use of drug eluting stents has decreased the restenosis rate by up to 50%. One should also keep in mind that the incidence of clinical restenosis is significantly lower than angiographic restenosis. In one large study of bare metal stents, the incidence of clinical in-stent restenosis was 50% lower than the angiographic in-stent restenosis (defined as >50% diameter stenosis). In-stent restenosis of greater than 70% was more commonly associated with symptoms. Additionally, aggressive medical therapy and risk factor modification have further improved the outcomes of patients with CAD by

TABLE 8-1 Indications for Stress MPI in Patients After Revascularization

	SCORE
Appropriate Indications	
Symptomatic patients evaluated for ischemic symptoms	8
Asymptomatic patients evaluated for incomplete revascularization when additional revascularization is feasible	7
Asymptomatic patients ≥ 5 years after CABG	7
Uncertain Indications	
Asymptomatic patients ≥ 2 years after PCI	6
Asymptomatic patients < 5 years after CABG	5
Inappropriate Indications	
Asymptomatic patients <2 years after PCI	3
Before participation in cardiac rehabilitation	3

Appropriateness scores are based on a score from 1 to 9, based on consensus of experts. Scores of 7 to 9 are considered appropriate indications, scores of 4 to 6 are considered uncertain indications, and scores of <4 are considered inappropriate indications. *(Modified from Brindis RG, et al. JACC 46: 1587-1605, 2005.)*

decreasing the rate of CAD progression and decreasing the rate of cardiac events.

Ischemic symptoms that occur within 48 hours of PCI are usually related to periprocedural events, such as acute closure, distal embolization, coronary vasospasm, no reflow, jailing of side branches, or acute stent thrombosis. Stress MPI is not helpful in this situation. Ischemic symptoms within 1 month of PCI are more commonly related to sub-acute stent thrombosis and less likely from in-stent restenosis. Patients presenting with typical symptoms within 6 months after PCI are usually evaluated with coronary angiography. Stress MPI is performed in patients with PCI who present with atypical symptoms or with typical symptoms beyond 6 to 9 months after PCI. Routine evaluation of asymptomatic patients after PCI is not endorsed by the various guidelines. Routine stress MPI of asymptomatic patients after PCI should be reserved for high risk patients such as those with multivessel PCI, suboptimal PCI, incomplete revascularization, previous sudden cardiac death, proximal LAD PCI, prior silent ischemia, and hazardous occupation.

Graft disease, or failure after CABG, remains an important reason of symptom recurrence or other adverse cardiac events. Although internal mammary artery (IMA) grafts have a 10-year patency rate that approaches 90%, saphenous vein grafts have patency rates of around 75% and 40% at 5 and 10 years, respectively. As with PCI, stress testing in patients with prior CABG should be performed in conjunction with imaging. In a study that assessed graft stenosis after CABG, the sensitivity of the exercise ECG alone for detecting any graft stenosis was 31% compared to 80% with exercise MPI, with comparable specificities of 93% and 87%, respectively. The relationship between graft patency and perfusion pattern is far more complicated than in patients with native vessel disease. The presence of a patent graft does not guarantee a normal perfusion pattern and neither does the presence of graft disease guarantee an abnormal perfusion pattern. The size of the vessel and the status of other branches in the same territory are important factors that affect this relationship. This, most likely, explains the lower sensitivity of the test in such patients. It is imperative to review both the coronary angiogram and the MPI and not to rely on reports that often are not very helpful. Stress MPI is indicated in patients with CABG with recurrent symptoms during the 5-year window following CABG. Routine and periodic testing in patients 5 years following CABG is appropriate except in a select group of high-risk patients.

| **Case 8-1** | **Stress Testing Before and After PCI (Figure 8-1)** |

A 52-year-old African American man with HTN, obesity, GERD, and CAD underwent exercise MPI in 2008 for evaluation of chest pain. The images showed a large area of ischemia in the territory of the LCX artery with normal LVEF (Figure 8-1, *A, B*). Coronary angiography showed mild to moderate disease in the LAD and RCA and severe stenoses in the LCX artery (Figure 8-1, *C*). He underwent PCI of the LCX with two drug-eluting stents. He had recurrent atypical chest pains in 2010 and was evaluated with a regadenoson MPI. He had no ECG changes and the perfusion pattern and EF were normal (not shown). He was continued on medical therapy and did not undergo repeat coronary angiography.

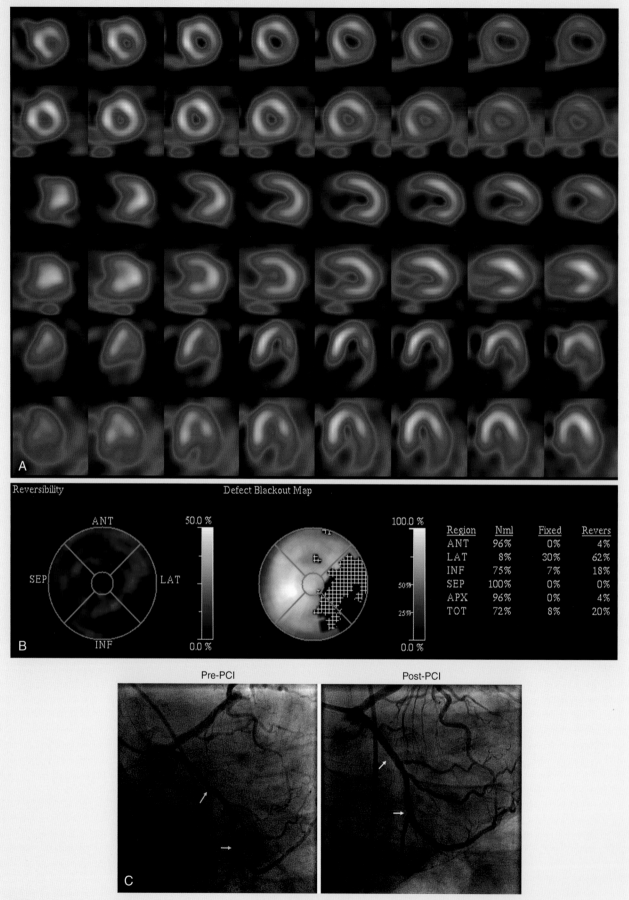

■ **Figure 8-1** Exercise MPI in 2008 showing large LCX ischemia **(A)**. The polar maps are shown in **B**. Coronary angiogram showing mild to moderate LAD and RCA disease **(C)** and severe stenosis of mid and distal LCX *(yellow arrows)*. Mid and distal LCX post-PCI with 2 drug eluting stents *(white arrows)* **(C)**. Post-PCI MPI was normal (not shown).

Case 8-2   **Stress Testing After PCI for Acute MI (Figure 8-2)**

A 31-year-old white man with type 1 DM and dyslipidemia sustained an anterior ST elevation MI in October 2009. Coronary angiography showed thrombotic occlusion of the mid LAD and mild disease in the RCA and LCX (Figure 8-2, *A*). He underwent PCI of the LAD with deployment of a drug-eluting stent (Figure 8-2, *B*). Two-dimensional echocardiography showed moderate LV dysfunction. In July 2010, he underwent an exercise MPI for evaluation of atypical chest pains. He exercised on the treadmill for 14 minutes and 30 seconds and stopped due to fatigue. The exercise ECG showed no ischemia. The perfusion images showed a large LAD scar (Figure 8-2, *C*). He had septal and apical dyskinesis and a mildly depressed rest LVEF of 46% (Figure 8-2, *D*, and Video 8-1). He was continued on medical therapy.

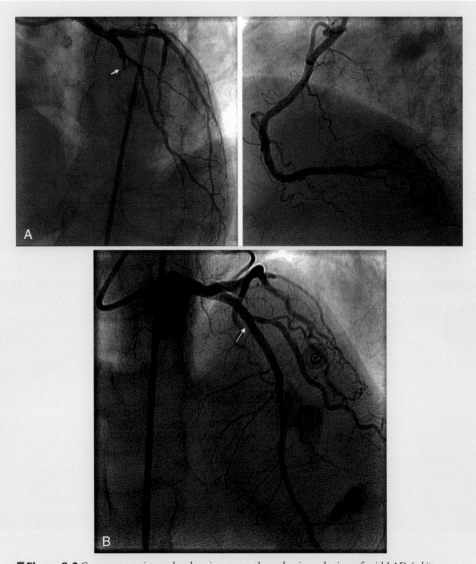

■ **Figure 8-2** Coronary angiography showing acute thrombotic occlusion of mid LAD *(white arrow)* and mild-to-moderate LCX and RCA disease **(A)**. The LAD post-PCI with a drug-eluting stent *(white arrow)* **(B)**.

(Continued)

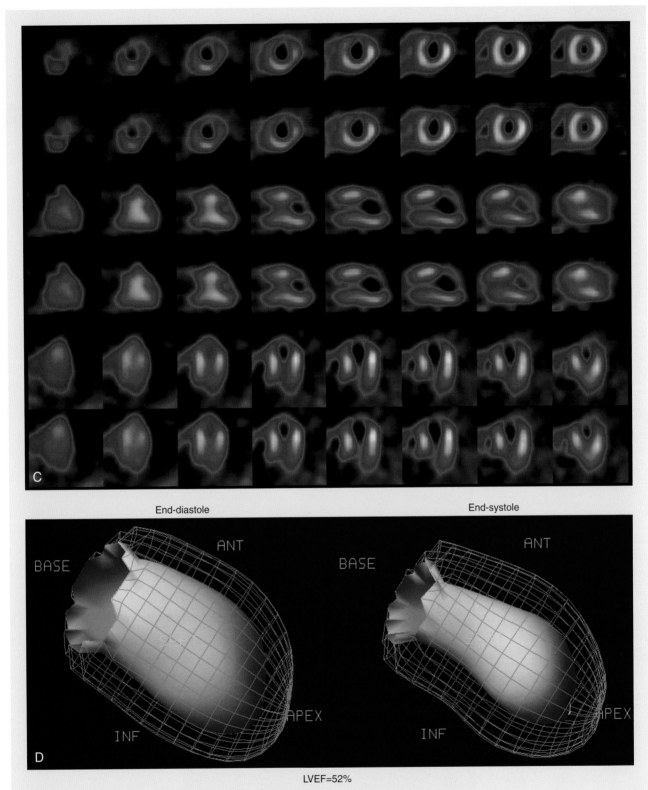

End-diastole   End-systole

LVEF=52%

■ **Figure 8-2—Cont'd** Exercise MPI showing a large LAD scar **(C)** with regional wall motion abnormality (**D** and Video 8-1).

Case 8-3   **Stress Testing After Multiple PCIs for Recurrent Symptoms (Figure 8-3)**

An 83-year-old white man with HTN, dyslipidemia, chronic kidney disease, peptic ulcer disease, and CAD with a history of MI and multiple PCIs of the LAD, RCA, and LCX underwent regadenoson MPI for evaluation of recurrent chest pain. The stress ECG was negative for ischemia. The SPECT images showed a large area of ischemia in the LAD and LCX territories (Figure 8-3, *A*). The wall motion and EF were

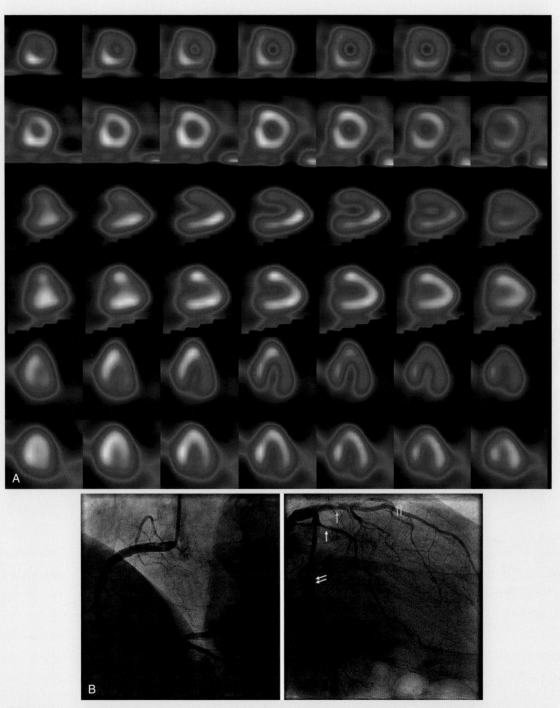

■ **Figure 8-3** Regadenoson MPI showing a large ischemia in the distribution of the LAD and LCX **(A)**. The coronary angiogram is shown in **B**. The RCA has mild disease. The LAD has severe proximal stenosis *(yellow arrow)* and the first diagonal is totally occluded proximal *(yellow double arrows)*. First and second obtuse marginal branches have severe stenoses *(white single* and *double arrows)*.

normal. Coronary angiography showed a patent RCA stent with minimal RCA disease, severe stenosis of the proximal LAD, and an occluded second diagonal (in-stent) with left to left collaterals. The LCX had severe stenoses of the first and second obtuse marginal branches (Figure 8-3, *B*). The patient underwent successful CABG.

Case 8-4	Area at Risk Assessment During Transient Balloon Occlusion (Figure 8-4)

A 63-year-old woman underwent adenosine MPI for evaluation of chest pain and shortness of breath. The images showed LAD ischemia. She underwent coronary angiography, which showed severe proximal LAD stenosis. At the time of coronary angioplasty and while the balloon was inflated, Tc99m-sestamibi was injected intravenously. After successful angioplasty (before the era of stenting), SPECT images were obtained. The perfusion abnormality was in the same location and the same extent as that seen in the prior adenosine images, but was more severe. The coronary flow reserve ratio improved immediately after the angioplasty. The angioplasty model provides a unique opportunity to examine the relationship between coronary anatomy, flow, and perfusion (Figure 8-4).

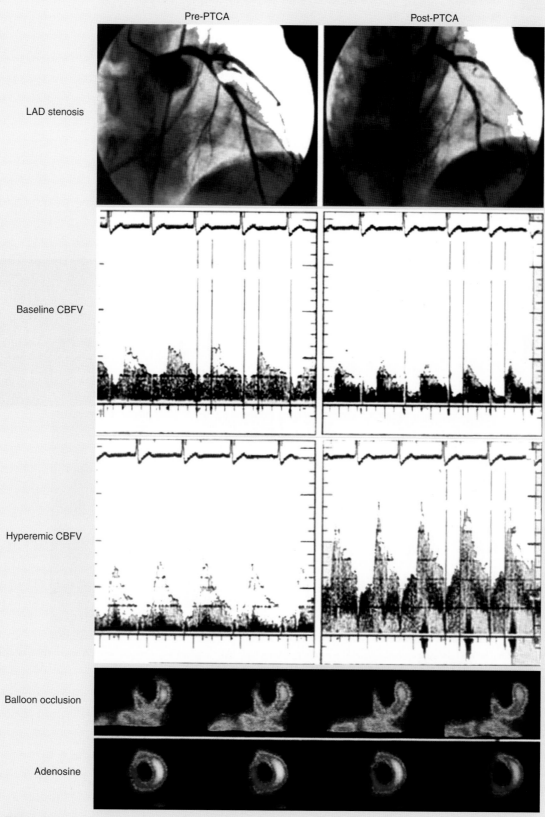

■ **Figure 8-4** The coronary angiogram before and after angioplasty of a severe proximal LAD stenosis, the coronary flow velocity at rest and during adenosine-induced hyperemia (before and after angioplasty), and selected slices of SPECT images obtained during transient balloon occlusion and in a prior study obtained with adenosine stress. The flow velocity improved after angioplasty. The perfusion abnormality is more severe (as would have been predicted) during balloon occlusion than adenosine stress, but the areas at jeopardy are comparable.

Case 8-5   **Ischemia Due to Native Downstream Disease Despite Patent Stents (Figure 8-5)**

A 67-year-old man with HTN, dyslipidemia, paroxysmal atrial fibrillation, and CAD with prior PCIs of the LAD, LCX, and RCA underwent a follow-up stress MPI because he had experienced silent ischemia with prior interventions. He exercised on the treadmill for 7 minutes and stopped due to fatigue. The ECG showed 1-mm ST depression in the lateral leads. The polar maps showed distal apical ischemia (Figure 8-5, *A*). The wall motion and the LVEF were normal. Coronary angiography showed patent RCA, LCX, and LAD stents and a diffusely diseased small distal LAD (Figure 8-5, *B*) that was responsible for the apical perfusion defect. He was continued on medical therapy.

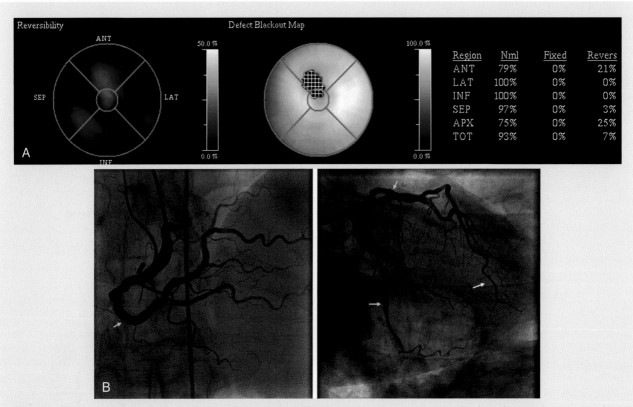

■ **Figure 8-5** Exercise MPI showing a small area of ischemia in the distal LAD **(A)**. Coronary angiography showed patent RCA, LAD, and LCX stents *(yellow arrows)* but diffuse disease in the small distal LAD *(white arrow)* **(B)**.

Case 8-6 Ischemia Due to Jailed Septal Perforator Branch After PCI of LAD (Figure 8-6)

A 48-year-old man with HTN, dyslipidemia, prior tobacco abuse, Hodgkin's lymphoma, prior inferior ST elevation MI, and PCI of the RCA and LAD (Figure 8-6, *A, B*) underwent exercise MPI prior to employment with the National Guard. He exercised on the treadmill for 10 minutes and stopped due to fatigue. The ECG showed no ischemic changes. The SPECT images showed a small area of ischemia in the basal septum and apex (Figure 8-6, *C*). The wall motion and the LVEF were normal. He was continued on medical therapy.

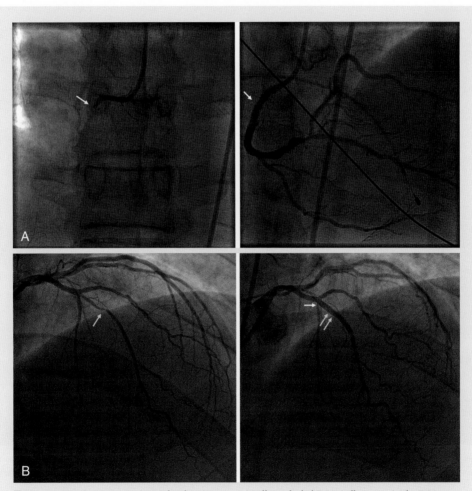

■ **Figure 8-6** Coronary angiography showing a proximally occluded RCA *(yellow arrow)*. The RCA post-PCI with a drug eluting stent *(white arrow)* **(A)**. Coronary angiography showed severe mid LAD stenosis *(yellow arrow)* **(B)**. Coronary angiography post-LAD PCI showed patent stent *(double yellow arrows)* but jailed septal perforator branch with severe ostial stenosis *(white arrow)* **(B)**.

(Continued)

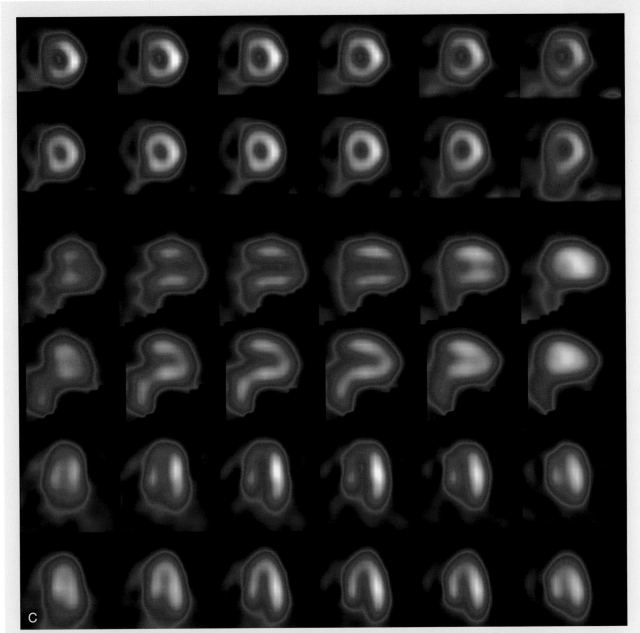

■ **Figure 8-6—Cont'd** Note that the distal LAD is very small and diffusely diseased. Exercise MPI showing small area of ischemia in the distribution of the septal perforator branch of the LAD involving the basal septum, although there is also an apical abnormality **(C)**.

COMMENTS (Cases 8-1 to 8-6)

The sensitivity and specificity of stress MPI to detect restenosis after balloon angioplasty alone were ~80% from various pooled studies. The sensitivity and specificity for identification of in-stent restenosis improved to 100% and 82% in territories without prior MI. Of note, side branch stenosis was seen in some patients without significant in-stent restenosis but with ischemia on the MPI. Downstream lesions due to diffuse disease are another reason for abnormal MPI, despite patent stents. The limitations of coronary angiography in predicting

flow limitations, discussed earlier, are compounded after PCI and CABG.

In a study of 365 patients who underwent stress MPI >6 months after PCI with bare metal stents, 23% of patients had target vessel ischemia, 62% of whom had silent ischemia. Patients with silent ischemia had a higher event rate (cardiac death, MI, and revascularization) compared to those without ischemia (32% vs. 17%) though they had a lower event rate than those with symptomatic ischemia (52%).

In another study of 370 patients who underwent exercise MPI at least 1 month after coronary stenting, 23%

had ischemia. The 30-month hard event (death or MI) rate was 9.1% in those without ischemia versus 17% in those with ischemia. The presence of ischemia was a significant multivariate predictor of events in both asymptomatic and symptomatic patients. In another study of 152 patients who underwent stress SPECT within 5 months of stenting with bare metal stents, the event rate was 3% in those with no ischemia compared to 28% in those with ischemia. The results of these studies are limited to bare metal stenting and cannot be extrapolated to patients with drug-eluting stents.

In a study of 322 consecutive patients who underwent exercise SPECT 4 to 6 months after incomplete PCI, the perfusion results provided significant independent prognostic information for future risk of cardiac events. The annual event rate was <2% in patients with normal scans versus 8.5% in patients with markedly abnormal scans.

| Case 8-7 | **Stress Testing Before and After CABG (Figure 8-7)** |

An 80-year-old woman with HTN underwent CABG in 2006 because of severe angina. A prior adenosine MPI showed a large ischemic area (Figure 8-7, *top*). Coronary angiography showed severe left main, LAD, LCX, and RCA disease with an LVEF of 61%. She experienced atypical chest pains several months following CABG. A repeat adenosine MPI showed normal perfusion pattern with normal LVEF and wall motion (Figure 8-7, *bottom*).

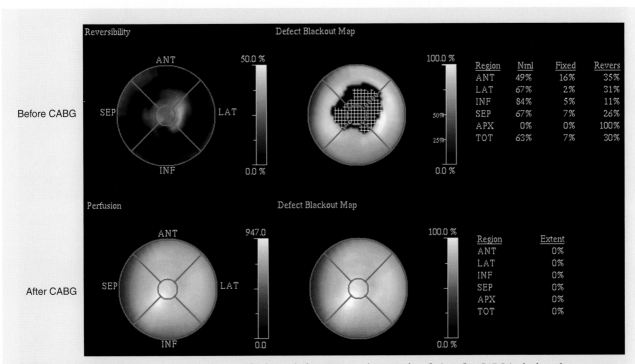

■ **Figure 8-7** Adenosine MPI showing a large area of ischemia before CABG and a normal perfusion after CABG (only the polar maps are shown).

Case 8-8   **Ischemia Due to Jeopardized Branches From Proximal LAD Despite Patent LIMA (Figure 8-8)**

A 57-year-old white male with HTN, DM, dyslipidemia, hypothyroidism, and prior CABG underwent exercise MPI for evaluation of recurrent angina. He exercised on the treadmill for 10 minutes and stopped due to angina and fatigue. The exercise ECG showed 2-mm flat ST depression in the inferior and lateral leads. The SPECT images showed ischemia in the distribution of the basal septum (Figure 8-8, *A, B*). The LVEF was 58%. Coronary angiography showed occlusion of the LAD and RCA and severe LCX disease. The LIMA to LAD (Figure 8-8, *C*), the SVG to RCA, and the SVG to the LCX-OM1 grafts were patent. There were jeopardized branches in the proximal LAD between the proximal occlusion and before the LIMA anastomosis.

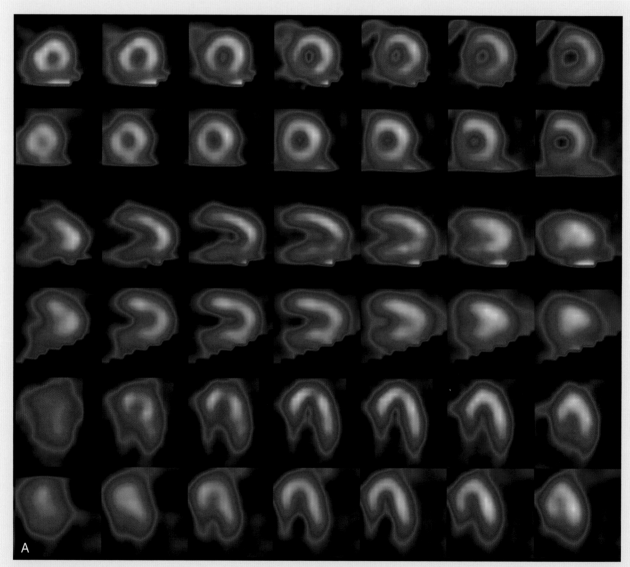

■ Figure 8-8 Exercise MPI (with polar maps) showing small area of ischemia in the distribution of the LAD involving the basal septum and sparing the apex and distal anterior wall and septum **(A, B)**. This pattern is very suggestive of patent LIMA but indicates jeopardized branches before the LIMA anastomosis. Coronary angiography showed occluded LAD and RCA and severe LCX disease. The LIMA to LAD graft was patent **(C)**, but there are jeopardized branches before the LIMA anastomosis. The double white arrows show faint collaterals from the LAD to small RCA branches. The vein grafts to the RCA and LCX-OM1 were patent as well (not shown).

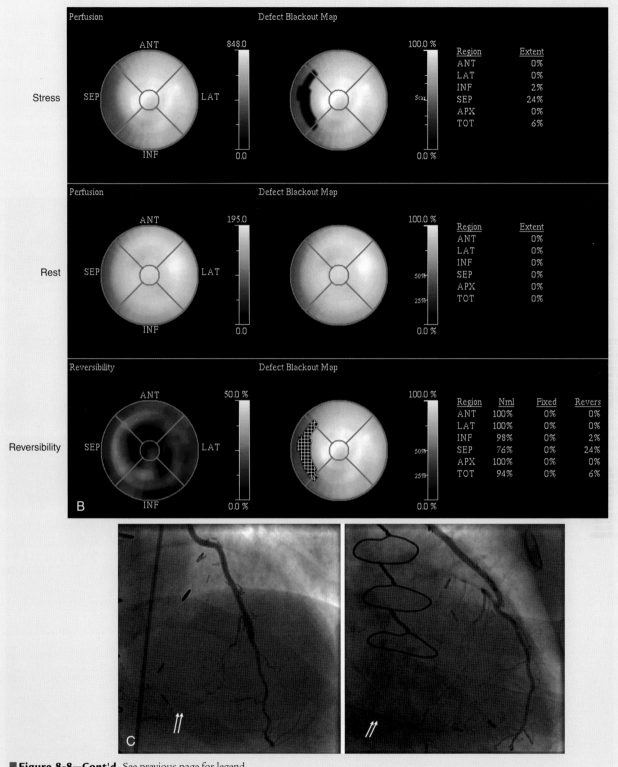

■**Figure 8-8—Cont'd.** See previous page for legend.

Case 8-9	Septal Motion Abnormality but Normal Thickening After Uncomplicated CABG (Figure 8-9)

A 67-year-old man with dyslipidemia, Parkinson's disease, prior MI, and three-vessel CABG was referred for regadenoson MPI for evaluation of dyspnea on exertion. He had no chest pain or ECG during the stress test. He had normal perfusion with an LVEF of 72% (Figure 8-9, *A*). There was a septal wall motion abnormality but the wall thickening was normal (Figure 8-9, *B*). The patient was continued on medical therapy.

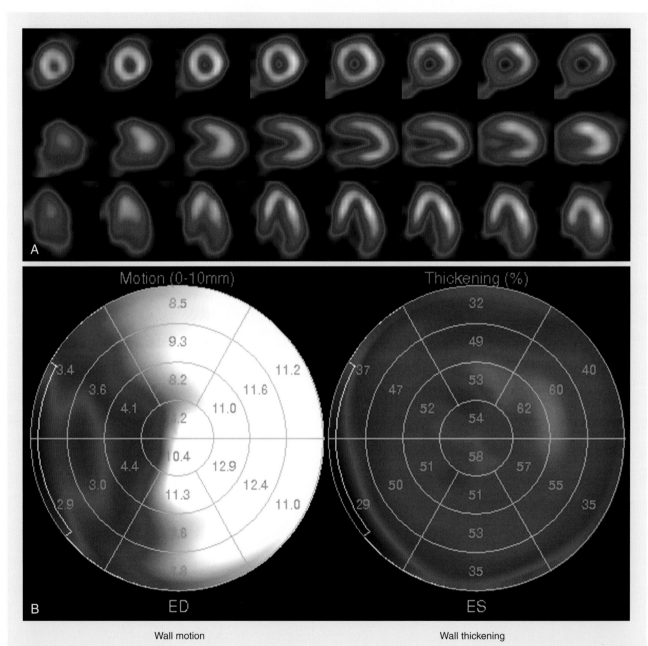

Wall motion   Wall thickening

■ **Figure 8-9** Regadenoson MPI showing normal perfusion (**A**). The gated SPECT images show abnormal motion but normal thickening consistent with post-CABG changes (**B**).

Case 8-10   Ischemia Due to Downstream Disease Despite Patent Grafts
(Figure 8-10)

A 65-year-old woman with DM, HTN, dyslipidemia, peripheral vascular disease, depression, and prior CABG was referred for stress MPI for evaluation of recurrent chest pain. She had no chest pain or ECG changes during adenosine stress. The perfusion images showed a large area of ischemia in the distribution of the LAD and RCA territories with an LVEF of 75% and normal wall thickening (Figure 8-10, *A*). Subsequent coronary angiography showed severe native three-vessel disease (Figure 8-10, *B*). The LIMA to LAD graft and the sequential vein grafts to the PDA and LCX marginal were patent, though the PDA was occluded beyond the graft anastomosis. There was diffuse disease downstream from the graft anastomoses (Figure 8-10, *B*, *C*). The patient was continued on intensified medical therapy.

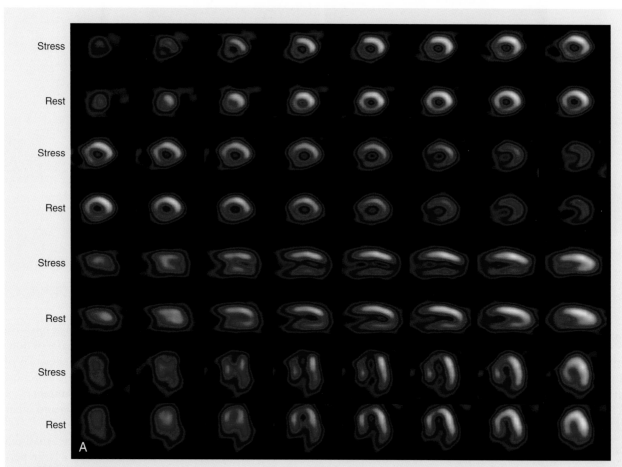

■ Figure 8-10 Adenosine stress/rest MPI showing a large area of ischemia in the distribution of the LAD and RCA **(A)**.

(Continued)

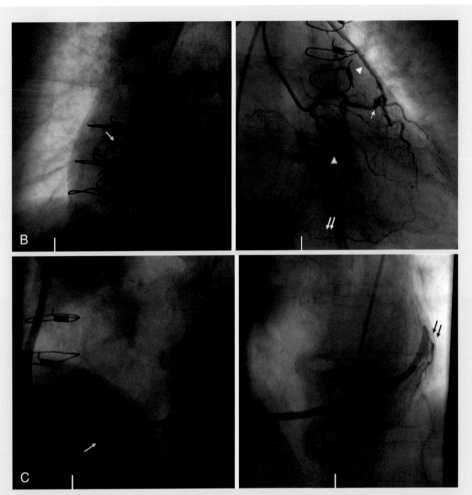

■ **Figure 8-10—Cont'd** Coronary angiogram showing totally occluded RCA *(yellow arrow)* and severe LAD *(white arrow)* and LCX *(yellow arrowhead)* disease **(B)**. Note the patent LIMA to LAD graft *(white arrowhead)*, the diffuse distal LAD disease and the mature collaterals to the RCA *(double white arrows)* **(B)**. C shows a patent sequential vein graft to PDA and obtuse marginal, though the PDA is occluded beyond the graft anastomosis *(yellow arrow)*. The graft supplies a small obtuse marginal *(double black arrows)*.

COMMENTS (Cases 8-7 to 8-10)

In a study of 50 patients with CABG who underwent stress MPI for evaluation of typical and atypical chest pain, the sensitivity of thallium SPECT for detection of >50% graft stenosis was 83%. The sensitivity of thallium-201 SPECT for correctly localizing the graft stenosis site was 82% for the LAD, 92% for the RCA, and 75% for the LCX. In another study of 27 patients who underwent stress SPECT after CABG, the sensitivity of SPECT for detecting >75% stenosis in a graft, distal vessel, or un-grafted vessel was 77%. In another study, thallium MPI had an 80% sensitivity, 88% specificity, and 86% overall accuracy in detecting bypass graft disease. In 109 patients who underwent both adenosine thallium-201 SPECT and coronary angiography at 6.7 ± 4.8 years after CABG, significant graft stenoses were present in 68 patients. Perfusion defects were present in 65 patients resulting in a sensitivity of 96%. Significant stenoses were present in 107 of 283 grafts. The overall specificity of SPECT

was 61%. Around 70% of the apparently false-positive perfusion defects could be explained on the basis of non-bypassed native diseased vessels or by the presence of fixed defects in patients with prior MI. As is evident most of these studies are old and involve small numbers of patients and the results are limited by selection and other confounding factors.

In 411 patients who underwent exercise thallium SPECT within 2 years of CABG, 26% had a large per-fusion defect and only 12% had evidence of ischemia proximal to a graft insertion site. The 5-year event-free (cardiac death or MI) rate was 93% for patients without angina and a normal image or a small perfusion defect versus 71% for patients with angina and a medium or large perfusion defect. In 294 patients who underwent exercise thallium SPECT ≥5 years after CABG, the 31-month event rate (death or nonfatal MI) was 14%. Abnormal perfusion and increased lung thallium uptake increased the odds of cardiac events by 80% and 10% respectively. In a study of 255 patients who underwent stress SPECT within 5 years after CABG, the annual mortality and total event rates were 7.5% and 9.5% with presence of multivessel ischemia and increased lung thallium uptake, 3.4% and 4.3% with either abnormality, and 0.6% and 1.7% with neither abnormalities (p = .01). In a study of 1765 patients who underwent dual-isotope SPECT MPI at 7.1 ± 5.0 years after CABG, the annual cardiac mortality in patients with moderate or large abnormalities was 2.1% in symptomatic patients ≤5 years post-CABG and 3.1% in patients >5 years post-CABG irrespective of symptoms. The annual cardiac mortality was 0% in symptomatic patients ≤5 years post-CABG and 0.7% in patients >5 years post-CABG, irrespective of symptoms in the remaining patients. In 873 asymptomatic patients with CABG (at a mean of 7 years) who underwent exercise thallium SPECT, perfusion defects were present in 58% of patients. Reversible perfusion defects were predictive of all-cause mortality (12% vs. 5%) and death or MI (13% vs. 7%). In multivariate analysis, perfusion defects remained predictive of death (adjusted relative risk 2.78, 95% CI 1.44-5.39) and death or MI (2.63, 1.49-4.66). Impaired exercise capacity (≤6 METs) was also an independent multivariate predictor of death and death or MI.

SELECTED READINGS

Acampa W, Evangelista L, Petretta M, et al: Usefulness of stress cardiac single-photon emission computed tomographic imaging late after percutaneous coronary intervention for assessing cardiac events and time to such events, *Am J Cardiol* 100:436–441, 2007.

Acampa W, Petretta M, Florimonte L, et al: Prognostic value of exercise cardiac tomography performed late after percutaneous coronary intervention in symptomatic and symptom-free patients, *Am J Cardiol* 91:259–263, 2003.

Chin ASL, Goldman LE, Eisenberg MJ: Functional testing after coronary artery bypass graft surgery: a meta-analysis, *Can J Cardiol* 19:802–808, 2003.

Cottin Y, Rezaizadeh K, Touzery C, et al: Long-term prognostic value of 201Tl single-photon emission computed tomographic myocardial perfusion imaging after coronary stenting, *Am Heart J* 141:999–1006, 2001.

Cutlip DE, Chauhan MS, Baim DS, et al: Clinical restenosis after coronary stenting: perspectives from multicenter clinical trials, *J Am Coll Cardiol* 40:2082–2089, 2002.

Deluca AJ, Cusack E, Aronow WS, et al: Sensitivity, specificity, positive predictive value, and negative predictive value of the dipyridamole sestamibi stress test in predicting graft occlusion or > or = 50% new native coronary artery disease in men versus women and in patients aged > or = 65 years versus < 65 years who had prior coronary artery bypass grafting, *Am J Cardiol* 94:625–626, 2004.

Dori G, Denekamp Y, Fishman S, et al: Exercise stress testing, myocardial perfusion imaging and stress echocardiography for detecting restenosis after successful percutaneous transluminal coronary angioplasty: a review of performance, *J Intern Med* 253:253–262, 2003.

Fitzgibbon GM, Kafka HP, Leach AJ, et al: Coronary bypass graft fate and patient outcome: angiographic follow-up of 5,065 grafts related to survival and reoperation in 1,388 patients during 25 years, *J Am Coll Cardiol* 28:616–626, 1996.

Galassi AR, Grasso C, Azzarelli S, et al: Usefulness of exercise myocardial scintigraphy in multivessel coronary disease after incomplete revascularization with coronary stenting, *Am J Cardiol* 97:207–215, 2006.

Georgoulias P, Demakopoulos N, Tzavara C, et al: Long-term prognostic value of Tc-99m tetrofosmin myocardial gated-SPECT imaging in asymptomatic patients after percutaneous coronary intervention, *Clin Nucl Med* 33:743–747, 2008.

Georgoulias P, Tzavara C, Demakopoulos N, et al: Incremental prognostic value of (99m)Tc-tetrofosmin myocardial SPECT after percutaneous coronary intervention, *Ann Nucl Med* 22:899–909, 2008.

Giedd KN, Bergmann SR: Myocardial perfusion imaging following percutaneous coronary intervention: the importance of restenosis, disease progression, and directed reintervention, *J Am Coll Cardiol* 43:328–336, 2004.

Hendel RC, Berman DS, Di Carli MF, et al: ACCF/ASNC/ACR/AHA/ASE/SCCT/SCMR/SNM 2009 Appropriate Use Criteria for Cardiac Radionuclide Imaging: A Report of the American College of Cardiology Foundation Appropriate Use Criteria Task Force, the American Society of Nuclear Cardiology, the American College of Radiology, the American Heart Association, the American Society of Echocardiography, the Society of Cardiovascular Computed Tomography, the Society for Cardiovascular Magnetic Resonance, and the Society of Nuclear Medicine, *J Am Coll Cardiol* 53:2201–2229, 2009.

Khoury AF, Rivera JM, Mahmarian JJ, et al: Adenosine thallium-201 tomography in evaluation of graft patency late after coronary artery bypass graft surgery, *J Am Coll Cardiol* 29:1290–1295, 1997.

Klocke FJ, Baird MG, Lorell BH, et al: ACC/AHA/ASNC guidelines for the clinical use of cardiac radionuclide imaging—executive summary: a report of the American College of Cardiology/American Heart Association Task Force on Practice Guidelines (ACC/AHA/ASNC Committee to Revise the 1995 Guidelines for the Clinical Use of Cardiac Radionuclide Imaging), *J Am Coll Cardiol* 42:1318–1333, 2003.

Kósa I, Blasini R, Schneider-Eicke J, et al: Myocardial perfusion scintigraphy to evaluate patients after coronary stent implantation, *J Nucl Med* 39:1307–1311, 1998.

Lakkis NM, Mahmarian JJ, Verani MS: Exercise thallium-201 single photon emission computed tomography for evaluation of coronary artery bypass graft patency, *Am J Cardiol* 76:107–111, 1995.

Lauer MS, Lytle B, Pashkow F, et al: Prediction of death and myocardial infarction by screening with exercise-thallium testing after coronary-artery-bypass grafting, *Lancet* 351:615–622, 1998.

Milavetz JJ, Miller TD, Hodge DO, et al: Accuracy of single-photon emission computed tomography myocardial perfusion imaging in patients with stents in native coronary arteries, *Am J Cardiol* 82:857–861, 1998.

Nallamothu N, Johnson JH, Bagheri B, et al: Utility of stress single-photon emission computed tomography (SPECT) perfusion imaging in predicting outcome after coronary artery bypass grafting, *Am J Cardiol* 80:1517–1521, 1997.

Palmas W, Bingham S, Diamond GA, et al: Incremental prognostic value of exercise thallium-201 myocardial single-photon emission computed tomography late after coronary artery bypass surgery, *J Am Coll Cardiol* 25:403–409, 1995.

Pfisterer M, Emmenegger H, Schmitt HE, et al: Accuracy of serial myocardial perfusion scintigraphy with thallium-201 for prediction of graft patency early and late after coronary artery bypass surgery, A controlled prospective study, *Circulation* 66:1017–1024, 1982.

Rajagopal V, Gurm HS, Brunken RC, et al: Prediction of death or myocardial infarction by exercise single photon emission computed tomography perfusion scintigraphy in patients who have had recent coronary artery stenting, *Am Heart J* 149:534–540, 2005.

Solodky A, Assali AR, Mats I, et al: Prognostic value of myocardial perfusion imaging in symptomatic and asymptomatic patients after percutaneous coronary intervention, *Cardiology* 107:38–43, 2007.

Takeuchi M, Miura Y, Toyokawa T, et al: The comparative diagnostic value of dobutamine stress echocardiography and thallium stress tomography for detecting restenosis after coronary angioplasty, *J Am Soc Echocardiogr* 8:696–702, 1995.

Zellweger MJ, Lewin HC, Lai S, et al: When to stress patients after coronary artery bypass surgery? Risk stratification in patients early and late post-CABG using stress myocardial perfusion SPECT: implications of appropriate clinical strategies, *J Am Coll Cardiol* 37:144–152, 2001.

Zellweger MJ, Weinbacher M, Zutter AW, et al: Long-term outcome of patients with silent versus symptomatic ischemia six months after percutaneous coronary intervention and stenting, *J Am Coll Cardiol* 42:33–40, 2003.

Zhang X, Liu X, He Z, et al: Long-term prognostic value of exercise 99mTc-MIBI SPET myocardial perfusion imaging in patients after percutaneous coronary intervention, *Eur J Nucl Med Mol Imaging* 31:655–662, 2004.

Chapter 9

Patients with Acute Coronary Syndrome

Gilbert J. Zoghbi, Jaekyeong Heo, and Ami E. Iskandrian

KEY POINTS

- Acute coronary syndrome encompasses a wide spectrum of clinical presentations, including UA, non–ST elevation MI, and ST elevation MI.

- Patients with ST elevation MI are preferably treated with primary PCI or thrombolytic therapy.

- Rest MPI can be used to assess infarct size, area at risk, and the impact of various interventions to modify infarct size.

- Rest MPI can be used to identify culprit vessels if the tracer is injected during pain.

- Stress MPI has no role during an acute presentation.

- Stress MPI is clearly helpful in risk stratification of stabilized patients after the first 24 to 48 hours after acute onset.

- Such patients include those who were treated conservatively, those who were treated with thrombolytic therapy, or those who were treated with PCIs but had either less than ideal angiographic result or incomplete revascularization.

- Vasodilator MPI can be used 24 to 48 hours after acute presentation in the absence of angina, heart failure, or serious arrhythmia within the past 24 hours.

- Depending on patient selection, the stress MPI abnormalities could be mild, absent, or severe and extensive.

- The MPI findings could be used as effective tools to further triage patients toward coronary interventions or optimal medical management.

BACKGROUND

The ACSs encompass UA, NSTEMI, and STEMI. In 2006, 1,365,000 patients were discharged from U.S. hospitals with a diagnosis of ACS. Of the total discharges, 810,000 patients had an MI, with nearly one third being STEMI. Patients with STEMI are treated emergently, and preferably with PCI or with thrombolytic (fibrinolytic) therapy if PCI is not readily available. Patients with STEMI who are treated with thrombolytic therapy or conservatively and who have high-risk clinical features or who are unstable should undergo coronary angiography with intent to revascularize. Stable patients who received thrombolytic therapy or who were treated conservatively can undergo stress MPI for risk stratification and particularly to assess LV function, infarct size, and residual ischemia in the infarct and remote zones.

The use of clinical information, biomarkers, and ECG results, as well as risk stratification models (such as the TIMI or GRACE risk score or the PURSUIT model), can be used in the early risk stratification of patients with UA or NSTEMI. Rest MPI can also be used in the evaluation of these patients in the emergency department (ED) and will be discussed in Chapter 14. Patients with UA or NSTEMI with high-risk features, such as elevated cardiac biomarkers, ST segment depression, hemodynamic instability, reduced LV function, signs or symptoms of HF, recurrent or persistent angina despite optimal medical therapy, new or worsening mitral regurgitation, sustained ventricular arrhythmias, PCI within 6 months, prior CABG, high-risk TIMI or GRACE score, or high-risk findings on noninvasive testing, are preferably treated with an invasive strategy that includes coronary angiography and revascularization with either PCI or CABG.

Stress MPI can be used in the evaluation and risk stratification of patients at low to intermediate risk who have UA or NSTEMI, those with STEMI who have received thrombolytic therapy, and patients who were treated with coronary interventions with either less than optimal results by angiography or those who have had incomplete revascularization. Stress MPI should be performed in patients who have been free of ischemic symptoms, serious arrhythmias, or HF for a minimum of 12 to 24 hours. High-risk features on stress MPI carry >3% annual mortality rate and include a resting LVEF <35%, exercise LVEF <35%, large reversible perfusion defect, multiple reversible perfusion defects of moderate size, large fixed perfusion defect with LV dilation or with increased lung uptake (if imaged with thallium-201), or a Duke treadmill risk score of ≤−11. Rest MPI can also be used for infarct sizing in patients who are post-MI. Appropriateness criteria for stress MPI in patients with ACS are listed in Table 9-1.

Although some of the guidelines recommend exercise treadmill testing as the stress test of choice and reserve stress testing with MPI for those with uninterruptable ECG or those who cannot exercise, exercise treadmill testing as a stand-alone test is rarely used in real practice. Vasodilator stress MPI has been the modality of choice in patients with MI as it allows early stress testing compared to exercise stress testing.

TABLE 9-1 Indications for MPI in Patients With Acute Chest Pain

	SCORE
Appropriate Indications	
Possible ACS (stress MPI)	
No ischemic ECG changes, LBBB, or paced rhythm + low risk TIMI score + borderline, equivocal, or minimally elevated troponin	9
No ischemic ECG changes, LBBB, or paced rhythm + low risk TIMI score + negative troponin	8
No ischemic ECG changes, LBBB, or paced rhythm + high risk TIMI score + negative troponin	8
No ischemic ECG changes, LBBB, or paced rhythm + high risk TIMI score + borderline, equivocal, or minimally elevated troponin	8
Possible ACS (rest MPI)	
No ischemic ECG changes, LBBB, or paced rhythm + initial negative troponin + recent or ongoing chest pain	7
Elevated troponin without additional evidence of ACS	7
UA/NSTEMI (within 3 months)	
No prior coronary angiography + hemodynamically stable + no recurrent angina + no signs of CHF (to evaluate for inducible ischemia)	9
STEMI (within 3 months)	
No prior coronary angiography + hemodynamically stable + no recurrent angina + no signs of CHF (to evaluate for inducible ischemia)	8
Inappropriate Indications	
Definite ACS	1
STEMI within 3 months + PCI with complete revascularization + no recurrent symptoms	2
STEMI within 3 months + hemodynamic instability, signs of cardiogenic shock or mechanical complications	1
ACS + post-revascularization + asymptomatic (evaluation prior to hospital discharge)	1
Before participation in cardiac rehabilitation	1

Appropriateness scores are based on a score from 1 to 9, based on consensus of experts. Scores of 7 to 9 are considered appropriate indications, scores of 4 to 6 are considered uncertain indications, and scores of <4 are considered inappropriate indications.

Case 9-1   **Rest Imaging With Tracer Injection During Chest Pain (Figure 9-1)**

A 56-year-old African American woman with history of HTN and GERD presented to the ED with 2 weeks of intermittent retrosternal chest pains that initially occurred with exertion but progressed to occurring at rest. The initial ECG and cardiac markers in the ED were unremarkable. She was injected with 33 mCi of Tc-99m sestamibi at rest while she was still having chest pain. The rest SPECT images with attenuation correction revealed abnormal perfusion in the LAD territory with an LVEF of 65% and normal wall motion (Figure 9-1, *A*). Subsequent coronary angiography showed a 99% proximal LAD stenosis involving the first diagonal branch with right to left collaterals (Figure 9-1, *B, C*). The RCA and LCX had mild disease (Figure 9-1, *B*). The LAD was stented with a drug-eluting stent (Figure 9-1, *C*).

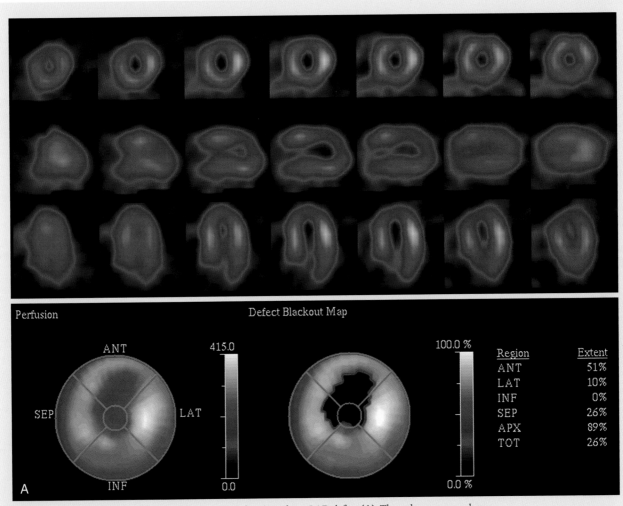

■ **Figure 9-1** Rest SPECT images during chest pain showing a large LAD defect **(A)**. The polar maps are shown.

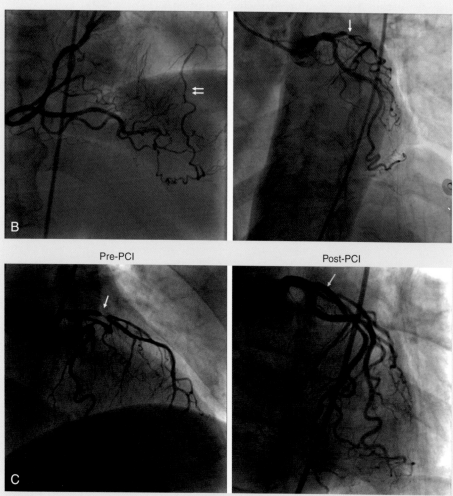

Pre-PCI   Post-PCI

■ **Figure 9-1—Cont'd** Coronary angiogram showing mild RCA and LCX disease **(B)** and a severe proximal LAD stenosis *(white arrow)* **(B, C)** with collaterals from the RCA to LAD *(double white arrows)*. The LAD post-PCI with a drug eluting stent is also shown *(yellow arrow)* **(C)**.

COMMENTS

Gated rest SPECT imaging in the ED can be used in the evaluation of patients who present with cardiac symptoms without significant ECG changes or abnormal cardiac biomarkers. Rest imaging can detect an MI earlier than the rise in cardiac markers. A normal rest MPI has a 99% negative predictive value to rule out an MI and a 97% negative predictive value for future cardiac events. The sensitivity and specificity of rest MPI to detect acute MI ranged from 90% to 100% and 60% to 78%, respectively, in various studies. The sensitivity and specificity of rest MPI to detect CAD ranged from 73% to 100% and 79% to 93%, respectively.

In one study, the injection of technetium-99m sestamibi during chest pain had a sensitivity and specificity of 96% and 79% for the detection of significant CAD compared to 35% and 74% for the ECG. The respective sensitivity and specificity of rest MPI were 65% and 84% when the tracer was injected while patients were free of chest pain. The site of the perfusion defect correlated with the most severe coronary artery on angiography in 88% of patients. In another study, acute MI, as defined by an elevated CK-MB, was present in only 15% of patients who had an abnormal rest MPI, while the rest of the patients had other endpoints, such as significant CAD or revascularization. In a study of rest MPI in 479 patients presenting with chest pains, 45 patients had abnormal scans. The 30-day event rate was 22% (11% MI and 20% PCI) in those with abnormal scans and 0.7% (0.3% MI and 0.6% PCI) in the 434 patients with normal scans. The three patients with normal scans and cardiac events had tracer injected >2 hours after the resolution of the chest pain episode.

In conclusion, rest MPI is not diagnostic in patients with prior MI and does not exclude the presence of CAD. Rest MPI is more diagnostic when the tracer is injected during the episode of chest pain and has a high negative predictive value for cardiac events. Obviously, the MPI abnormality might reflect ischemia rather than necrosis, which may explain why MPI abnormalities precede biomarker elevation or why they can occur without biomarker elevation.

Case 9-2   **Stress Testing After Medical Stabilization of ACS (Figure 9-2)**

A 65-year-old white woman with a history of DM, dyslipidemia, tobacco abuse, and prior stroke presented to the ED with a 2-day history of generalized weakness and lethargy. She was found to have acute renal failure with tripling of creatinine level. Initial ECG showed inferior and lateral injury and infarction (Figure 9-2, *A*). The cardiac markers were elevated upon presentation, with subsequent downward trend. She was treated medically given her atypical presentation. She underwent further evaluation with adenosine MPI. She had nonspecific ECG changes with adenosine stress. The SPECT images showed a large mixed defect in the inferior and lateral walls (mostly scar) (Figure 9-2, *B*). The LVEF was 37%. She was treated medically and did well.

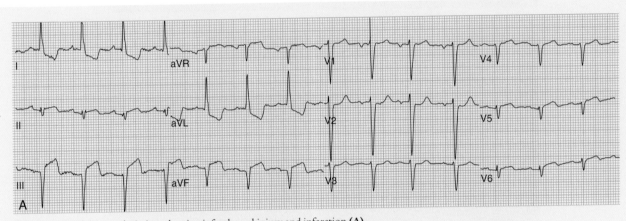

■ **Figure 9-2** ECG on admission, showing inferolateral injury and infarction **(A)**.

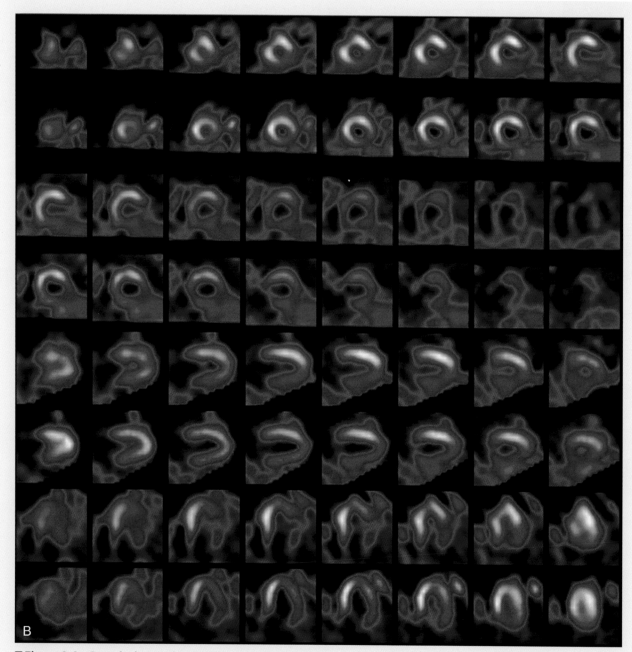

■ **Figure 9-2—Cont'd** Adenosine/rest MPI showing a large mixed defect (mostly scar) in the distribution of the RCA **(B)**.

Case 9-3   **Rest Imaging for Infarct Sizing After PCI for Acute MI (Figure 9-3)**

An 83-year-old white man with a history of HTN, hyperlipidemia, and DM presented to the ED with new onset chest pain of 4 hours' duration. He had an anterior STEMI. He was taken emergently to the catheterization laboratory where coronary angiography revealed acute occlusion of the proximal LAD (Figure 9-3, *A*). He underwent PCI of the LAD with a bare metal stent with restoration of TIMI 3 flow though the LAD was small and diffusely diseased distally. Echocardiography revealed severe LV dysfunction with LV apical clot. He underwent rest Tc-99m sestamibi SPECT that showed a large scar in the LAD territory (Figure 9-3, *B*, and Video 9-1) with severely depressed LVEF and apical aneurysm. ECG shows persistent anterior ST elevation and anterior scar (Figure 9-3, *C*).

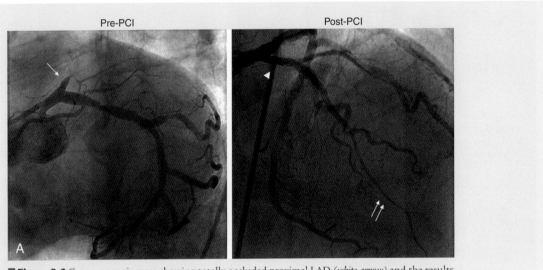

Pre-PCI   Post-PCI

■ **Figure 9-3** Coronary angiogram showing totally occluded proximal LAD *(white arrow)* and the results after PCI *(white arrowhead)*. Note the diffuse disease in the small distal LAD *(double white arrows)* **(A)**.

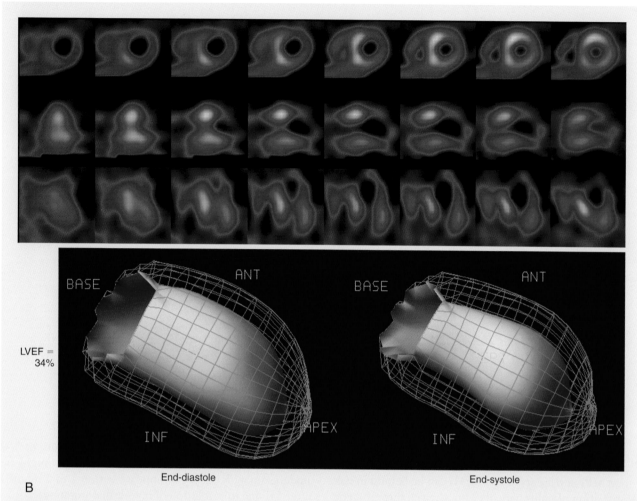

B

End-diastole

End-systole

■**Figure 9-3—Cont'd** Rest SPECT images showing a large LAD scar with LV apical aneurysm, also seen on the 3D images and the video (**B,** and Video 9-1).

(Continued)

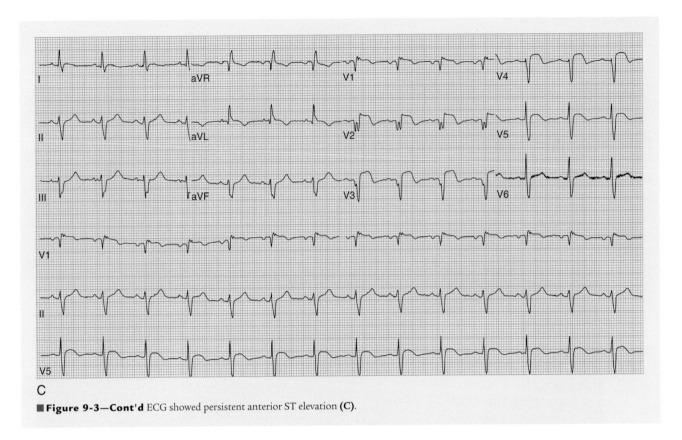

■ **Figure 9-3—Cont'd** ECG showed persistent anterior ST elevation (**C**).

COMMENTS (Cases 9-2 and 9-3)

Stress MPI in patients with STEMI can be helpful in risk stratification of stable patients who received thrombolytic therapy or who were treated conservatively. Stress MPI can provide information regarding infarct size, LVEF, LV volumes, remodeling, and residual myocardial ischemia; all of which have been shown to be predictive of outcomes.

In one study of 618 patients who were randomized to thrombolysis with streptokinase or conventional treatment, patients who had an infarct size of >20% had a significantly higher long-term mortality compared to those who had small (<10%) or moderate (10% to 20%) sized infarcts. In another study, 274 patients presenting with acute MI underwent SPECT imaging on arrival to the hospital. Patients with an infarct size of >12% of the LV had a 2-year mortality rate of 7% compared to 0% in those who presented with an infarct size of <12% of the LV.

LVEF remains one of the most important predictors of survival post-MI. In one study of 866 patients with acute MI who underwent radionuclide imaging before discharge, univariate analyses showed an exponential increase in 1-year cardiac mortality as LVEF decreased to <40%. The 1-year mortality rate was 10% in those with an LVEF of 20% to 39% and approached 50% in those with an LVEF <20%. Other studies also showed significantly higher mortality rates with an LVEF of 35% to 40%. An LVEF of 40% to 50% carries a 1-year mortality of 1% to 2%. The LVEF determined early after MI might be underestimated, but it can improve within 1 to 2 months after MI due to resolution of myocardial stunning.

LV volumes post-MI have also been also shown to affect survival, especially when the LVEF is <50%. Survival decreased significantly as the end-systolic volume increased to >95 ml and to >130 ml.

The positive predictive accuracy of exercise MPI, dipyridamole MPI, and adenosine MPI for prediction of long-term cardiac events from pooled studies (death, MI, and UA) was 37%, 30%, and 50%, respectively, and the negative predictive values were 93%, 94%, and 97%, respectively. In a study of patients who had an acute MI and who underwent submaximal exercise MPI without revascularization, the 1-year cardiac event rate was 7% in patients without ischemia compared to 19% in those who had an ischemic defect. The event rate increased from 12% in those with one or two ischemic defects to 38% in those with three or more ischemic defects. Similar results have been observed with vasodilator MPI.

In a study of adenosine MPI that was performed in stable patients after acute MI without revascularization, cardiac events occurred in 33% of patients over a 15.7-month period; ischemic defect size and LVEF were predictors of outcome by multivariate analysis. In another study, 126 stable patients underwent adenosine MPI at a mean of 4.5 ± 2.9 days after acute MI. Patients were divided into three risk groups: low risk (<20% perfusion defect), intermediate risk (≥ 20% perfusion defect with <10% ischemia), and high risk (≥20% perfusion defect with > 10% ischemia). The cardiac event rates at 1 year were 19%, 28%, and 78%, respectively. Significant multivariate predictors for events were female gender (relative risk [RR] = 2.90), LVEF (RR = 1.34), and ischemic defect size (RR = 1.46). These results were further confirmed in the prospective multicenter INSPIRE trial that enrolled 728 stable survivors of acute MI, who underwent adenosine MPI within 10 days of MI. Total cardiac events and death/reinfarction occurred in 5.4% and 1.8% of the low-risk group, in 14% and 9.2% of the intermediate-risk group, and in 18.6% and 11.6% of the high-risk group. Each 10% absolute increment in total or ischemic defect size increased the unadjusted RR for any event by 37% and 64%, respectively. LVEF also was predictive of cardiac events and of death/reinfarction. An LVEF >50% predicted a 1-year event rate of 5% that increased to 27% with an LVEF <20%. Stepwise logistic regression showed that the total perfusion defect size was the most important independent risk factor for cardiac events, followed by ischemic defect size, followed by LVEF. The total perfusion defect size was the only significant predictor of death or reinfarction.

Case 9-4   Imaging in a Patient With Multivessel CAD (Figure 9-4)

A 42-year-old African-American woman with ESRD, DM, dyslipidemia, HTN, severe LV dysfunction, and coronary artery disease with prior PCI of the RCA presented with worsening shortness of breath. Her physical examination and chest radiograph were suggestive of HF. The cardiac markers were mildly elevated. She underwent regadenoson MPI that showed ischemia in the lateral wall with an LVEF of 35% (Figure 9-4, *A*). Coronary angiography showed a patent mid-RCA stent with severe stenosis of a small posterolateral branch, moderate LCX, and first marginal disease (Figure 9-4, *B*) and severe stenosis of a first diagonal (Figure 9-4, *C*). Evaluation of the LCX and first marginal with a pressure wire revealed a fractional flow reserve of 0.86. The LCX was left alone, and PCI of the first diagonal with a bare metal stent was performed (Figure 9-4, *C*).

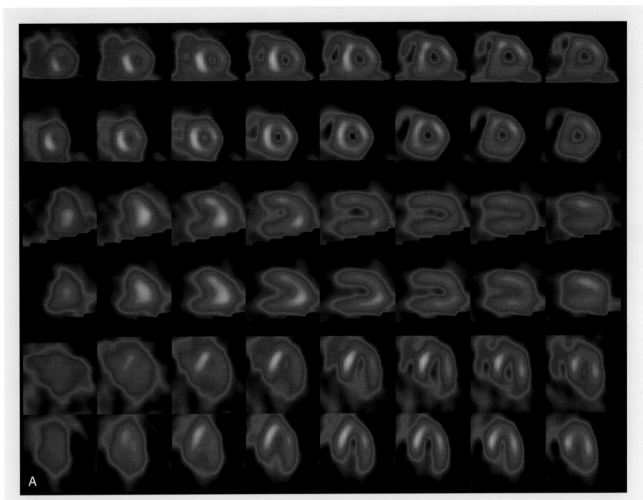

■ **Figure 9-4** Regadenoson MPI showing ischemia in the lateral wall **(A)**.

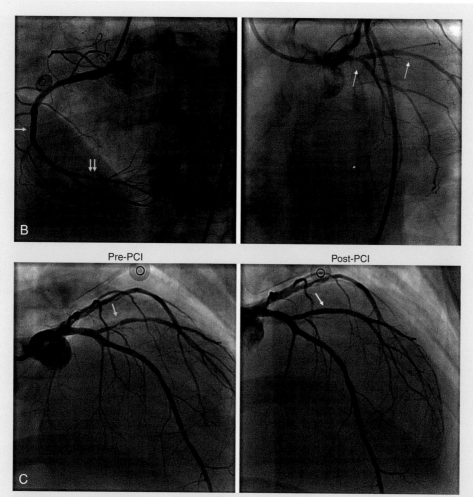

Pre-PCI   Post-PCI

■ **Figure 9-4—Cont'd** Coronary angiogram showed a patent mid-RCA stent *(yellow arrow)*, severe stenosis of a small posterolateral branch *(double yellow arrows)*, and moderate LCX and first obtuse marginal disease *(white arrows)* **(B)**. **C,** Severe first diagonal disease *(yellow arrow)*. The diagonal after PCI with a bare metal stent is also shown *(white arrow)*.

Case 9-5   **Ischemia Due to Side Branch Disease After CABG (Figure 9-5)**

A 74-year-old white man with HTN, dyslipidemia, DM, cerebrovascular disease, ischemic cardiomyopathy, and history of multivessel disease with prior CABG and multiple PCIs 4 years earlier (LCX, marginal branches, and distal LAD via left internal mammary artery graft) presented with atypical chest pain a few months following his most recent PCI. He underwent exercise MPI for further evaluation. He walked on the treadmill for 9 minutes 30 seconds with no ECG changes. The SPECT images showed a small area of ischemia in a diagonal distribution with an LVEF of 71% and normal wall motion (Figure 9-5). He was continued on medical therapy.

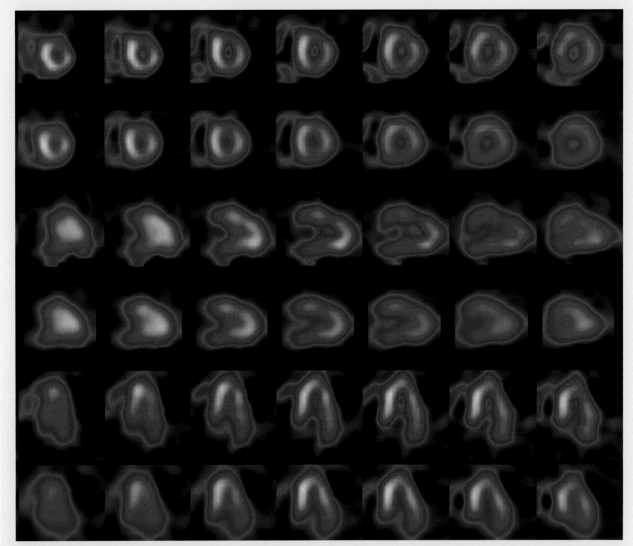

■**Figure 9-5** Exercise SPECT showing a small area of ischemia in the distribution of a diagonal branch of the LAD involving the anterolateral region of the LV myocardium.

COMMENTS (Cases 9-4 and 9-5)

Stress MPI can be used for evaluation and risk stratification in patients presenting with UA or NSTEMI who are initially treated with a noninvasive strategy. The INSPIRE trial enrolled 728 stable patients with acute MI (40% NSTEMI). All patients were initially assigned to a conservative strategy. Patients with low risk (perfusion defect size <10%) and intermediate risk (perfusion defect size <20% and ischemic defect size <10%) were treated medically. Patients with high risk (perfusion defect size ≥20% and ischemia defect size >10%) and LVEF <35% underwent coronary angiography with the intent to revascularize. Patients at high risk and with an LVEF >35% were randomized to optimal medical management versus revascularization with optimal medical management. The 1-year death or reinfarction rate was 1.8% in the low-risk group independent of the clinical risk. There

was no difference in the cardiac event rates in low- and intermediate-risk patients who subsequently underwent revascularization. However, the cardiac event rate in the high-risk patients who underwent revascularization was 10% compared to 32% in those who did not undergo revascularization. The results of this study confirm that revascularization will not improve outcomes if there is a small-sized residual ischemic region.

In patients with known CAD, as in Case 9-5, stress MPI can be used for evaluation of recurrent symptoms. The annual cardiac event rate increases with the extent of perfusion abnormalities and ranges from 0.6%/year with normal scans to 8.5%/year with high-risk scans among all patients studied. In patients with known CAD, the 1-year cardiac event rate approaches 2% in those with low-risk scans and 12% in those with high-risk scans. The event rates were significantly reduced in patients with moderately to severely abnormal MPI studies with revascularization compared to optimal medical management, though there was no significant difference in event rates in those with normal or mildly abnormal MPI studies who were treated medically or with revascularization.

SELECTED READINGS

Risk stratification and survival after myocardial infarction, *N Engl J Med* 309:331–336, 1983.

Anderson JL, Adams CD, Antman EM, et al: ACC/AHA 2007 guidelines for the management of patients with unstable angina/non-ST-Elevation myocardial infarction: a report of the American College of Cardiology/American Heart Association Task Force on Practice Guidelines (Writing Committee to Revise the 2002 Guidelines for the Management of Patients With Unstable Angina/Non-ST-Elevation Myocardial Infarction) developed in collaboration with the American College of Emergency Physicians, the Society for Cardiovascular Angiography and Interventions, and the Society of Thoracic Surgeons endorsed by the American Association of Cardiovascular and Pulmonary Rehabilitation, and the Society for Academic Emergency Medicine, *J Am Coll Cardiol* 50:e1–e157, 2007.

Bilodeau L, Théroux P, Grégoire J, et al: Technetium-99m sestamibi tomography in patients with spontaneous chest pain: correlations with clinical, electrocardiographic and angiographic findings, *J Am Coll Cardiol* 18:1684–1691, 1991.

Cerqueira MD, Maynard C, Ritchie JL, et al: Long-term survival in 618 patients from the Western Washington Streptokinase in Myocardial Infarction trials, *J Am Coll Cardiol* 20:1452–1459, 1992.

Dakik HA, Wendt JA, Kimball K, et al: Prognostic value of adenosine Tl-201 myocardial perfusion imaging after acute myocardial infarction: results of a prospective clinical trial, *J Nucl Cardiol* 12:276–283, 2005.

Hendel RC, Berman DS, Di Carli MF, et al: ACCF/ASNC/ACR/AHA/ASE/SCCT/SCMR/SNM 2009 Appropriate Use Criteria for Cardiac Radionuclide Imaging: A Report of the American College of Cardiology Foundation Appropriate Use Criteria Task Force, the American Society of Nuclear Cardiology, the American College of Radiology, the American Heart Association, the American Society of Echocardiography, the Society of Cardiovascular Computed Tomography, the Society for Cardiovascular Magnetic Resonance, and the Society of Nuclear Medicine, *J Am Coll Cardiol* 53:2201–2229, 2009.

Iskandrian A, Garcia E, editors: *Nuclear Cardiac Imaging: Principles and Applications*, ed 4, New York, 2008, Oxford University Press.

Kontos MC, Jesse RL, Schmidt KL, et al: Value of acute rest sestamibi perfusion imaging for evaluation of patients admitted to the emergency department with chest pain, *J Am Coll Cardiol* 30:976–982, 1997.

Kushner FG, Hand M, Smith SC, et al: 2009 focused updates: ACC/AHA guidelines for the management of patients with ST-elevation myocardial infarction (updating the 2004 guideline and 2007 focused update) and ACC/AHA/SCAI guidelines on percutaneous coronary intervention (updating the 2005 guideline and 2007 focused update) a report of the American College of Cardiology Foundation/American Heart Association Task Force on Practice Guidelines, *J Am Coll Cardiol* 54:2205–2241, 2009.

Lloyd-Jones D, Adams RJ, Brown TM, et al: Executive summary: heart disease and stroke statistics–2010 update: a report from the American Heart Association, *Circulation* 121:948–954, 2010.

Mahmarian JJ, Dakik HA, Filipchuk NG, et al: An initial strategy of intensive medical therapy is comparable to that of coronary revascularization for suppression of scintigraphic ischemia in high-risk but stable survivors of acute myocardial infarction, *J Am Coll Cardiol* 48:2458–2467, 2006.

Mahmarian JJ, Mahmarian AC, Marks GF, et al: Role of adenosine thallium-201 tomography for defining long-term risk in patients after acute myocardial infarction, *J Am Coll Cardiol* 25:1333–1340, 1995.

Mahmarian JJ, Shaw LJ, Filipchuk NG, et al: A multinational study to establish the value of early adenosine technetium-99m sestamibi myocardial perfusion imaging in identifying a low-risk group for early hospital discharge after acute myocardial infarction, *J Am Coll Cardiol* 48:2448–2457, 2006.

Miller TD, Christian TF, Hopfenspirger MR, et al: Infarct size after acute myocardial infarction measured by quantitative tomographic 99mTc sestamibi imaging predicts subsequent mortality, *Circulation* 92:334–341, 1995.

Schaeffer MW, Brennan TD, Hughes JA, et al: Resting radionuclide myocardial perfusion imaging in a chest pain center including an overnight delayed image acquisition protocol, *J Nucl Med Technol* 35:242–245, 2007.

Travin MI, Dessouki A, Cameron T, et al: Use of exercise technetium-99m sestamibi SPECT imaging to detect residual ischemia and for risk stratification after acute myocardial infarction, *Am J Cardiol* 75:665–669, 1995.

Chapter 10

Risk Stratification Prior to Noncardiac Surgery

Fadi G. Hage, Fahad M. Iqbal, and Ami E. Iskandrian

KEY POINTS

- Cardiac risk in patients undergoing noncardiac surgery is a reflection of patient-related risk factors and risk inherent to the surgical procedure.

- Interventions are rarely indicated to simply lower perioperative risk unless such interventions are needed irrespective of the upcoming surgery.

- Perioperative cardiac assessment often presents the opportunity for the modification of long-term cardiac outcomes that are unrelated to the planned surgical intervention.

- Patients with acute coronary syndromes, decompensated heart failure, significant arrhythmias, and severe valvular heart disease should be managed for their cardiac condition according to current guidelines with a delay or cancellation of the planned surgery until their cardiac status is stabilized.

- The perioperative risk increases in proportion to the number of clinical risk factors that a patient has, including ischemic heart disease, compensated heart failure, cerebrovascular disease, DM, and CKD.

- MPI can be used for risk stratification in order to guide decision-making in patients undergoing intermediate- or high-risk surgeries who have clinical risk factors.

- A stress MPI showing normal LV perfusion and function predicts low cardiac risk in patients undergoing high-risk vascular surgery.

- Patients with ESRD who are at high cardiovascular risk should undergo stress testing prior to renal transplantation. Perfusion abnormalities are associated with higher risk for adverse outcomes but the value of coronary revascularization in this population is not well-defined.

- Abnormal LVEF is a strong predictor of mortality in ESRD patients awaiting renal transplantation, although it may improve after transplantation.

- A normal stress MPI predicts a benign outcome in patients with end-stage liver disease undergoing orthotopic liver transplantation and who are at high risk of cardiovascular complications.

BACKGROUND

The risk of perioperative cardiac events, including MI, heart failure, serious arrhythmias, or death, in patients undergoing noncardiac surgery depends on multiple factors. Careful clinical evaluation may help patient triage, such as to proceed forward with the planned surgery, to cancel the surgical procedure, have it replaced by a less risky procedure, or to have additional tests to assess risk or procedures to modify the risk. The evaluation often presents the opportunity for the assessment and modification of long-term cardiac outcomes that are unrelated to the planned surgical intervention.

The updated American College of Cardiology/American Heart Association Guidelines provide a much-needed evidence-based framework for the assessment of cardiac risk in patients undergoing noncardiac surgery and for decision making in these patients. These guidelines have undergone significant modifications over the years in light of emerging new information. The underlying premise of the guidelines is that the perioperative risk is a reflection of three factors: patient-related risk factors, functional capacity, and the risk inherent to the surgical procedure (assuming the surgical skill and perioperative care are excellent). It is important to note that the guidelines emphasize at the outset that coronary interventions are rarely indicated to simply lower perioperative risk unless such interventions are needed irrespective of the planned surgery.

With respect to patient-related risk factors, active cardiac conditions that indicate major clinical risk mandate intensive management and may result in delay or cancellation of surgery unless the surgery itself is emergent. These include acute coronary syndromes (including recent MI <1 month before planned surgery), decompensated heart failure, serious arrhythmias, and severe valvular heart disease (including severe aortic and mitral stenoses). For all other patients, risk is assessed based on the Revised Cardiac Risk Index, which consists of five high-risk factors: ischemic heart disease, compensated heart failure, cerebrovascular disease, DM, and CKD (serum creatinine ≥2 mg/dL). The perioperative risk increases in proportion to the number of high-risk factors in a given patient. The functional capacity of the patient is a good overall measure of patient-related risk and can be readily determined using a treadmill stress test or, more commonly, estimated by what daily tasks the patient can perform. As a general rule, 4 METs (metabolic equivalent) correspond to walking 4 blocks on level ground or walking up one or two flights of stairs.

Regarding the risk that is inherent to the surgical procedure, the guidelines group surgical procedures into three categories: vascular surgery is considered the highest-risk category, intermediate-risk procedures include intraperitoneal and intrathoracic, head and neck, orthopedic, and prostate procedures. Carotid endarterectomy is also considered an intermediate-risk procedure. Low-risk procedures include superficial, ambulatory, cataract, breast, and endoscopic surgeries.

The first step of the evaluation is to determine the urgency of the surgical procedure. If the surgery is emergent, it should proceed without wasting time on further evaluation. Perioperative medical management and surveillance may be appropriate, while risk stratification can be delayed to the postoperative period, where it can be helpful for improving long-term prognosis. The perioperative risk associated with low-risk procedures is low even in high-risk patients. Therefore, patients should proceed with low-risk procedures irrespective of other considerations unless they have active cardiac conditions that require immediate attention, as detailed earlier.

Patients who are to undergo intermediate- or high-risk surgical procedures and have a good functional capacity with no symptoms (>4 METs) can also proceed with the planned procedure. The decision-making process is more complicated in patients with low functional capacity and in those with unknown functional capacity; these patients probably could proceed with surgery if they have no risk factors based on the Revised Cardiac Risk Index.

In many of the remaining patients, noninvasive testing is often performed. The role of beta-blocker therapy has evolved over time, including timing on when to start therapy, flexible dosing based on heart rate and blood pressure response, and the risk profile of patients. In general, such therapy is better started weeks before, rather than the day before, the planned surgery and is most beneficial in patients with high perioperative risk.

Stress MPI can identify low-risk patients who can proceed with surgery and a high-risk group that requires intensive medical therapy, coronary angiography, or coronary revascularization.

In this chapter, we will demonstrate the value of MPI in the assessment of perioperative risk in particular patients undergoing noncardiac surgery. We will stress the prognostic information that can be gained and how it can be used to influence the decision-making process.

| Case 10-1 | Stress Testing Before Vascular Surgery in a Diabetic Patient (Figure 10-1) |

A 60-year-old man with hyperlipidemia, DM, and CKD presented with progressive lower extremity claudication. Evaluation confirmed the presence of severe right iliac artery stenosis and moderate left iliac disease. He was started on aspirin and a statin and plans were made for revascularization. Preoperative evaluation included regadenoson MPI, which showed a large ischemic area in the distribution of the LCX and RCA (Figure 10-1, *A, B*). The LVEF was preserved. Coronary angiography revealed complete occlusion of the second obtuse marginal (OM2) branch of the LCX and severe stenosis of the distal RCA. The occluded OM2 filled retrograde via collaterals from the LAD (Figure 10-1, *C*). The patient was treated with medical therapy for CAD, including a beta-blocker and risk factor modifications. He underwent peripheral vascular revascularization with no complications.

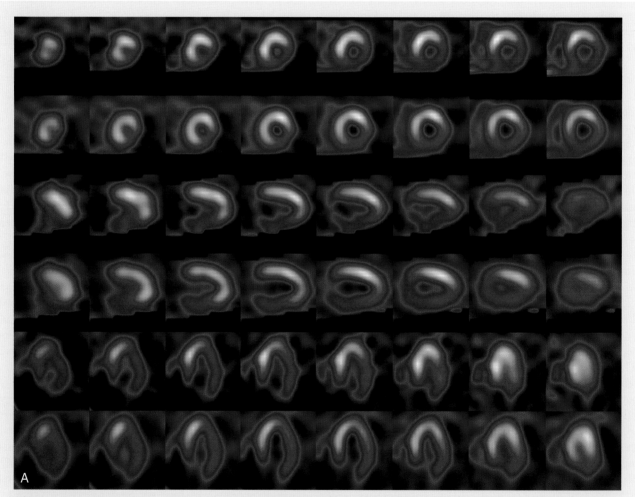

■ **Figure 10-1 A** and **B,** Regadenoson MPI and polar maps showing a large partially reversible perfusion abnormality in the RCA and LCX territories. The LVEF is 69%.

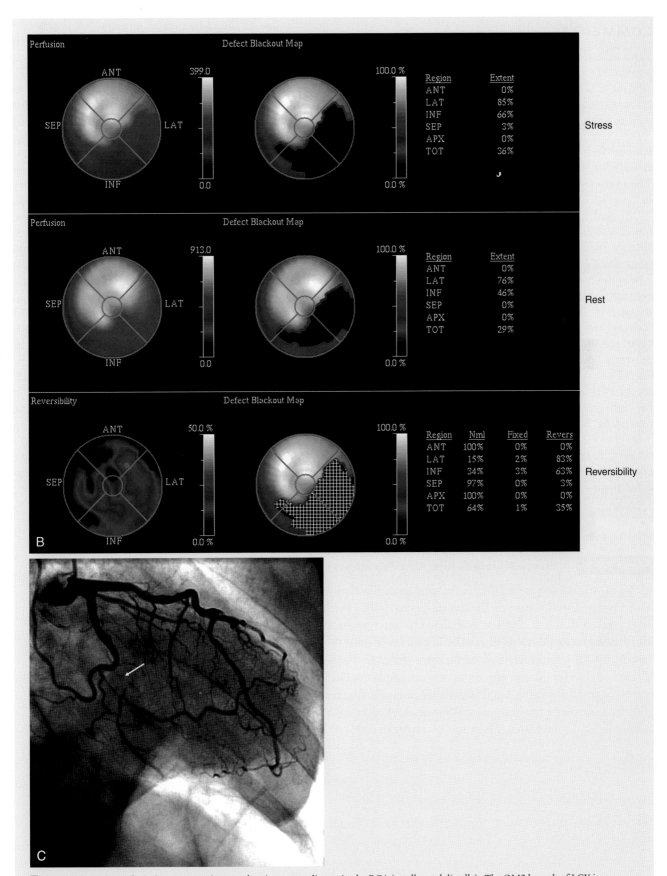

■ **Figure 10-1—Cont'd. C,** Coronary angiogram showing severe disease in the RCA (small vessel distally). The OM2 branch of LCX is occluded *(arrow)* and fills via collaterals from the LAD. There is only mild disease in the LAD and its branches.

COMMENTS

Since atherosclerosis is a systemic disease, patients with peripheral vascular disease are at high risk of having significant CAD. Risk stratification with stress MPI is indicated in patients undergoing vascular surgery who have a poor or unknown functional capacity and have at least one clinical risk factor from the Revised Cardiac Risk Index. Patients with normal MPI, and those with small areas of abnormality (ischemia or scar), are considered low risk. The presence of a large area of abnormality is indicative of high risk of perioperative cardiac events.

Medical management of CAD in patients who are found to be at high risk is reasonable. Patients who are already receiving beta-blockers and/or statin medications should be continued on these medications (class I recommendation). For patients undergoing vascular surgery and not on a statin, it is reasonable to start such therapy in the perioperative period (class IIa). Beta-blockers can also be started in patients undergoing vascular surgery who are at high cardiac risk due to the presence of CAD, myocardial ischemia on stress testing, or one or more clinical risk factors (class IIa). In the recent POISE trial that randomized 8351 intermediate- to high-risk patients undergoing noncardiac surgery (including vascular surgery) to placebo or fixed-dose metoprolol 2 to 4 hours before surgery and 6 hours after surgery, fewer patients in the metoprolol arm experienced the primary endpoint (a composite of cardiovascular death, nonfatal MI, and nonfatal cardiac arrest)

mostly due to the reduction of nonfatal MI (3.6% versus 5.1%, $p = .0008$). The potential dangers of such an approach were highlighted by the higher risk of death in the metoprolol group (3.1% versus 2.3%, $p = .03$). It is, therefore, better to start beta-blocker therapy in advance of the planned surgery and titrate the dose for the particular patient rather than to initiate this therapy a few hours ahead of surgery and at a fixed dose.

The indications for perioperative coronary revascularization are generally consistent with those for the general population with CAD. In this regard, coronary revascularization aims to improve long-term prognosis rather than to solely decrease the risk of perioperative cardiac events. Multiple randomized studies have, therefore, failed to show an advantage of prophylactic coronary revascularization in the perioperative period. In the CARP study, coronary revascularization did not decrease long-term mortality (2.7 years after randomization) in patients at increased risk for cardiac complications who were undergoing vascular surgery. In the DECREASE V study, prophylactic coronary revascularization in high-risk cardiac patients with extensive stress-induced ischemia undergoing major vascular surgery did not provide a survival advantage after 2.8 years of follow-up.

In our patient, the OM branch was collateralized and occluded and the RCA disease was distal. Therefore, no coronary intervention was deemed necessary. The message here is that not all patients with abnormal MPI require coronary angiography and not all patients who have coronary angiography require coronary revascularization.

Case 10-2   **Stress Testing Before Aortic Aneurysm Repair (Figure 10-2)**

A 76-year-old woman with DM, paroxysmal atrial fibrillation, and CKD presented with a progressively enlarging thoracoabdominal aortic aneurysm measuring 6.6 cm at its greatest diameter. She was considered for operative aortic aneurysm repair. Her functional capacity was limited by degenerative joint disease. She underwent vasodilator MPI, which showed normal myocardial perfusion and normal LVEF (Figure 10-2). Her postoperative course was complicated by gastrointestinal bleeding and atrial fibrillation with rapid ventricular response. She received blood transfusions and rate controlling medications and was discharged from the hospital for physical rehabilitation 10 days later. There was no evidence of MI or heart failure.

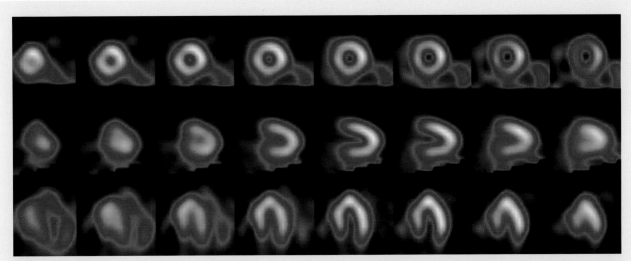

■ **Figure 10-2** Regadenoson stress-only MPI images showing a normal myocardial perfusion pattern. Rest imaging was not performed. The LVEF measured 68%.

COMMENTS

In the meta-analysis by Shaw et al. (10 studies, 1,994 vascular surgery candidates), 40% of patients had ischemia, 24% had scar, and 36% had normal perfusion on MPI. The corresponding rates for cardiac death or MI were 9%, 7%, and 1%, respectively. In a more recent review of vascular surgery trials by Dahlberg and Leppo, 42% of patients had ischemia on MPI. The positive predictive value for perioperative cardiac events (death or MI) was 12%, a normal perfusion was present in 38% of patients, and the negative predictive accuracy was 99%.

Case 10-3   **Stress Testing Before Vascular Surgery in a Patient With Prior CABG (Figure 10-3)**

A 71-year-old man with known peripheral vascular disease presented with bilateral lower extremity pain. The pain was initially related to exertion but is now occurring at rest and has progressively worsened over the past 4 weeks. He has a history of prior peripheral vascular surgery and had presented 5 weeks earlier with graft thrombosis, which was managed with fibrinolytic therapy. Evaluation included computed tomography angiography, which showed complete occlusion of the graft extending from the right common femoral artery to the right popliteal artery and of the two grafts arising from the left common femoral artery to the left superficial femoral and popliteal arteries. The patient is known to have CAD (treated with CABG 13 years earlier), DM, hypertension, hyperlipidemia, and paroxysmal atrial fibrillation. He underwent adenosine MPI for risk stratification. The stress images (Figure 10-3, *A, top*) showed partially reversible perfusion defects in the anterior and lateral segments of the myocardium. Coronary angiography showed severe disease in the native coronary arteries with an occluded graft to OM branch (Figure 10-3, *B*). The coronary anatomy was not amenable to coronary intervention or repeat CABG. He underwent high-risk peripheral revascularization after optimization of medical therapy. He tolerated the surgery well and had no perioperative complications.

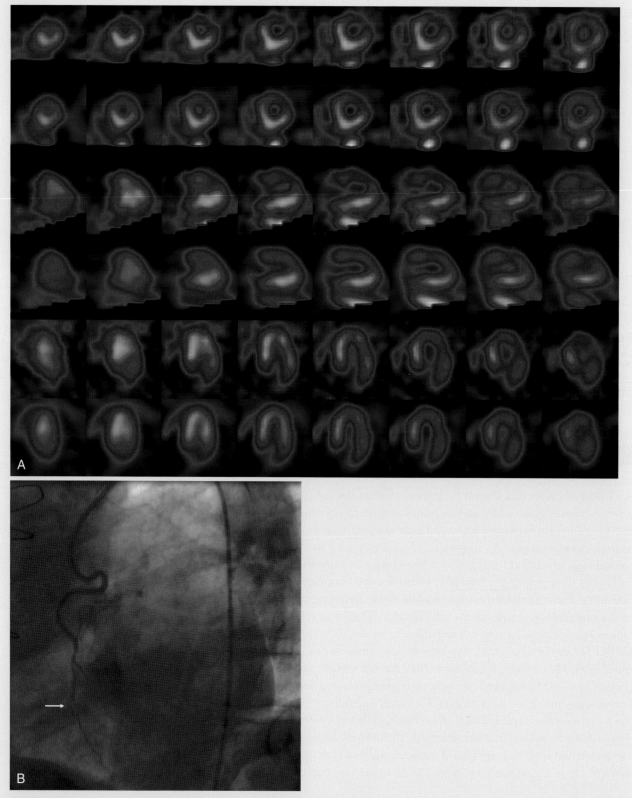

■ **Figure 10-3** Regadenoson MPI showing partially reversible perfusion abnormalities in LAD and LCX territories **(A)**. The LVEF was decreased. Coronary angiography showed severe 3-vessel CAD. The LIMA to LAD graft is patent but there is severe disease in the LAD distal to the LIMA anastomosis, explaining the LAD ischemia seen on the MPI. The vein graft to the RCA is patent with moderate disease distal to the anastomosis *(arrow)*. The vein graft to the OM is occluded **(B)**.

COMMENTS

This patient with a large perfusion abnormality and depressed LVEF is at high perioperative cardiac risk. The clinical condition warranted an emergency revascularization procedure to prevent lower extremity gangrene. Thus, in some patients, the risk-benefit ratio favors proceeding with planned vascular surgery, despite the known risk.

Case 10-4   **Stress Testing Before Renal Transplantation (Figure 10-4)**

A 56-year-old man with ESRD secondary to hypertension who was also known to have DM, hyperlipidemia, and CAD underwent evaluation for renal transplantation. Adenosine MPI showed ischemia in all three vascular territories with transient ischemic dilation (Figure 10-4, *A*). The patient underwent coronary angiography, showing severe three-vessel CAD. He underwent CABG with complete revascularization prior to renal transplantation. He had no complication during his deceased-donor renal transplantation or on long-term follow-up.

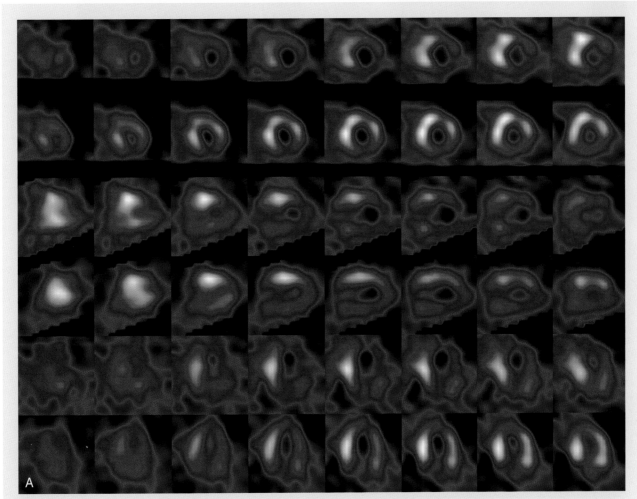

■ **Figure 10-4** Adenosine/rest MPI and polar maps showing a large perfusion abnormality in the distribution of the three major vessels **(A, B)**.

(Continued)

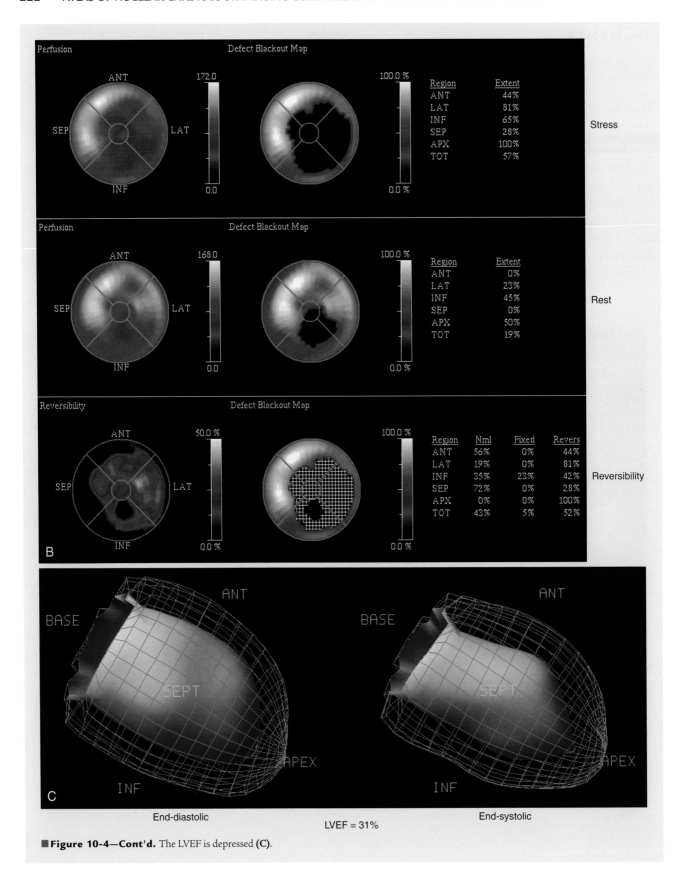

■**Figure 10-4—Cont'd.** The LVEF is depressed **(C)**.

COMMENTS

Patients with ESRD undergo rigorous assessment of perioperative risk prior to renal transplantation. CKD, and especially ESRD, is associated with an increased risk of cardiovascular morbidity and mortality; cardiovascular disease accounts for almost one-half of all deaths in patients with ESRD. Thus, screening for CAD prior to renal transplantation is appropriate in all ESRD candidates who are more than 50 years old, and in younger patients who have DM or other clinical risk factors for CAD. These patients undergo stress testing with imaging to evaluate for the presence of CAD and to gauge the perioperative and long-term risk. Unfortunately, there are little data on whether coronary revascularization in asymptomatic patients improves outcome. We studied 3698 ESRD patients who were evaluated for possible renal transplantation at our institution, of whom 60% underwent stress MPI per the above guidelines. One of every five patients who underwent MPI had abnormal perfusion (5% scar, 15% ischemia). The presence of a perfusion abnormality in this study was a strong predictor of mortality on long-term follow-up. In patients who underwent MPI and coronary angiography, MPI provided more powerful prognostic data than coronary angiography. In our retrospective analysis, coronary revascularization did not impact survival except in patients with three-vessel CAD with no prior bypass surgery. Clearly, this area requires more randomized controlled trials in order to establish evidence-based guidelines for interventions, but patients with high-risk scans (similar to the patient presented here) will likely benefit from coronary angiography and revascularization prior to transplantation since their perioperative risk is substantial. Another important consideration is that the current waiting time for deceased nonrelated renal transplantation after being placed on the transplant list is measured in years rather than months due to the shortage of organs. These patients should therefore receive treatments that improve long-term prognosis irrespective of their transplantation status.

Case 10-5   **Decision-making for a Patient With Severe LV Dysfunction Before Renal Re-transplantation (Figure 10-5)**

A 45-year-old man with ESRD secondary to Goodpasture's syndrome and malignant hypertension underwent a living-related donor kidney transplant from his father 15 years ago but had rejection several years later and is now presenting for evaluation for re-transplantation. He underwent regadenoson MPI, which showed normal myocardial perfusion but severely depressed LVEF (Figure 10-5, *A, B*). Transthoracic echocardiography showed depressed LV and RV functions with diffuse hypokinesis and moderate to severe mitral and tricuspid regurgitation with evidence of pulmonary hypertension (Figure 10-5, *C*). He was managed with heart failure treatment, including strict blood pressure control utilizing a beta-blocker and angiotensin-converting enzyme inhibitor and more stringent hemodialysis to remove fluid overload. Subsequent right-heart catheterization with invasive hemodynamic measurements revealed normal LV filling pressure, mild reduction in cardiac output, and much improved pulmonary artery pressure. He subsequently underwent renal transplantation with no complications. The LVEF improved 4 months after the procedure.

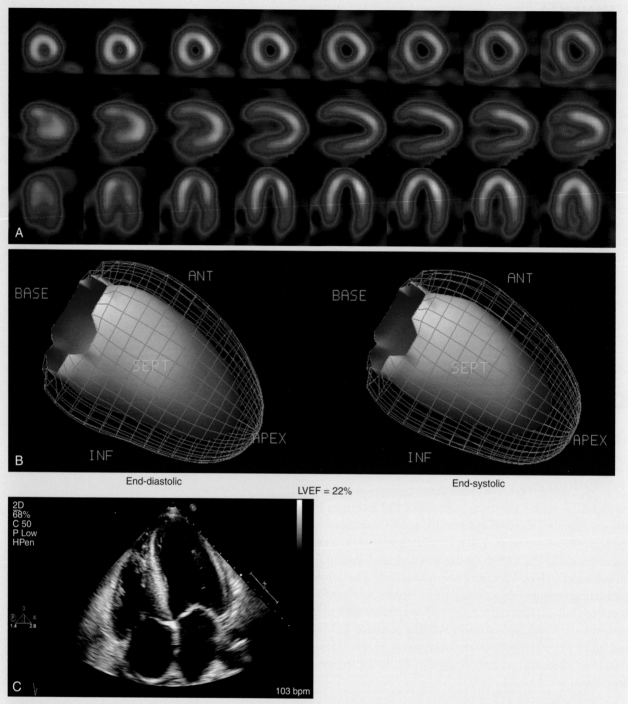

■ **Figure 10-5** Regadenoson only MPI showing a normal myocardial perfusion pattern with dilated LV cavity **(A)**. The LVEF is severely depressed **(B)**. Transthoracic echocardiogram showing depressed biventricular systolic function with EF of 25% and diffuse hypokinesis. **C,** Doppler ultrasound showed an estimated pulmonary artery systolic pressure of 63 mm Hg. Right heart catheterization done after optimizing the treatment of heart failure showed right atrial pressure of 8 mm Hg, pulmonary capillary artery pressure of 10 mm Hg, cardiac index of 2.24 L/min/m², and pulmonary artery pressure of 41/14 mm Hg.

COMMENTS

Although almost one-half of mortality in ESRD is cardiovascular related, more than 60% of this cardiovascular mortality (26% of all-cause mortality) is related to sudden cardiac death. It is unclear what the contribution of CAD is to sudden death in ESRD. Some have suggested that most of the sudden death is associated with LV structural changes and autonomic dysfunction, which are unrelated to CAD. In our study of 3698 ESRD patients evaluated for possible renal transplantation, a depressed LVEF was the strongest predictor of mortality on long-term follow-up. After a follow-up of 30 ± 15 months accumulating 622 deaths (17%), there was a stepwise relationship of increased mortality with decreasing LVEF. After adjusting for age, gender, race, abnormal stress MPI, tobacco smoking, LV hypertrophy, DM, obesity, and socioeconomic status, each 1% decrease in the LVEF accounted for a 2.7% increase in mortality. In a separate analysis, a blunted heart rate response to adenosine (a measure of autonomic dysfunction) was a strong and independent predictor of mortality in this population and provided more powerful prognostic information than the presence and severity of CAD by angiography. It is unclear what interventions will improve survival in ESRD patients with depressed LVEF, but current accepted treatments for heart failure provide a reasonable starting point. Renal transplantation itself has been shown to improve LVEF as in our patient and, therefore, patients with depressed LVEF should still be considered for transplantation, despite the elevated perioperative risk.

> **Case 10-6**   **Shortness of Breath in Patient With Prior PCI Requiring Major Surgery (Figure 10-6)**

A 76-year-old man with known CAD with prior coronary stent placements (3 and 5 years ago) and DM was hospitalized for progressively worsening lower back pain that has recently limited his walking. He has a history of fixation and fusion surgery of the lumbosacral spine several years ago. His angina is generally manifested as shortness of breath on exertion. Although he denied any cardiac symptoms, he has had limited physical activity due to back pain, limiting his functional status. Vasodilator MPI showed evidence of ischemia in the distribution of the LCX with normal LVEF (Figure 10-6, *A, B*). He underwent coronary angiography, which revealed severe in-stent stenosis of the proximal dominant LCX, which was treated with another bare metal stent. The patient underwent the planned surgical procedure, including removal of internal fixation hardware and spinal decompression with fixation and fusion 2 months later. He had no cardiac complications.

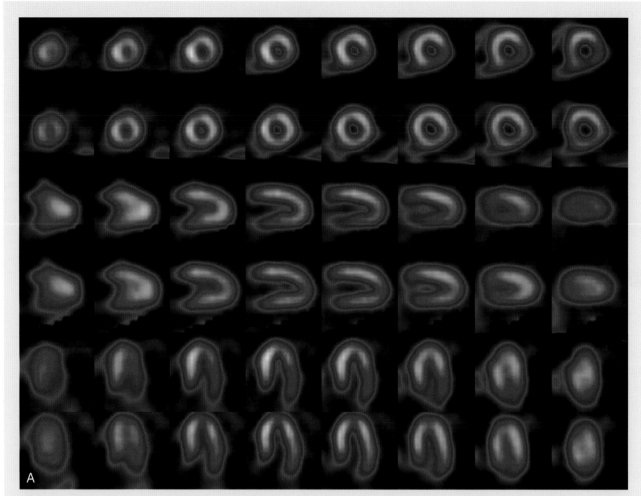

■ **Figure 10-6** Regadenoson/rest MPI showing a reversible perfusion abnormality in the distribution of LCX **(A)**.

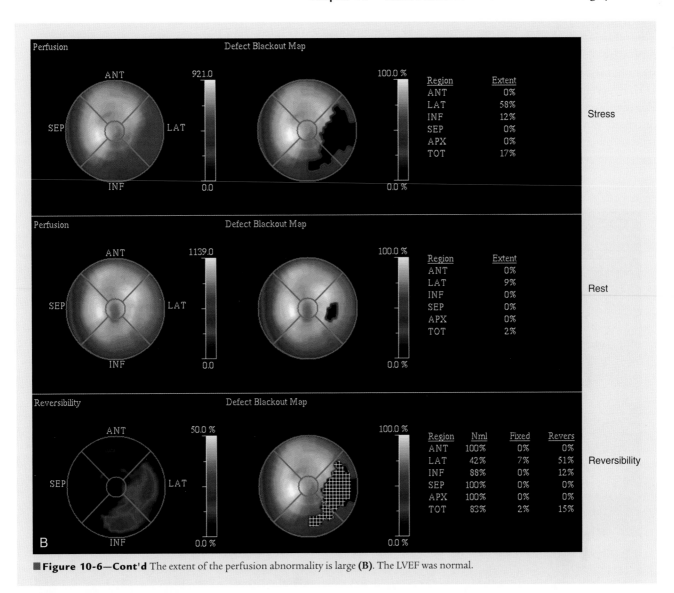

■**Figure 10-6—Cont'd** The extent of the perfusion abnormality is large **(B)**. The LVEF was normal.

COMMENTS

Risk assessment (with MPI) of patients undergoing intermediate-risk surgery who have known risk factors is debatable (class IIb). Nevertheless, most physicians favor risk assessment in such patients. Our patient had two clinical risk factors (known CAD, stents >2 years old, and DM). Further, his angina is not expressed as chest pain. It is reasonable to proceed with coronary angiography and revascularization prior to his back surgery as the perfusion

abnormality was large. Clearly, treatment with a drug-eluting stent in such a scenario is less than ideal due to the risk of stent thrombosis with the discontinuation of dual antiplatelet therapy in the first 6 months (preferably 1 year). In this patient, such a prolonged delay was not an option. Brief discontinuation of clopidogrel (while continuing aspirin) therapy 6 weeks after bare metal PCI is associated with a low risk of complications and is thus considered acceptable. Balloon angioplasty alone would have been another option.

| Case 10-7 | Stress Testing Before Liver Transplantation (Figure 10-7) |

A 60-year-old woman with end-stage liver disease due to advanced nonalcoholic steatohepatitis underwent evaluation for possible liver transplantation. She had DM, hypertension, and hyperlipidemia and was obese, but not known to have CAD. Regadenoson MPI showed evidence of a large area of scar and ischemia in the distribution of the LAD and RCA territories (Figure 10-7, *A*). She was considered a poor candidate for liver transplantation due to extensive vascular calcifications in the mesenteric arteries. Coronary angiography showed three-vessel CAD.

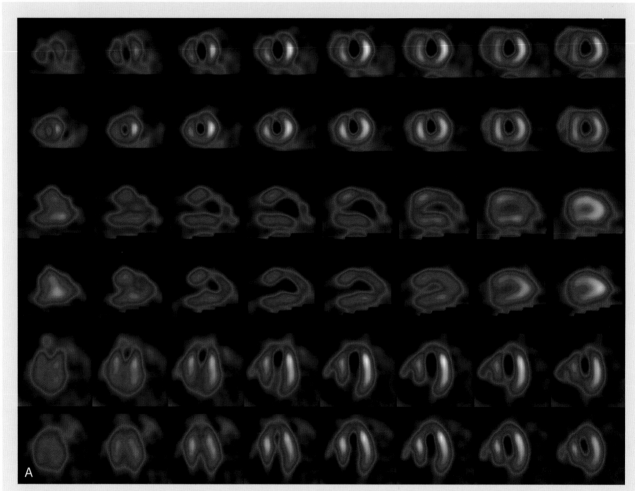

■ **Figure 10-7** Regadenoson/rest MPI showing extensive partially reversible perfusion defects in the LAD and RCA territories **(A)**.

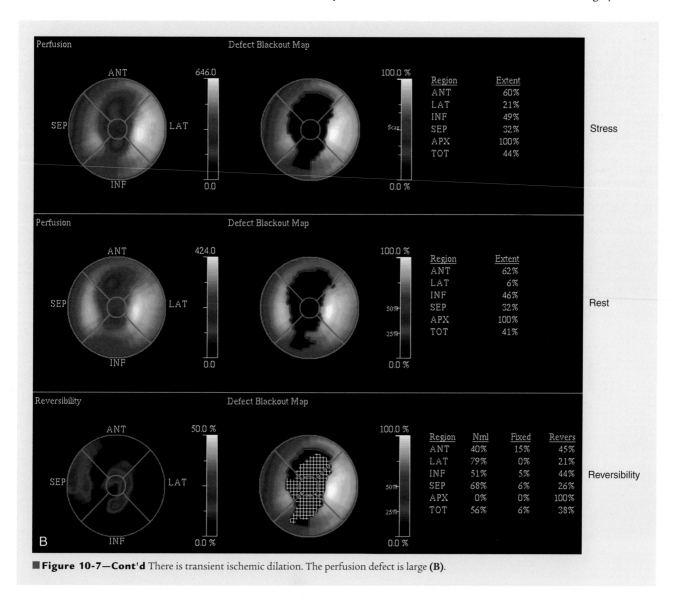

■ **Figure 10-7—Cont'd** There is transient ischemic dilation. The perfusion defect is large **(B)**.

COMMENTS

Patients with end-stage liver disease undergoing orthotopic liver transplantation are at high-risk of cardiovascular complications. Patients with CAD and those with CAD risk factors experience an even higher risk of perioperative complications. There is great interest in better risk stratification in patients awaiting liver transplantation. Unlike renal transplantation, there are no clear guidelines as to who should undergo formal cardiac evaluation, but generally patients older than 45 years of age with CAD risk factors are referred for stress testing. In a recent study that evaluated 30-day outcomes in 403 patients who underwent liver transplants, 7% had myocardial infarctions and 9% died in the perioperative period. A normal stress test was associated with a lower risk of death (odds ratio 0.31, $p = .03$). Another study in 339 patients who underwent liver transplantation (87 patients with preoperative MPI) reported 10% mortality over a mean follow-up of 21 months (3% in the perioperative period), with most deaths being noncardiac. Five

(1%) myocardial infarctions occurred during follow-up, with only one happening in the perioperative period. In this report, a normal MPI study had a 99% negative predictive value for perioperative cardiac events and a 96% negative predictive value for late cardiac events. Thus, survival in these patients seems to depend on occurrence of noncardiac events such as sepsis and rejection. Unlike this patient, most stress MPIs in our experience show normal perfusion, which is likely due to patient selection.

SELECTED READINGS

Becker RC, Scheiman J, Dauerman HL, et al: Management of platelet-directed pharmacotherapy in patients with atherosclerotic coronary artery disease undergoing elective endoscopic gastrointestinal procedures, *J Am Coll Cardiol* 54:2261–2276, 2009.

Devereaux PJ, Yang H, Yusuf S, et al: Effects of extended-release metoprolol succinate in patients undergoing noncardiac surgery (POISE trial): a randomised controlled trial, *Lancet* 371:1839–1847, 2008.

Fleisher LA, Beckman JA, Brown KA, et al: ACC/AHA 2007 Guidelines on Perioperative Cardiovascular Evaluation and Care for Noncardiac Surgery: Executive Summary: A Report of the American College of Cardiology/American Heart Association Task Force on Practice

Guidelines (Writing Committee to Revise the 2002 Guidelines on Perioperative Cardiovascular Evaluation for Noncardiac Surgery) Developed in Collaboration With the American Society of Echocardiography, American Society of Nuclear Cardiology, Heart Rhythm Society, Society of Cardiovascular Anesthesiologists, Society for Cardiovascular Angiography and Interventions, Society for Vascular Medicine and Biology, and Society for Vascular Surgery, *J Am Coll Cardiol* 50:1707–1732, 2007.

Fleisher LA, Beckman JA, Brown KA, et al: 2009 ACCF/AHA focused update on perioperative beta blockade incorporated into the ACC/AHA 2007 guidelines on perioperative cardiovascular evaluation and care for noncardiac surgery, *J Am Coll Cardiol* 54:e13–e118, 2009.

Hage FG, Smalheiser S, Zoghbi GJ, et al: Predictors of survival in patients with end-stage renal disease evaluated for kidney transplantation, *Am J Cardiol* 100:1020–1025, 2007.

Hage FG, Venkataraman R, Zoghbi GJ, et al: The scope of coronary heart disease in patients with chronic kidney disease, *J Am Coll Cardiol* 53:2129–2140, 2009.

Iskandrian A, Garcia E, editors: *Nuclear Cardiac Imaging: Principles and Applications*, ed 4, New York, 2008, Oxford University Press.

Kasiske BL, Cangro CB, Hariharan S, et al: The evaluation of renal transplantation candidates: clinical practice guidelines, *Am J Transplant* 1:3–95, 2001.

McFalls EO, Ward HB, Moritz TE, et al: Coronary-artery revascularization before elective major vascular surgery, *N Engl J Med* 351:2795–2804, 2004.

Poldermans D, Schouten O, Vidakovic R, et al: A clinical randomized trial to evaluate the safety of a noninvasive approach in high-risk patients undergoing major vascular surgery: the DECREASE-V Pilot Study, *J Am Coll Cardiol* 49:1763–1769, 2007.

Safadi A, Homsi M, Maskoun W, et al: Perioperative risk predictors of cardiac outcomes in patients undergoing liver transplantation surgery, *Circulation* 120:1189–1194, 2009.

Shaw LJ, Eagle KA, Gersh BJ, et al: Meta-analysis of intravenous dipyridamole-thallium-201 imaging (1985 to 1994) and dobutamine echocardiography (1991 to 1994) for risk stratification before vascular surgery, *J Am Coll Cardiol* 27:787–798, 1996.

Venkataraman R, Hage FG, Dorfman TA, et al: Relation between heart rate response to adenosine and mortality in patients with end-stage renal disease, *Am J Cardiol* 103:1159–1164, 2009.

Venkataraman R, Hage FG, Dorfman T, et al: Role of myocardial perfusion imaging in patients with end-stage renal disease undergoing coronary angiography, *Am J Cardiol* 102:1451–1456, 2008.

Zoghbi GJ, Patel AD, Ershadi RE, et al: Usefulness of preoperative stress perfusion imaging in predicting prognosis after liver transplantation, *Am J Cardiol* 92:1066–1071, 2003.

Chapter 11

MPI of Special Patient Groups

Fadi G. Hage, Eva V. Dubovsky, and Ami E. Iskandrian

KEY POINTS

- Current guidelines do not recommend routine screening with stress MPI in asymptomatic individuals. Obviously, some exceptions are expected.

- Although patients with DM are considered at high risk for cardiovascular events, there is a spectrum of risk in these patients and MPI is a useful tool for risk stratification in this population. Recent data from prospective studies show that the risk of cardiac events is actually small in asymptomatic but well-treated patients.

- Patients with CKD are also a subgroup at high risk for cardiac events. LV hypertrophy, especially septal hypertrophy, is common and may affect the perfusion pattern by downscaling of the lateral wall.

- Perfusion pattern and LVEF on MPI are powerful predictors of outcome in patients with ESRD being considered for renal transplantation.

- Women have unique characteristics that need to be recognized, such as atypical clinical presentations, small hearts, breast attenuation, a greater need for vasodilator stress testing, smaller coronary vessels, and more microvascular disease. Women with an ischemic ECG response during stress but normal perfusion tend to have a benign course.

- Vasodilator stress testing might be the stress test modality of choice in elderly patients, who are more likely than younger patients to fail to achieve target heart rates during treadmill exercise testing.

- In patients with LBBB, the rest MPI should be normal in the absence of prior myocardial infarction (MI). The exercise (or dobutamine or any other stress agent that is associated with high heart rate) MPI might show reversible defects that mimic LAD disease, even in the absence of angiographic LAD disease, in about 40% of patients. These are not seen with vasodilator stress where the heart rate is not high. Any abnormality outside the LAD zone should not be ascribed to LBBB. Vasodilator stress, rather than exercise or dobutamine, should therefore be the stress modality of choice in such patients.

- In patients with LBBB, the gated images often show abnormal septal wall motion but normal thickening. The presence of the wall-thickening abnormality together with a perfusion defect suggests that the septal scar is responsible for the LBBB and not the reverse.

- In morbidly obese patients, a higher tracer dose and a longer imaging time could ensure high-quality images. Otherwise, the images would be of poor quality and difficult to interpret.

- Some, but not all, arrhythmias can interfere with gating and produce falsely low LVEF. This is another reason why gating should be done on both the rest and stress images.

BACKGROUND

Certain groups of patients might pose challenges in the performance and interpretation of MPI. Most, if not all, of the groups discussed in this chapter are not "zebras" that are encountered every now and then, but rather are part and parcel of everyday practice. These patient groups include asymptomatic patients, those with DM, CKD (especially those at end-stage on dialysis [ESRD]), women, the elderly, morbidly obese patients, and patients with LBBB, and arrhythmias. Some of their unique features are discussed in this chapter.

| Case 11-1 | Stress Testing in a Patient With Diabetes and Shortness of Breath (Figure 11-1) |

A 74-year-old woman with type 2 DM for more than 30 years but no past medical history of CAD, is referred for stress MPI because of a recent history of progressive shortness of breath and unusual fatigue. She also has chronic obstructive pulmonary disease, dyslipidemia, hypertension, and osteoporosis, and has had hip surgery in the past. There is a strong family history of CAD. Adenosine/rest gated SPECT MPI showed a large area of reversible perfusion abnormality (Figure 11-1, *A, B*). Coronary angiography subsequently revealed severe stenosis in the LAD with occlusion of the LCX. The LVEF was normal (Figure 11-1, *C*). Mature collaterals to the LCX were evident. She was treated with a drug-eluting stent to the LAD plus optimization of medical therapy. Her symptoms resolved.

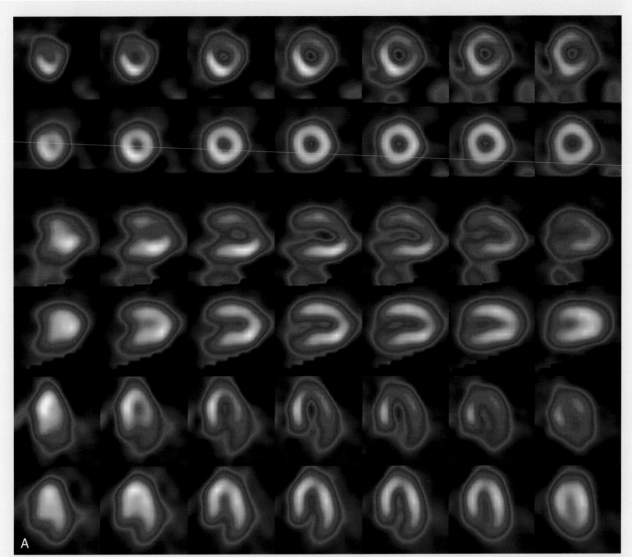

■ **Figure 11-1** Adenosine/rest SPECT MPI showing a large reversible perfusion abnormality in the anterior and lateral walls and apex **(A)**.

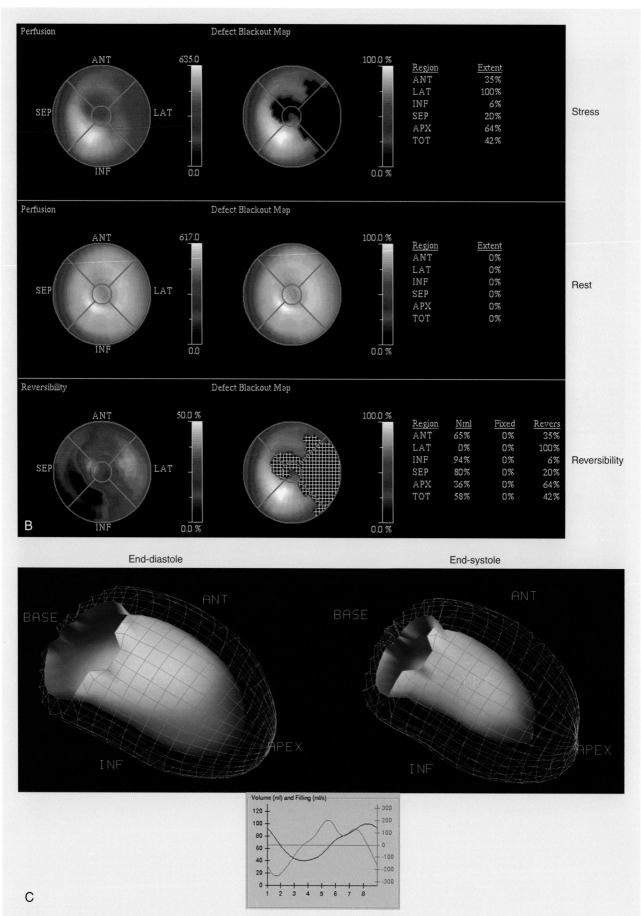

Figure 11-1—Cont'd The extent of the perfusion abnormality on polar maps **(B)**. The LVEF measured 58% on the gated images **(C)**.

Comments

Although it is widely acknowledged that DM constitutes a CAD-equivalent based on studies that demonstrated that DM patients without known CAD have an equivalent cardiac risk to patients without DM but with prior MI, there is a spectrum of risk for DM patients and the presence of CAD increases cardiovascular risk substantially. As a general rule, the diagnostic accuracy of MPI is similar in patients with and without DM. The presence and extent of myocardial ischemia is a powerful predictor of future cardiovascular events. Nevertheless, there is a residual risk associated with DM such that patients with DM with an abnormal MPI have a higher cardiovascular risk than patients without DM with an abnormal MPI. More significantly, patients with DM with a normal MPI are also at higher risk than patients without DM with normal results. Recent data from the BARI2D trial showed that residual ischemia is decreased following coronary revascularization with the addition of optimal medical management compared to optimal medical management alone. DM also affects LV function; the LV volume is higher and the EF is slightly lower in patients with DM compared to those without DM. Abnormalities in diastolic LV function are even more common and may occur earlier.

Case 11-2 Stress Testing in a Patient With Severe CKD (Figure 11-2)

A 60-year-old man with stage IV CKD secondary to long-standing uncontrolled hypertension is referred for stress MPI prior to high-risk peripheral vascular surgery. The rest ECG showed severe LVH. The perfusion pattern after regadenoson was normal, but there was marked septal hypertrophy producing downscaling of the lateral wall on both the stress and rest images (Figure 11-2, only stress images are shown). The gated images showed normal EF and wall motion/thickening. He underwent surgery with no complications.

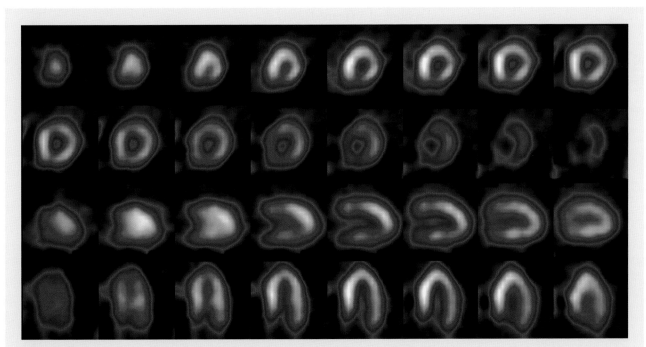

■ **Figure 11-2** Regadenoson SPECT MPI. The perfusion is normal, but the septum is the brightest region of the myocardium, causing downscaling of the lateral wall. The rest images (not shown) had a similar pattern. The LVEF is normal.

COMMENTS

CKD is increasingly being recognized as an important risk factor for cardiovascular disease, and current guidelines consider patients with CKD to be in the highest CAD risk category for risk factor management. The risk of cardiovascular events is known to increase with progressively decreasing eGFR. Moreover, most patients with CKD succumb to cardiovascular death before initiating hemodialysis (stage 5 CKD). The presence and extent of perfusion abnormalities on MPI have been shown to be predictive of risk, but those with a normal MPI are at a higher risk than patients without CKD and a normal MPI. This could be due to the effect of CKD on cardiac structure and function that are independent of coronary perfusion. By the time the renal function deteriorates to stage V, most patients would already have developed LVH and/or LV dysfunction. The LVH in ESRD involves the septum more than the lateral wall. The reasons are not known, but we believe that the LV diastolic dysfunction (due to LVH) produces pulmonary hypertension and this, together with volume overload, produces right ventricular hypertrophy. Thus, the septum is subjected to both LVH and right ventricular hypertrophy/volume overload. This unique feature (also seen in patients with hypertrophic cardiomyopathy) may give the appearance of a lateral wall perfusion abnormality on MPI and misdiagnosis of LCX scar or ischemia. As in patients with severe hypertrophy, the EF might be underestimated because of improper tracking of the endocardial borders. Analysis of the cine slices often show cavity obliteration and should be interpreted as normal.

| Case 11-3 | Stress Testing Before Renal Transplantation in a Patient With Known Heart Disease (Figure 11-3) |

A 61-year-old man with ESRD secondary to IgA nephropathy is referred for stress MPI before renal transplantation. He underwent coronary artery bypass grafting and aortic valve replacement a year ago and has been on hemodialysis for 6 years. Adenosine MPI showed a large mixed (scar and ischemia) perfusion abnormality (Figure 11-3, *A, B*). The LVEF was severely depressed on the gated images (Figure 11-3, *C*). Coronary angiography revealed severe CAD and poor runoff. He was denied renal transplantation and continued on hemodialysis.

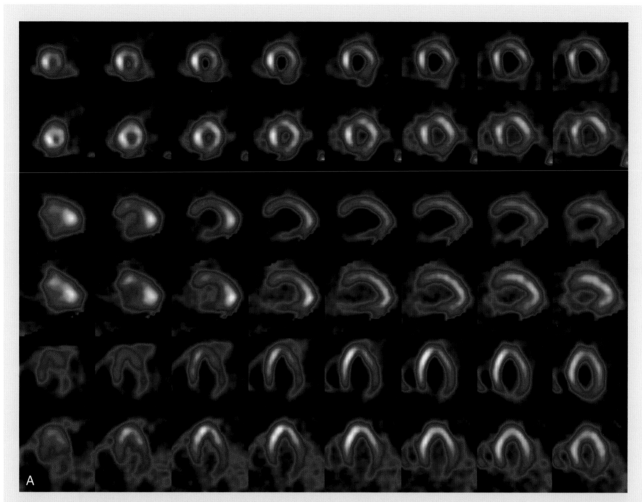

■Figure 11-3 Adenosine/rest MPI showing partially reversible perfusion defects in three vascular territories, with some residual scar in the inferior wall **(A)**.

(Continued)

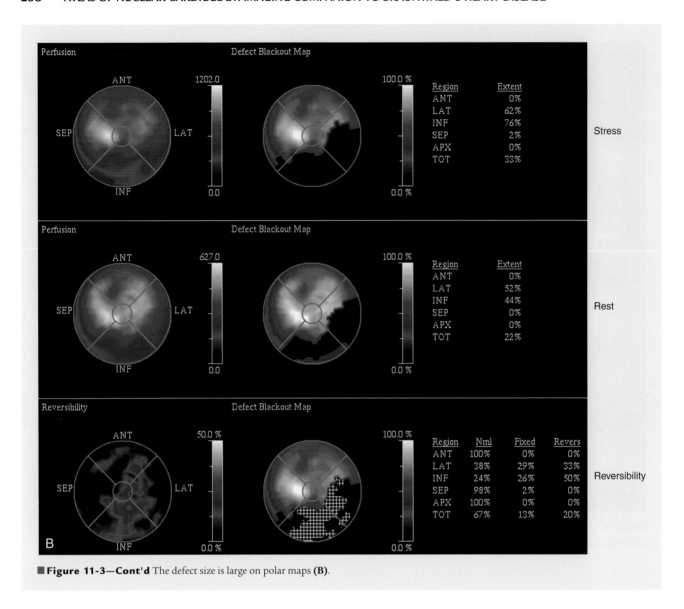

■Figure 11-3—Cont'd The defect size is large on polar maps **(B)**.

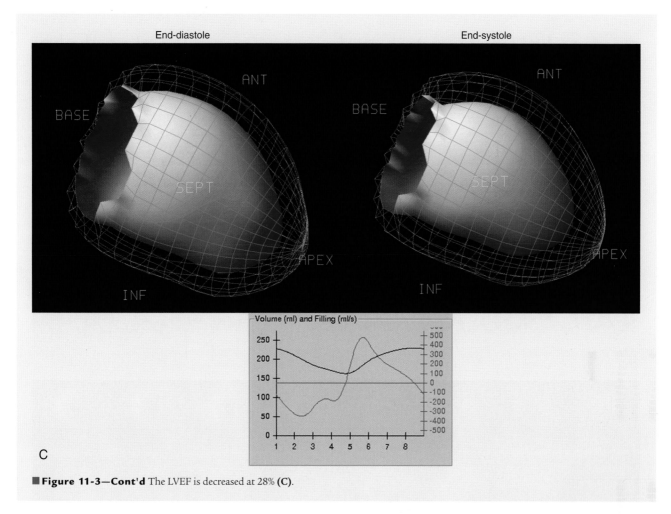

■ **Figure 11-3—Cont'd** The LVEF is decreased at 28% **(C)**.

Comments

Cardiovascular mortality accounts for almost one-half of all-cause mortality in patients with ESRD. There are multiple factors that contribute to the increased cardiovascular risk in these patients; an important process that accompanies decreased renal function is an alteration in calcium and phosphorus homeostasis that results in vascular and valvular calcification. In addition to increased vascular stiffness, this can result in valvular pathologies, such as aortic stenosis, as seen in this patient at an earlier than anticipated age.

Because of this increased risk, most renal transplantation centers use a cardiac evaluation protocol (our institution includes stress MPI in our protocol) in patients >50 years of age and in those with cardiac risk factors. In this population, perfusion abnormalities predict cardiovascular events and overall mortality despite the absence of symptoms. In fact, MPI provides more powerful prognostic data than coronary angiography. Further, a depressed LVEF is a strong predictor of mortality prior to transplantation. Despite this, the value of coronary revascularization has not yet been established in prospective randomized studies to improve survival, although retrospective data from large databases suggest that it may offer a benefit in patients with three-vessel disease, but not in those with less severe CAD.

Case 11-4   **Stress Testing After Calcium Score Study (Figure 11-4)**

A 56-year-old asymptomatic man with no known CAD underwent a screening EBCT for evaluation of cardiac risk. He has a history of hypertension with an intermediate Framingham Risk Score. The EBCT showed significant coronary artery calcifications in the LAD and RCA with a coronary artery calcium score of 800 Agatston units. He was started on an appropriate medical regimen plus regular exercise and weight loss. Two years later, he noted shortness of breath and chest tightness during exercise. He was referred for an exercise MPI. He exercised for 11 minutes on a treadmill and had chest tightness and ST depression (Figure 11-4, *A*). The LVEF was normal. The MPI showed a large area of ischemia (Figure 11-4, *B, C*). Coronary angiography showed severe LAD stenosis, which was treated with a drug-eluting stent.

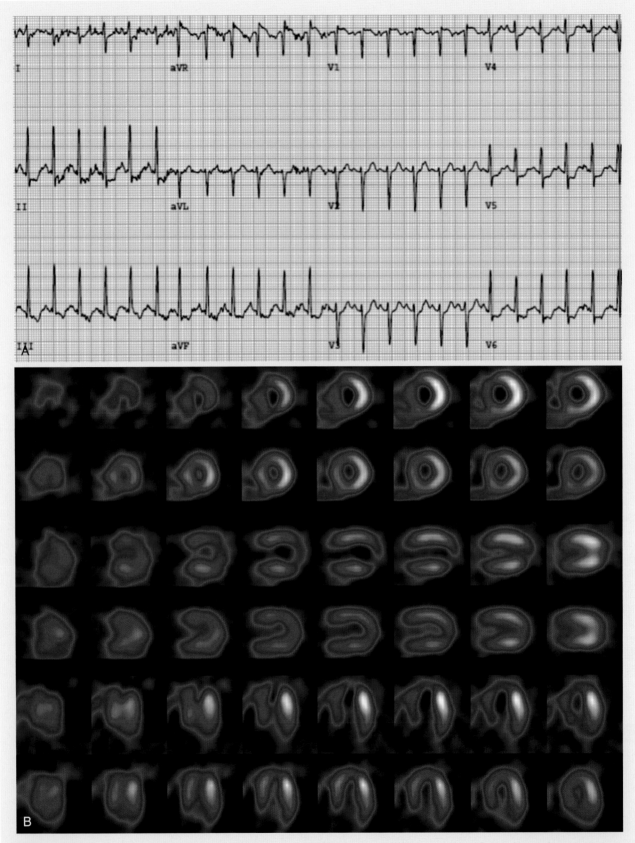

■Figure 11-4 Exercise ECG showing ST depression (A). Exercise/rest SPECT MPI showing a reversible perfusion abnormality in LAD territory (B).

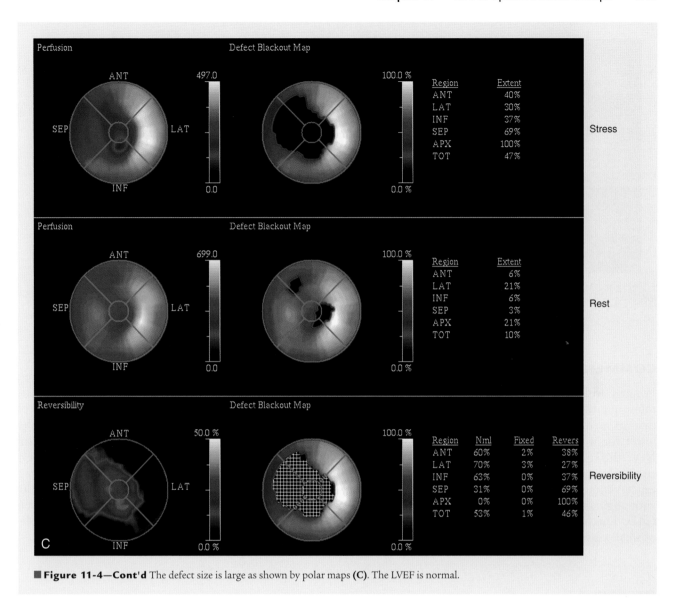

Perfusion   Defect Blackout Map

Region	Extent
ANT	40%
LAT	30%
INF	37%
SEP	69%
APX	100%
TOT	47%

Stress

Perfusion   Defect Blackout Map

Region	Extent
ANT	6%
LAT	21%
INF	6%
SEP	3%
APX	21%
TOT	10%

Rest

Reversibility   Defect Blackout Map

Region	Nml	Fixed	Revers
ANT	60%	2%	38%
LAT	70%	3%	27%
INF	63%	0%	37%
SEP	31%	0%	69%
APX	0%	0%	100%
TOT	53%	1%	46%

Reversibility

■ **Figure 11-4—Cont'd** The defect size is large as shown by polar maps **(C)**. The LVEF is normal.

COMMENTS

Most patients who suffer acute MI and/or sudden cardiac death do not have a prior diagnosis of CAD. There is, therefore, great interest in developing screening tests and paradigms for asymptomatic individuals. Global risk scores, such as the Framingham Risk Score, can be used to risk stratify individuals into low-, intermediate-, and high-risk categories, but only a small proportion of cardiac events occur in high-risk individuals. Coronary calcium scoring is considered inappropriate for asymptomatic patients at low risk or at high risk and of some value in the subset of patients at intermediate risk. The Detection of Ischemia in Asymptomatic Diabetics study (DIAD) did not show a reduction in cardiac event rates in the asymptomatic DM group randomized to screening with MPI compared to standard care.

Case 11-5   **Stress Testing in a Patient With Atrial Fibrillation and Atypical Symptoms of Angina (Figure 11-5)**

A 50-year-old woman with DM, hypertension, dyslipidemia, and atrial fibrillation is referred for MPI prior to the initiation of flecainide therapy. She reports symptoms of palpitations and atypical chest tightness. She exercised for 10 minutes on the treadmill with no ECG changes and had a normal perfusion pattern and normal LVEF (Figure 11-5). She was started on flecainide, which controlled her symptoms.

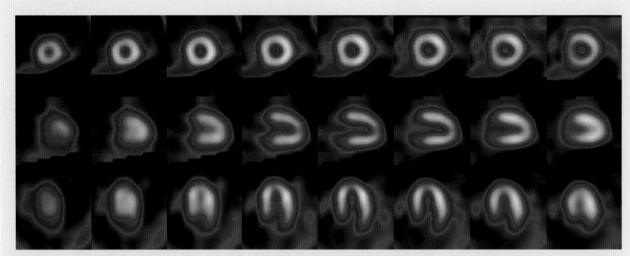

■**Figure 11-5** Exercise SPECT MPI showing a normal perfusion pattern. The exercise ST response was normal (not shown).

COMMENTS

Women with CAD often present with vague symptoms; typical symptoms occur much less frequently than in men. Furthermore, the prevalence of CAD is lower for women than men in age groups <70 years. Nevertheless, more women than men die from CAD, and CAD accounts for more deaths in women than all cancers combined. It is now apparent that not all women with angina and myocardial ischemia have obstructive CAD. This has been attributed to the higher prevalence of small vessel disease in women compared to men and

has been shown to have prognostic significance and, therefore, should not be disregarded as a false positive finding on MPI. The lower diagnostic accuracy of exercise ECG changes in women has emphasized the importance of imaging in this group. Atrial fibrillation in the absence of symptoms should not warrant stress MPI, according to current guidelines.

The interpreting physician should be aware of the peculiarities imposed by differences in body habitus when reading MPI scans of women. Breasts can cause significant tissue attenuation (see Chapter 3).

Case 11-6 **Stress Testing After Visit to Emergency Department (Figure 11-6)**

A 45-year-old woman with hypertension presented to the ED with a 3-hour episode of chest pain and shortness of breath that resolved spontaneously. There were no ischemic ECG changes and two sets of biomarkers were negative. She was discharged home and scheduled for exercise stress testing 2 days later. She exercised for 7 minutes on the treadmill, but stopped due to fatigue. The ECG showed ST depression during exercise (Figure 11-6, *A*). MPI revealed a normal perfusion pattern and a normal LVEF (Figure 11-6, *B*). She was managed conservatively and had no cardiac events on long-term follow-up.

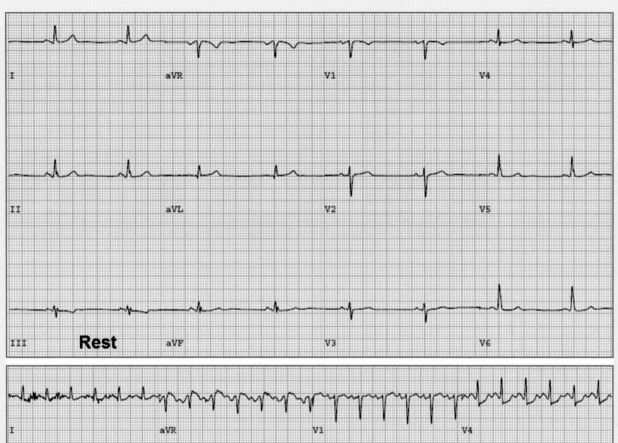

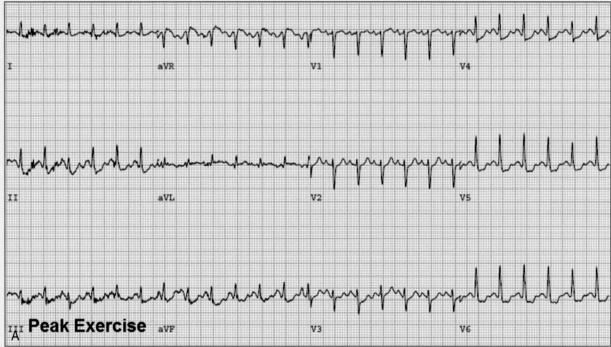

■**Figure 11-6** Exercise ECG showing ST depression **(A)**.

(Continued)

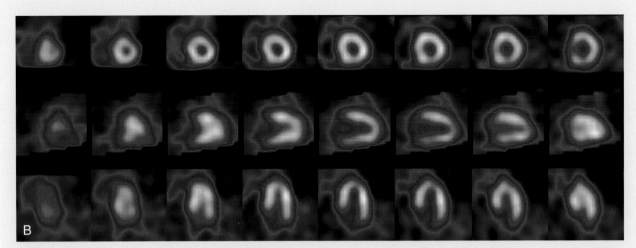

■ **Figure 11-6—Cont'd** The exercise SPECT MPI image shows a normal perfusion pattern **(B)**.

COMMENTS

Ischemic ECG changes in response to exercise are more likely to be false positive in women than in men. This is thought to be related to a digoxin-like effect of estrogen on the ECG. ST segment depression, therefore, does not add prognostic data to perfusion imaging since most patients with ST depression have perfusion abnormalities, and patients with normal perfusion and ST depression have a benign course. Similarly, most patients with ST depression after adenosine infusion have reversible perfusion defects and, in our experience, patients with an ischemic ECG response to adenosine but normal MPI are at low risk for cardiovascular events on long-term follow-up.

Case 11-7   Stress Testing in the Elderly (Figure 11-7)

An 83-year-old man with DM, hypertension, and hyperlipidemia but no prior history of CAD was referred for an exercise MPI for evaluation of new onset chest pain. He exercised for 3½ minutes on the treadmill and stopped due to fatigue after reaching 65% of maximum predicted heart rate. He did not report any chest pain, there were no ischemic changes on the ECG, and perfusion was normal (Figure 11-7, *A*). Because of the submaximal exercise, he underwent a repeat MPI with adenosine. This showed an abnormal perfusion pattern (Figure 11-7, *B*).

Exercise/rest SPECT images

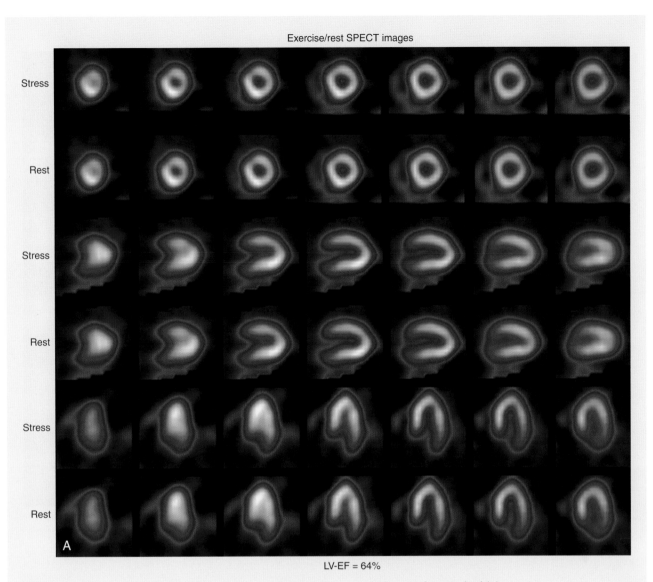

LV-EF = 64%

■**Figure 11-7** Exercise/rest SPECT MPI showing a normal perfusion pattern at submaximal exercise level **(A)**.

(Continued)

Adenosine/rest SPECT images

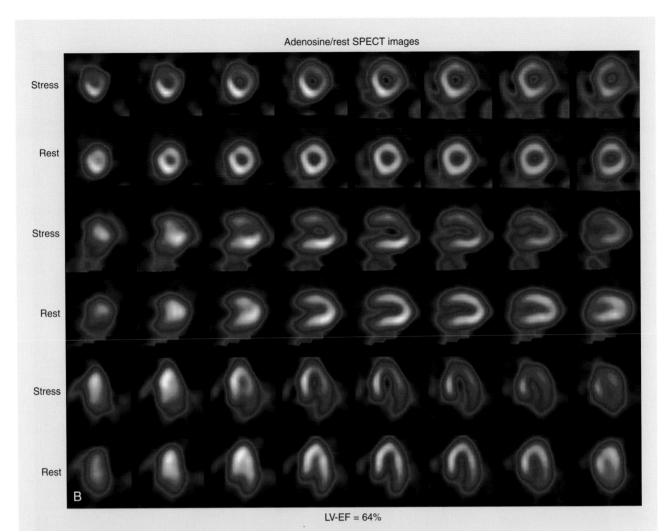

LV-EF = 64%

■**Figure 11-7—Cont'd** Repeat MPI after adenosine stress in the same patient shows a large perfusion abnormality in the LCX territory that is completely reversible at rest **(B)**.

Exercise (stress 1)/adenosine (stress 2) SPECT images

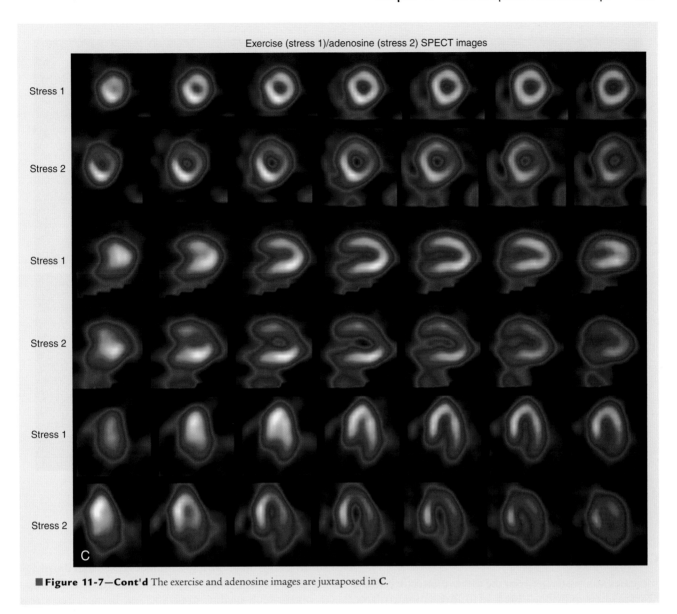

■**Figure 11-7—Cont'd** The exercise and adenosine images are juxtaposed in **C**.

COMMENTS

Many elderly patients are unable to reach their target heart rate on the treadmill because of various reasons. Submaximal exercise might conceal abnormal perfusion, potentially of a large degree. In such patients, vasodilator stress testing is preferred.

Case 11-8   **Stress Testing in Markedly Obese Patients (Figure 11-8)**

A 42-year-old morbidly obese woman (weight 450 lb) with DM, hypertension, and dyslipidemia presents with chest pain and shortness of breath. Adenosine MPI showed normal perfusion and LVEF (Figure 11-8). She was managed conservatively.

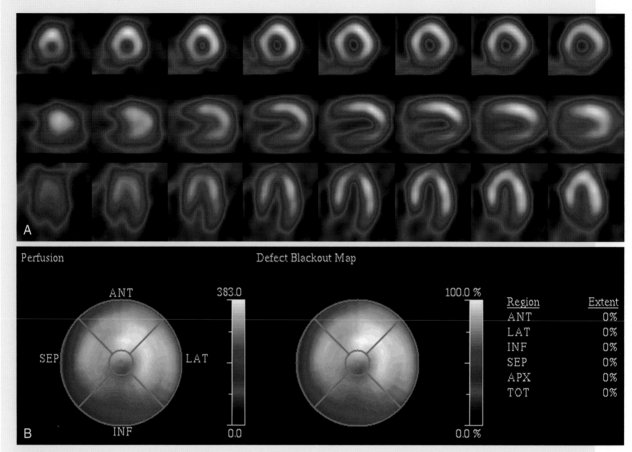

■**Figure 11-8 A,** Adenosine MPI of a morbidly obese patient showing a normal perfusion pattern and **B,** normal polar maps.

COMMENTS

Increased soft tissue between the camera/detector and the heart in obese individuals can lead to attenuation artifacts, poor count statistics, and noisy images. In this patient, a 40-mCi dose of Tc-99m sestamibi was used and the imaging time was increased by 5 minutes, which enabled us to obtain high-quality stress images. Because the stress images were normal, no rest imaging was performed.

Case 11-9   Stress Testing in LBBB (Figure 11-9)

An 82-year-old woman with hypertension, dyslipidemia, and mild dementia presented with chest pain and underwent exercise MPI. Her baseline ECG showed LBBB. She exercised for 4 minutes and stopped because of fatigue. The images showed inferior and lateral fixed defects (Figure 11-9, *A*). The EF was depressed (Figure 11-9, *B*).

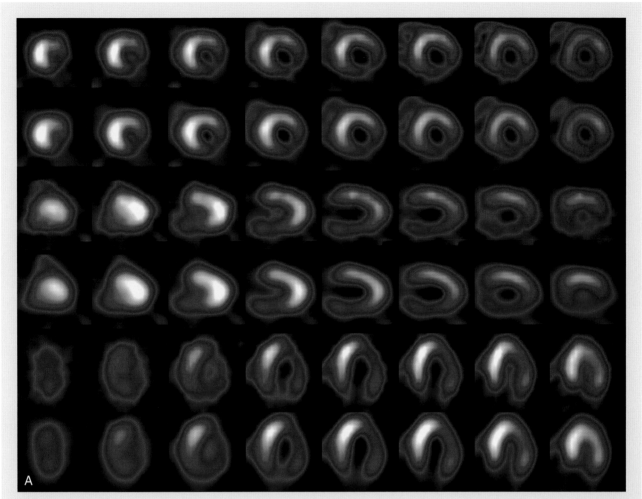

■ **Figure 11-9** Exercise/rest SPECT MPI showing a large fixed perfusion abnormality in LCX and RCA territories **(A)**.

(Continued)

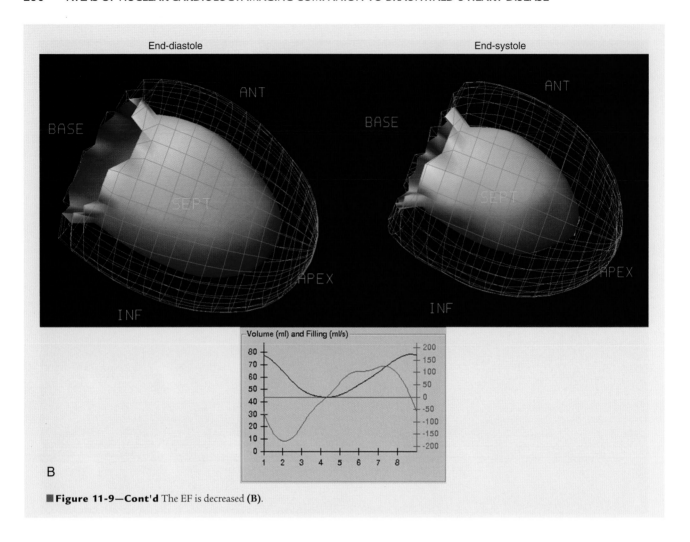

Figure 11-9—Cont'd The EF is decreased **(B)**.

COMMENTS

In this patient, the defects were fixed and not in the region of the LAD. Such defects are not related to LBBB, but are due to underlying CAD. The use of vasodilator stress would have been preferred (and has been routinely substituted for exercise testing in our institution for the past 15 years) and might have detected additional areas of reversible defects because the exercise was submaximal in this patient.

Case 11-10 **Stress Testing in a Patient With Ventricular Arrhythmias (Figure 11-10)**

A 55-year-old man with known CAD, prior MI, and recurrent nonsustained ventricular tachycardia underwent stress MPI for shortness of breath. He exercised for 4 minutes and stopped because of shortness of breath. The images showed a large multivessel scar. In the poststress images, the gating was poor because of multiple premature beats (Figure 11-10, *A*). Fortunately, there were only a few such beats during the rest study and the gating was improved (Figure 11-10, *B*).

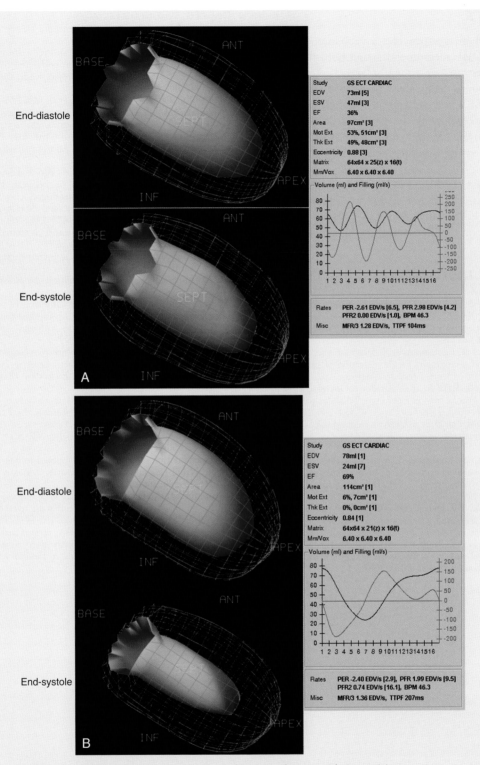

■ **Figure 11-10** The end-diastolic and end-systolic 3D gated images with time-activity curve showing poor gating **(A)** in the poststress images due to premature beats and proper gating in the rest images with higher EF **(B)**.

COMMENTS

Gating of MPI images provides a very important piece of information. We recommend gating both the rest and stress images because one set might be corrupted, typically by gating problems such as can be seen in patients with pacemakers, LBBB, low-voltage QRS complexes, or irregular rhythms (occasionally the gating is done for structures other than the LV, such as the liver or gallbladder or bowel loops!). Gating is still possible in most patients with atrial fibrillation or occasional premature beats. Poor gating almost always produces lower rather than higher EFs; therefore, we use the higher of the two measurements in our reporting. For quality control, we suggest inspection of the contours on the slices and the time-activity curves.

SELECTED READINGS

Berman DS, Kang X, Hayes SW, et al: Adenosine myocardial perfusion single-photon emission computed tomography in women compared with men. Impact of diabetes mellitus on incremental prognostic value and effect on patient management, *J Am Coll Cardiol* 41:1125–1133, 2003.

Burgstahler C, Beck T, Reimann A, et al: Diagnostic accuracy of multislice computed tomography for the detection of coronary artery disease in diabetic patients, *J Diabetes Complicat* 21:69–74, 2007.

Chung J, Abraszewski P, Yu X, et al: Paradoxical increase in ventricular torsion and systolic torsion rate in type I diabetic patients under tight glycemic control, *J Am Coll Cardiol* 47:384–390, 2006.

Go AS, Chertow GM, Fan D, et al: Chronic kidney disease and the risks of death, cardiovascular events, and hospitalization, *N Engl J Med* 351:1296–1305, 2004.

Haffner SM, Lehto S, Rönnemaa T, et al: Mortality from coronary heart disease in subjects with type 2 diabetes and in nondiabetic subjects with and without prior myocardial infarction, *N Engl J Med* 339:229–234, 1998.

Hage FG, Dubovsky EV, Heo J, et al: Outcome of patients with adenosine-induced ST-segment depression but with normal perfusion on tomographic imaging, *Am J Cardiol* 98:1009–1011, 2006.

Hage FG, Smalheiser S, Zoghbi GJ, et al: Predictors of survival in patients with end-stage renal disease evaluated for kidney transplantation, *Am J Cardiol* 100:1020–1025, 2007.

Hage FG, Venkataraman R, Zoghbi GJ, et al: The scope of coronary heart disease in patients with chronic kidney disease, *J Am Coll Cardiol* 53:2129–2140, 2009.

Hakeem A, Bhatti S, Dillie KS, et al: Predictive value of myocardial perfusion single-photon emission computed tomography and the impact of renal function on cardiac death, *Circulation* 118:2540–2549, 2008.

Hendel RC, Patel MR, Kramer CM, et al: ACCF/ACR/SCCT/SCMR/ASNC/NASCI/SCAI/SIR 2006 appropriateness criteria for cardiac computed tomography and cardiac magnetic resonance imaging: a report of the American College of Cardiology Foundation Quality Strategic Directions Committee Appropriateness Criteria Working Group, American College of Radiology, Society of Cardiovascular Computed Tomography, Society for Cardiovascular Magnetic Resonance, American Society of Nuclear Cardiology, North American Society for Cardiac Imaging, Society for Cardiovascular Angiography and Interventions, and Society of Interventional Radiology, *J Am Coll Cardiol* 48:1475–1497, 2006.

Htay T, Mehta D, Heo J, et al: Left ventricular function in patients with type 2 diabetes mellitus, *Am J Cardiol* 95:798–801, 2005.

Kang X, Berman DS, Lewin HC, et al: Incremental prognostic value of myocardial perfusion single photon emission computed tomography in patients with diabetes mellitus, *Am Heart J* 138:1025–1032, 1999.

Kang X, Berman DS, Lewin H, et al: Comparative ability of myocardial perfusion single-photon emission computed tomography to detect coronary artery disease in patients with and without diabetes mellitus, *Am Heart J* 137:949–957, 1999.

Korosoglou G, Humpert PM: Non-invasive diagnostic imaging techniques as a window into the diabetic heart: a review of experimental and clinical data, *Exp Clin Endocrinol Diabetes* 115:211–220, 2007.

Kwok Y, Kim C, Grady D, et al: Meta-analysis of exercise testing to detect coronary artery disease in women, *Am J Cardiol* 83:660–666, 1999.

O'Rourke RA, Brundage BH, Froelicher VF, et al: American College of Cardiology/American Heart Association Expert Consensus Document on electron-beam computed tomography for the diagnosis and prognosis of coronary artery disease, *J Am Coll Cardiol* 36:326–340, 2000.

Venkataraman R, Hage FG, Dorfman T, et al: Role of myocardial perfusion imaging in patients with end-stage renal disease undergoing coronary angiography, *Am J Cardiol* 102:1451–1456, 2008.

Young LH, Wackers FJT, Chyun DA, et al: Cardiac outcomes after screening for asymptomatic coronary artery disease in patients with type 2 diabetes: the DIAD study: a randomized controlled trial, *JAMA* 301:1547–1555, 2009.

Chapter 12

Applications in Patients With Heart Failure and Cardiomyopathy

Ami E. Iskandrian and Jaekyeong Heo

KEY POINTS

- Gated SPECT perfusion imaging is useful in differentiating ischemic cardiomyopathy from dilated cardiomyopathy.

- Gated SPECT perfusion imaging and RNA are useful in differentiating patients with HF with normal LVEF (diastolic HF) from patients with HF with depressed LVEF (systolic HF).

- The RVEF measured by RNA, provides important prognostic information in patients with HF.

- The perfusion pattern in dilated cardiomyopathy is often normal at stress and rest, but perfusion abnormalities can be seen in one-third of patients. The LV size is increased and the EF is depressed. The perfusion abnormality is best described as "patchy" and does not involve an entire vascular territory. The abnormality could be fixed or reversible (or both).

- The perfusion pattern in ischemic cardiomyopathy shows large perfusion defects involving one or more vascular territories; they can be fixed or reversible (or both). The LV cavity is dilated and the EF is depressed.

- Patients with hypertrophic cardiomyopathy have septal hypertrophy, which can produce perfusion defects in the lateral wall due to down-scaling.

- Reversible and fixed defects can be seen in some patients with hypertrophic cardiomyopathy in the absence of CAD; such findings should not be labeled as false positive despite the temptation to do so!

- Alcohol septal ablation in hypertrophic cardiomyopathy is followed by a small perfusion defect seen at the base of the septum, which often decreases in size over time.

- Incorrect tracking of the endocardial contour can produce a falsely low EF by gated SPECT despite a vigorous contraction pattern with cavity obliteration by visual analysis. Be aware!

- Phase analysis of gated SPECT perfusion images and of RNA can be used to assess LV dyssynchrony.

BACKGROUND

It is estimated that there are more than 5 million patients with HF in the United States and more than 500,000 new cases diagnosed each year. In 40% of these patients, the HF is due to diastolic dysfunction, known as diastolic HF or HF with preserved LVEF, and the remaining 60% have systolic HF with depressed EF (also known as HF with depressed EF). Most patients with HF also have CAD; by some estimates, as many as 90% (assessment of viability in patients with ICM is discussed in Chapter 15). Despite improvement in medical therapy and the use of ICDs and CRT, the morbidity and mortality in these patients remain high.

One of the classifications for HF is shown in Table 12-1. Patients with CAD and systolic HF are often categorized as having an ICM (a misnomer since ischemia may not be present in all patients), while those without CAD are lumped together under DCM. These patients often have no identifiable causes and the HF is presumed to be caused by hypertension, myocarditis, or genetic causes. Over the past few decades, many tracers, such as Tc-99m pyrophosphate, In-111–labeled pentetreotide (a somatostatin analog), In-111 antimyosin, Tc-99m Annexin-V, and Tc-99m–labeled glucarate, have been used to detect inflammation/necrosis but none of these is approved or currently used consistently in the United States.

ICM VERSUS DCM

Both DCM and ICM are characterized by a dilated LV cavity with wall motion/thickening abnormalities (WMAs) and a depressed EF. WMAs are often assumed to be regional in ICM and diffuse in DCM, but that distinction is often not reliable because, as the LV dilates, it also remodels and remote areas will exhibit WMAs as well. More often than not, the RV in DCM is also dilated and has a depressed EF because it is likely that the primary process (whatever it may be) that is affecting the LV, also affects the RV. However, this does not mean that RV function and size are always normal in ICM. On the contrary, it can also be abnormal in later stages of the disease when pulmonary hypertension and tricuspid regurgitation develop. Both MPI and RNA are quite helpful in these patients. MPI is used because these patients often have similar presentations, such as chest pain and shortness of breath on exertion. It also provides an incremental value in predicting new onset refractory HF.

TABLE 12-1 Classification of Various Types of Cardiomyopathies

Primary
Genetic
   Hypertrophic cardiomyopathy
   Arrythmogenic RV cardiomyopathy
   LV non-compaction
   Glycogen storage related
   Ion channel disorders
      Long QT syndromes
      Brugada
   Mixed
      Dilated cardiomyopathy
      Restrictive cardiomyopathy
Acquired
   Inflammatory
   Tako-tsubo
   Peripartum
Secondary

Case 12-1   **Patient With Dilated Cardiomyopathy and Shortness of Breath (Figure 12-1)**

A 55-year-old woman presents with chest pain, exertional dyspnea, and lack of energy of 1-year duration. She has hypertension, which is not well controlled. Her mother died of heart disease at the age of 50. The physical examination is unremarkable except for a BP of 145/95 mm Hg. The ECG shows nonspecific T-wave changes.

She exercised on the treadmill but became short of breath after 2 minutes and the stress test was switched to adenosine. The images are shown in Figure 12-1. Cardiac catheterizations showed LV end-diastolic pressure of 25 mm Hg and a normal coronary angiogram.

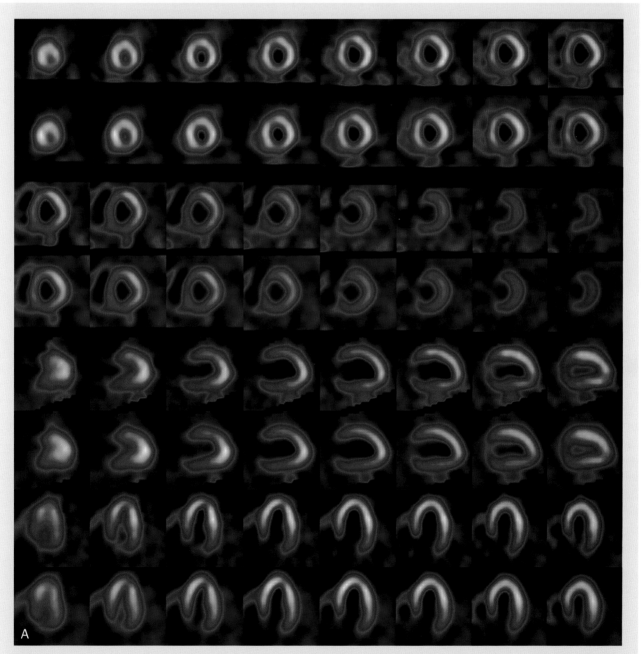

■ **Figure 12-1** Stress and rest gated SPECT MPI with Tc-99m sestamibi. The perfusion pattern is normal but the LV cavity is dilated **(A)**.

(Continued)

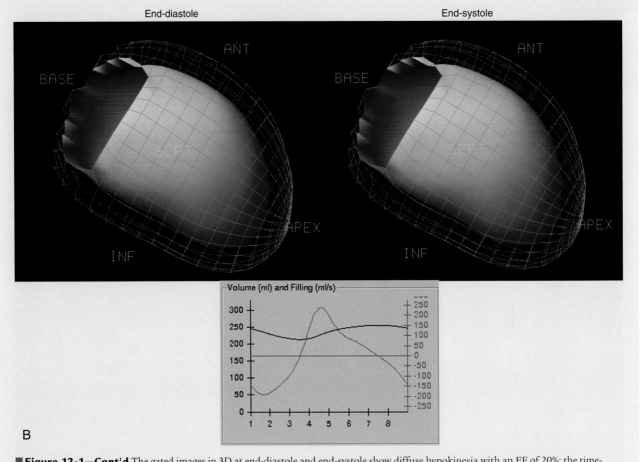

End-diastole   End-systole

B

■ **Figure 12-1—Cont'd** The gated images in 3D at end-diastole and end-systole show diffuse hypokinesia with an EF of 20%; the time-activity curve and its first derivative are also shown **(B)**. The dynamic images are shown in Video 12-1, A, B.

Case 12-2   **Patient With Dilated Cardiomyopathy and Chest Pains (Figure 12-2)**

A 44-year-old man was referred for stress testing because of chest pain and shortness of breath on exertion that had occurred for 2 years, but had worsened in the past 6 months. He was recently seen in the ED of another hospital for the same symptoms and was discharged home after evaluation showed no evidence of acute MI. He smokes and has hypertension. Physical examination is normal. The ECG shows left anterior hemiblock. He exercised for 6 minutes on the Bruce protocol and stopped because of shortness of breath at 80% of maximum predicted heart rate response. The images are shown in Figure 12-2. Subsequent cardiac catheterization showed elevated LV filling pressure, mild pulmonary hypertension, and 30% stenosis in the RCA.

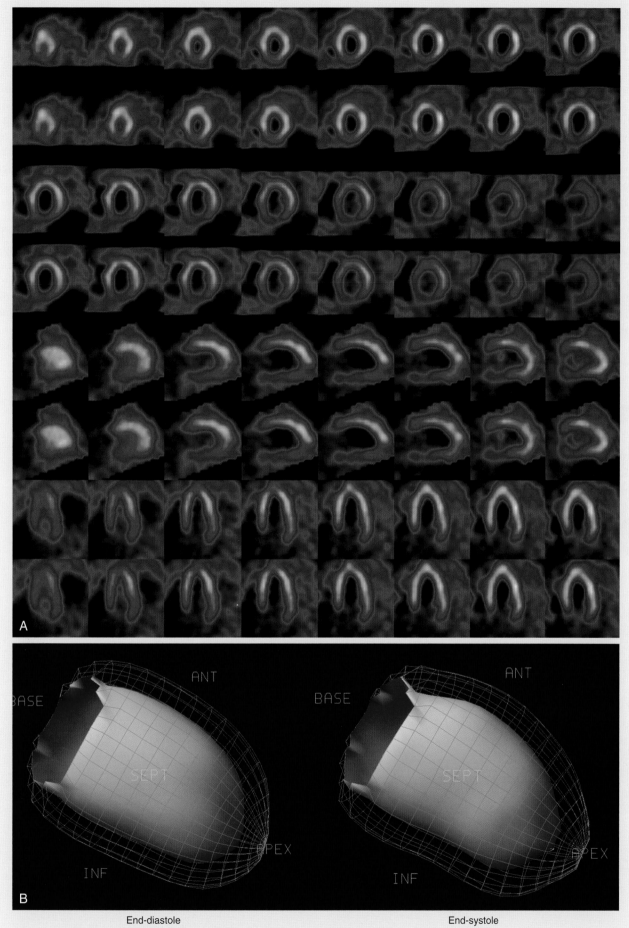

■**Figure 12-2** Stress and rest gated SPECT MPI with Tc-99m sestamibi. The stress images show small perfusion abnormality in both the stress and rest images **(A)**. The LV and RV cavities are enlarged. The gated 3D images in end-diastole and end-systole show diffuse wall motion abnormality with EF of 14% **(B)**. The dynamic images are shown in Video 12-2, **A, B.**

COMMENTS (Cases 12-1 and 12-2)

The images in these two patients illustrate part of the spectrum of perfusion patterns in patients with DCM. The perfusion pattern could be normal or show fixed or reversible defects (or both). Often attenuation abnormalities appear more prominent because of wall thinning and partial volume effect. Perfusion defects, when present, often involve small areas in multiple vascular territories consistent with the diffuse nature of the disease. The defects, therefore, are generally different from those seen in patients with CAD. Also, the decreases in EF and LV dilatation are out of proportion to the degree of the perfusion abnormality. Studies using positron emission tomography have shown a decrease in hyperemic MBF, as well as alteration in myocardial substrate utilization in such patients, even in the presence of normal coronary angiograms. Clearly, such abnormalities reflect microvascular dysfunction and microscarring.

Studies have linked such abnormalities to poor outcomes in these patients. In general, 70% of these patients will have a normal perfusion pattern, and the remaining 30% an abnormal pattern. It is improper to call these abnormalities false-positive scans because the epicardial arteries are normal. Both patients subsequently underwent coronary angiography, a not uncommon practice based on the premise that identification of CAD and coronary revascularization can alter the outcome in these patients. Based on the preceding discussion, one can make a good case for reserving coronary angiography for patients with an abnormal perfusion pattern. Skeptics might argue that balanced ischemia due to left main disease can go undetected in those with a normal perfusion pattern. This argument has a stronger appeal in patients with a small LV size and normal EF (see Chapter 6) than in patients with a dilated and poorly functioning LV. In patients with normal coronary angiograms, a rest study alone might be sufficient to exclude the possibility of prior MI due to occlusion and spontaneous recanalization of an otherwise normal coronary artery.

Case 12-3   **Patient With Ischemic Cardiomyopathy (Figure 12-3)**

A 79-year-old man presented with long-standing shortness of breath, which had progressively worsened in the last year. He had left leg pain with ambulation, which had also gotten progressively worse. The physical examination showed a displaced apical impulse with the soft murmur of mitral regurgitation and an S_3 gallop. The ECG showed LBBB. He underwent stress testing with adenosine without incident. The images are shown in Figure 12-3.

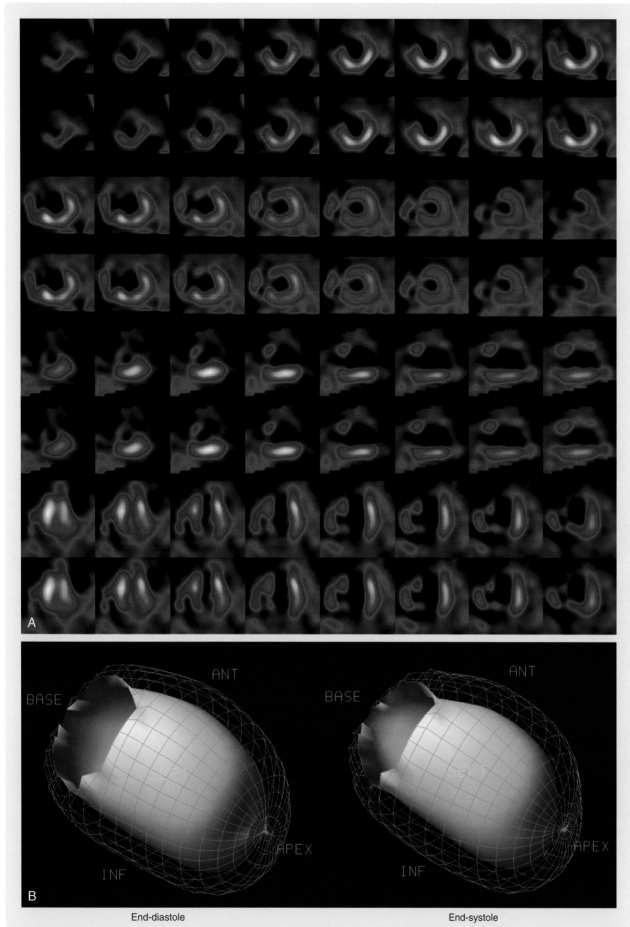

Figure 12-3 The stress and rest gated SPECT perfusion images **(A)**. There is a large severe fixed perfusion defect in the distribution of the left anterior descending artery with fixed LV cavity dilatation (not to be confused with transient LV dilatation). The gated 3D images in end-diastole and end-systole show severe wall motion abnormality with an EF of 33% **(B)**. The dynamic images are shown in Video 12-3, A, B.

Cases 12-4 and 12-5   Patient With Ischemic Cardiomyopathy
(Figures 12-4 and 12-5)

A 60-year-old woman presents with chest pain, shortness of breath, and a syncopal episode. She was previously diagnosed with HF, but has not seen a physician in years. She is obese (210 lbs) and has hypertension. She underwent stress and rest sestamibi imaging on two separate days, using adenosine as the stress agent. The images are shown in Figure 12-4.

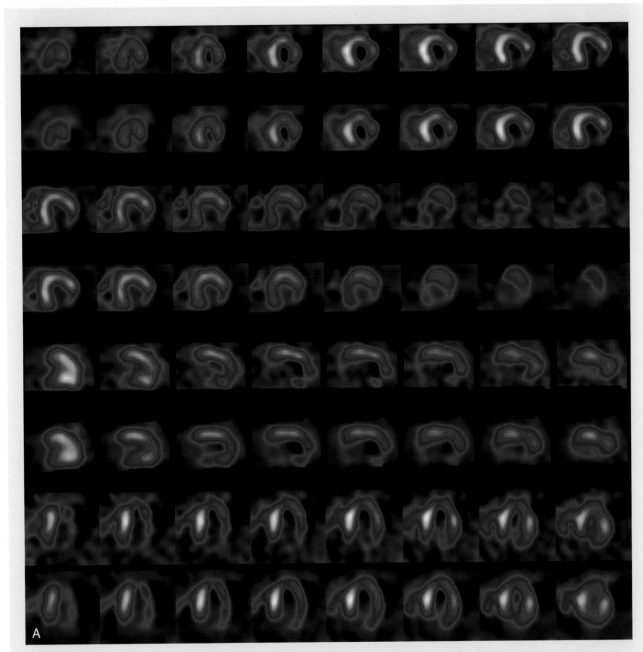

■ **Figure 12-4** The stress and rest gated SPECT perfusion images (**A**).

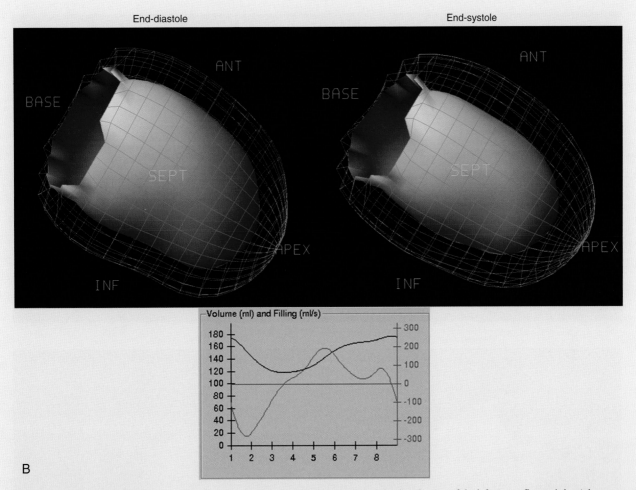

B

■ **Figure 12-4—Cont'd** There is a large and severe fixed perfusion abnormality in the distribution of the left circumflex and the right coronary arteries with fixed LV dilatation. The LV function (EF 34%) is abnormal on the 3D images; the volume time-activity curve and its first derivative are also shown **(B)**. The format is similar to Figures 12-1 through 12-3. The dynamic images are shown in Video 12-4, A, B.

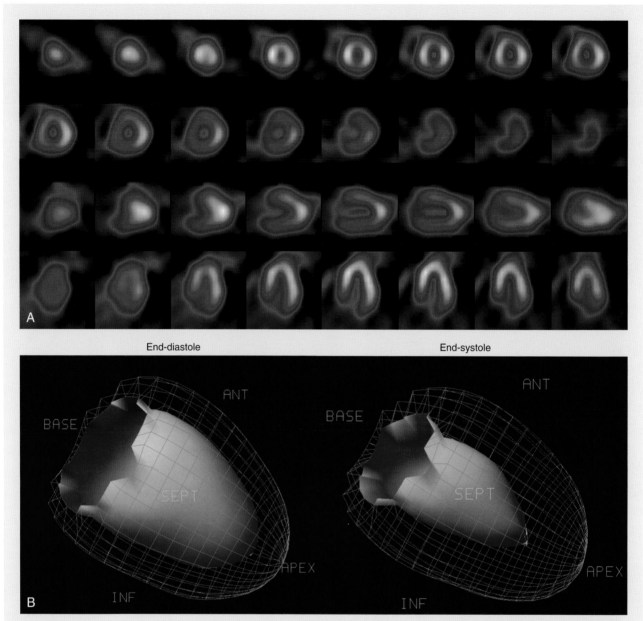

■ Figure 12-5 Stress-only images in a markedly obese patient showing normal perfusion pattern **(A)** and function **(B)**. The image quality is remarkably good. In fact, there was no need to perform resting imaging, which would have required a second visit for this patient who had traveled 80 miles from her home. She presented with shortness of breath, most likely due to morbid obesity. The dynamic images are shown in Video 12-5, **A, B**.

COMMENTS (Cases 12-3, 12-4, 12-5)

Both patients (Cases 12-3 and 12-4) have an ICM with large fixed defects, dilated LV cavity, severe WMAs, and a depressed EF. The RV function and size were normal. In the first patient, LBBB concealed the evidence of a prior infarction, and in the second patient, the location of the infarction was the reason Q waves were not present on the ECG. The WMA is diffuse, though more severe in areas with severe perfusion defects. The pattern in these two patients is quite different from the two patients with DCM discussed earlier.

Of note, image quality was high despite obesity. This patient is not an exception, and by adjusting the tracer dose and image acquisition time, good-quality images can be obtained, unlike with other imaging methods. An example of a good-quality normal image in a patient weighing 360 lbs is shown in Figure 12-5 (Case 12-5). This case also demonstrates the versatility of nuclear imaging where patient characteristics are not a hindrance. Also, because each patient has unique needs, the stress modality can be tailored to each patient's individual needs.

Case 12-6   Patient With Hypertrophic Cardiomypathy (Figure 12-6)

A 58-year-old man with chest pain and shortness of breath was referred for exercise testing. The angina was typical and had been stable for 8 months. He had no history of hypertension or known coronary risk factors. Family history was significant; his father died suddenly of heart disease at age 50. The physical examination was normal. The ECG showed left ventricular hypertrophy. He exercised for 5 minutes and stopped because of shortness of breath. The ECG showed 2-mm ST depression in V_4-V_6. The images are shown in Figure 12-6. The patient subsequently had a 2DE.

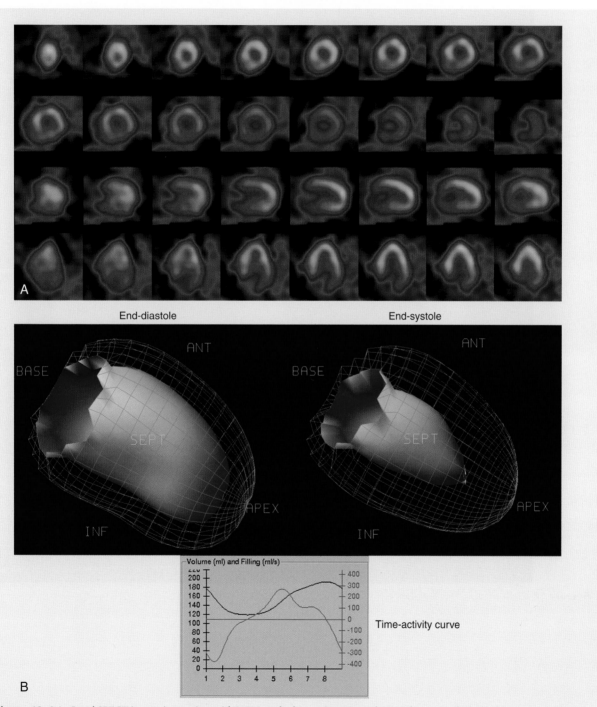

■**Figure 12-6 A,** Gated SPECT images in a patient with HCM. Only the rest images are shown. There is marked septal hypertrophy and down scaling of the other segments. **B,** The time-activity curve shows a depressed EF.

(Continued)

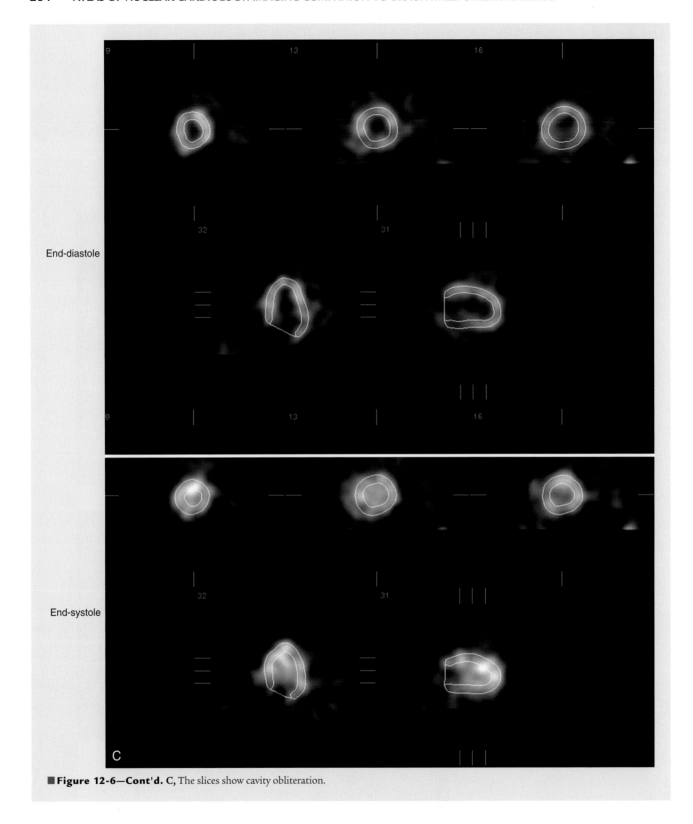

End-diastole

End-systole

■ **Figure 12-6—Cont'd. C,** The slices show cavity obliteration.

| **Cases 12-7 and 12-8** | **HCM Before and After Alcohol Septal Ablation (Figures 12-7 and 12-8)** |

The two patients were symptomatic and had obstructive HCM with large LV outflow tracts gradients. Both had alcohol septal ablation with marked improvement in symptoms. Rest sestamibi images were obtained before, 2 days after, and 3 months after ablation. These images are shown in Figures 12-7 and 12-8.

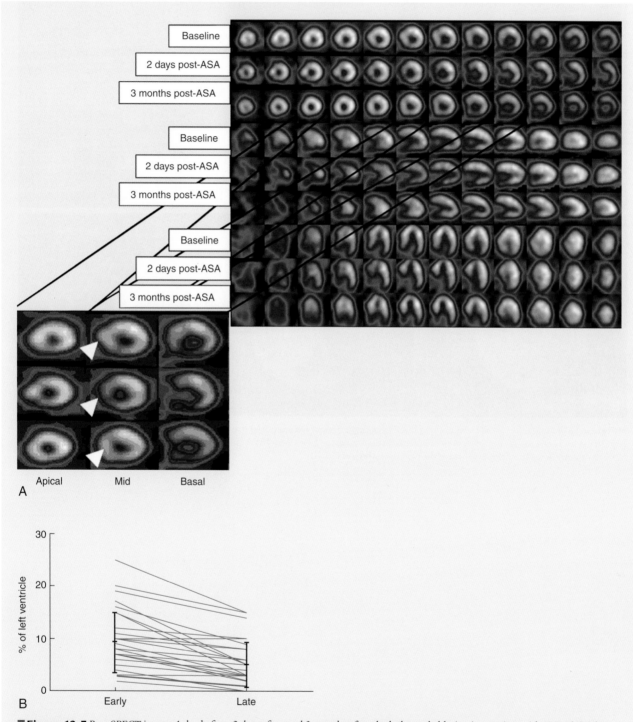

■ **Figure 12-7** Rest SPECT images 1 day before, 2 days after, and 3 months after alcohol septal ablation in a patient with HCM **(A)**. The baseline study shows septal hypertrophy. The early post ablation study shows a small defect at the base of the septum measuring 13% of the LV myocardium, as compared to a gender-matched polar map (derived from a group of patients with HCM before ablation). The late post-ablation images reveal a decrease in the size of the defect (8%). The serial changes in a large group of patients studied in our laboratory and previously reported are shown in **B**. *(Reproduced from Am J Cardiol 101:1328-1333, 2008.)*

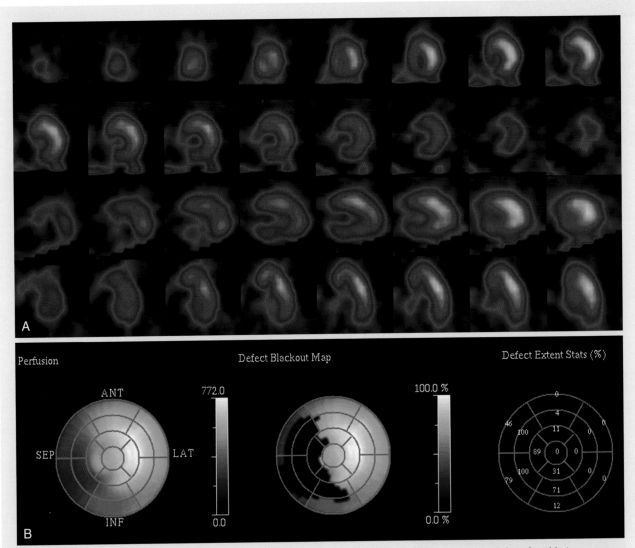

Figure 12-8 Similar format as in Figure 12-7 but in this single patient (very unusual in our experience), the defect after ablation was large, most likely due to spillover of alcohol into the left anterior descending artery **(A)**. This patient required a permanent pacemaker for AV block. The polar maps show the large size of the perfusion abnormality **(B)**.

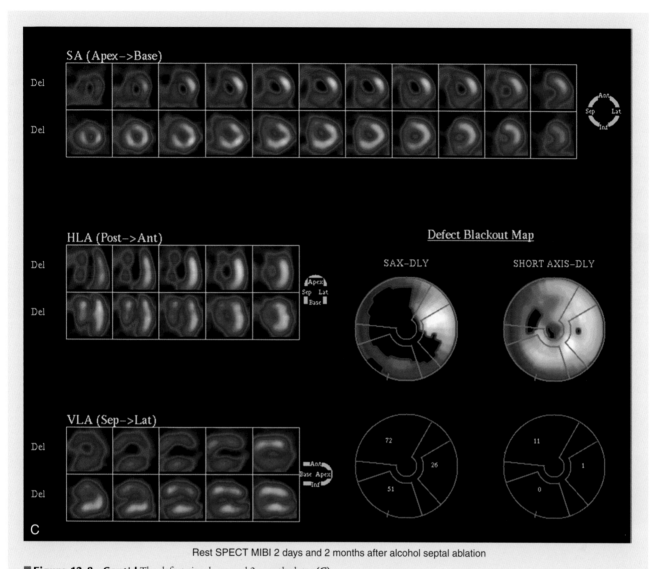

Rest SPECT MIBI 2 days and 2 months after alcohol septal ablation

■ **Figure 12-8—Cont'd** The defect size decreased 2 months later **(C)**.

Comments

Gated SPECT perfusion imaging has unique features and applications in patients with HCM. Many such patients, have no outflow tract obstruction and, therefore, the physical findings are of limited value. Because they can have angina, dyspnea, or syncope, they are often referred for stress imaging for suspected CAD. In some patients, this is when the initial diagnosis is implied or made. The disproportionate septal hypertrophy, so characteristic on 2DE, can also be seen on SPECT imaging. This is not to suggest that SPECT imaging should be used instead of 2DE for diagnosis; rather, reviewers should pay attention to septal hypertrophy and raise the possibility of HCM in the report. Septal hypertrophy can produce apparently fixed lateral wall defects due to downscaling. Automated programs often flag the lateral wall as abnormal, because

generally the lateral wall, not the septum, has the highest activity in normal subjects. In addition, patients with HCM can have fixed or reversible defects mimicking those found in patients with CAD in the absence of coronary disease. These perfusion defects reflect true ischemia and scarring due to microvascular dysfunction, increased medial thickness in arterioles, systolic bridging of septal perforators or main arteries, a disproportionate increase in the number of muscle cells to capillary density, and piecemeal necrosis and fibrosis. The perfusion defects are most commonly found in the hypertrophied septum, but can be seen in other areas as well.

In young patients, such ischemic abnormalities have been associated with an increased risk of sudden death. Obviously, in older patients, coexisting CAD can be another reason for symptoms and ischemia. We have seen examples where the software program gives an erroneously low EF even though visual inspection of the slices shows a vigorous contraction pattern and cavity obliteration. This is not unique to HCM, but can be seen in patients with other types of severe LV hypertrophy. We believe the problem is due to a lack of proper tracking of the endocardial contour; inspection of the contours shows that they are at the mid wall rather than close to the endocardial border (thickening decreases as one moves further away from the endocardial border). In such cases, we describe the vigorous contraction pattern with cavity obliteration and do not report the EF.

Alcohol septal ablation has been effective in relieving gradients and improving symptoms in selected patients with symptomatic obstructive HCM. After ablation, there is a small basal septal defect, which often decreases over time with preservation of LV function and size (see Figure 12-7, *A*). This is reassuring because of the fear that ablation could result in reverse LV remodeling and dysfunction and serious arrhythmias. In apical HCM, a variant of HCM, the hypertrophy involves the apex, which may downscale the activity elsewhere, giving the false impression of three-vessel disease.

Case 12-9   Tako-Tsubo Cardiomyopathy (Figure 12-9)

A 71-year-old woman underwent exercise sestamibi imaging for evaluation of chest pain. The physical examination and ECG were normal. The tracer was injected at 5 minutes of exercise when the patient experienced chest pain with ST depression (Figure 12-9, *A, B*). The pain and ST changes resolved with nitroglycerin.

The perfusion images 1 hour later were normal, but there was apical dyskinesia (Figure 12-9, *C–E*). Coronary angiography 3 hours later showed normal coronary arteries. The left ventriculogram was abnormal (Figure 12-9, *F*). A 2DE performed 1 month later showed normal LV function.

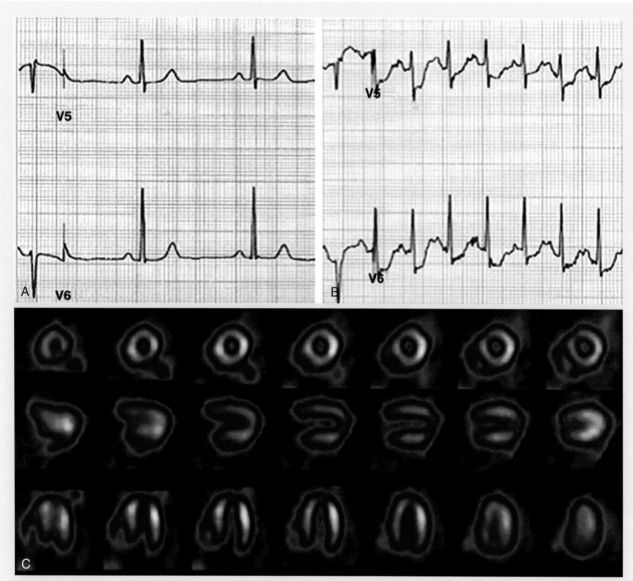

■ **Figure 12-9** The baseline electrocardiogram in leads V$_5$ and V$_6$ reveals normal sinus rhythm without ST-segment changes suggestive of ischemia **(A)**. The electrocardiogram during peak exercise and at the onset of substernal chest pressure shows 3 mm of ST-segment depression in V$_6$ **(B)**. The postexercise sestamibi perfusion images demonstrates normal perfusion pattern **(C)**.

(Continued)

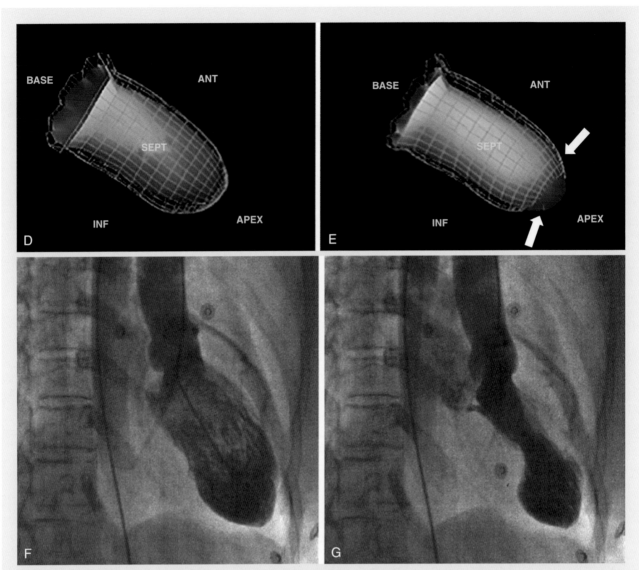

■ **Figure 12-9—Cont'd** 3D gated SPECT images at end-diastole **(D)** and end-systole **(E)**, revealing apical dyskinesia *(arrows)*. The contrast left ventriculogram at end-diastole and end-systole **(F, G)**, showing apical ballooning and basal hyperkinesis. *(From* J Am Coll Cardiol *49:1222–1225, 2007.)*

Comments

Tako-tsubo CM, also known as stress-induced CM, apical ballooning CM, or broken heart syndrome, is now a well-recognized entity of reversible CM. It mimics acute MI with characteristic findings on the left ventriculogram, similar to those in this patient involving the distal LV segments. Patients are often elderly women, and there is often an emotional or physical stress or use of high-dose beta-agonist involved. Many different variants have since been described with occurrences in younger patients (some cases of peripartum cardiomyopathy are now presumed to be such examples), men, and patients with coexisting CAD or without known stress. In some patients, the LV dysfunction involves the mid or even the basal LV segments and not the distal segments.

Most patients recover completely within a few days, but deaths have been reported, although serious ventricular arrhythmias are unusual. Unlike acute myocardial infarction due to CAD, the enzyme elevations are modest. In some patients, LV outflow tract obstruction develops due to a hyperdynamic contraction pattern involving the base to compensate for the apical dysfunction. This obstruction is aggravated by beta-agonists used to treat hypotension. The etiology is not certain but microvascular dysfunction, neurogenic factors, metabolic dysfunction, large vessel spasm, or a combination of these have all been suggested. Ironically, some patients with acute MI due to CAD are reported to have the same characteristic findings on their left ventriculograms. Recurrences are unusual but might be underreported. Presumably milder forms could occur but go undetected.

Case 12-10   LV Dyssynchrony (Figure 12-10)

A 51-year-old woman presented with HF symptoms despite optimal medical management (NYHA class III). She has had multiple prior infarctions and coronary revascularization procedures. The LVEF was 22%. The ECG showed LBBB. She was considered for implantation of an ICD and biventricular pacing device. A stress and rest MIBI was obtained before the procedure to assess residual ischemia and the need for repeat coronary angiography. A phase analysis was done to evaluate for LV dyssynchrony; the images are in Figure 12-10.

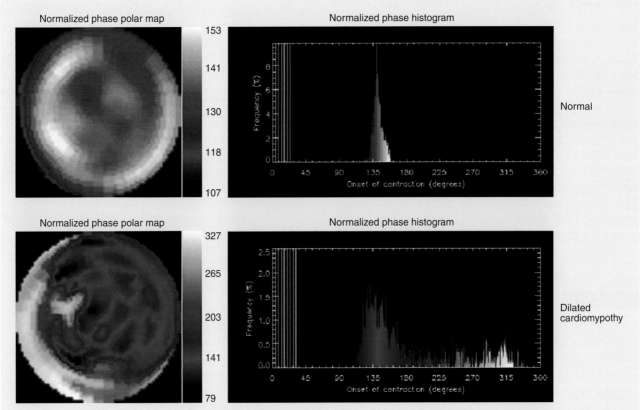

■ **Figure 12-10** The phase analysis of a patient with normal LV function *(top)* and a patient with LV dysfunction due to ischemic CM *(bottom)*. The phase standard deviation (SD) and bandwidth are larger in the patient with CM.

Comments

The use of phase analysis to assess LV dyssynchrony is a new and novel development in perfusion imaging. Phase analysis of MUGA has been around for many decades and the method has been modified and improved upon in recent years. The reality, however, is that phase analysis of gated SPECT is more appealing because many patients undergo MPI for a multitude of reasons. In such patients, the phase analysis is an additional piece of information, one that does not require any modification in how the gated SPECT images are acquired. It can also readily be applied to previously acquired images, unlike other imaging methods; it is also automated and thus highly reproducible.

LV dyssynchrony can be observed even in patients without LBBB, and there is ongoing concern about whether current criteria for biventricular pacing are too rigid as only patients with LBBB (and LV dysfunction) are qualified. We have observed patients with more severe dyssynchrony who are at higher risk of death, presumably sudden cardiac death. There is growing interest in the application of this emerging modality (see Chapter 17).

Case 12-11   **Peripartum Cardiomyopathy (Figure 12-11)**

A 22-year-old woman developed HF symptoms 2 weeks after delivering a healthy baby boy. She had no prior history of heart disease. The physical findings were consistent with volume overload and pulmonary congestion. The ECG showed poor R-wave progression across the precordial leads. The troponin level was minimally elevated. Rest gated SPECT sestamibi images were obtained and are shown in Figure 12-11.

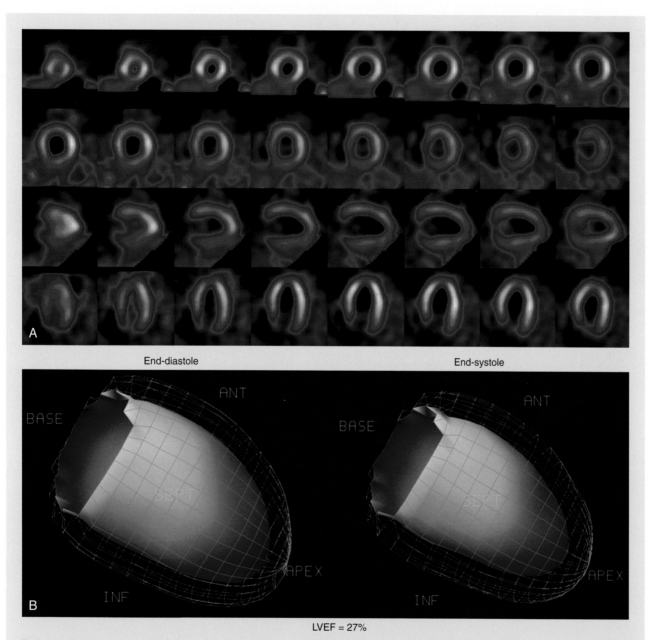

End-diastole   End-systole

LVEF = 27%

■ **Figure 12-11** The rest gated SPECT images in a patient with peripartum CM. The perfusion pattern is normal but the LV cavity is dilated **(A)** and the EF is reduced as depicted by 3D images at end-diastole and end-systole **(B)**. The dynamic images are shown in Video 12-6.

Comments

HF during pregnancy, or shortly after delivery, can be due to preexisting heart disease (for example, rheumatic heart disease), congenital heart disease, peripartum cardiomyopathy, or spontaneous coronary artery dissection. Some have suggested that tako-tsubo CM might also occur due to the stress of delivery. Rest perfusion imaging is quite helpful in differentiating these entities. With dissection (which usually involves the LAD), a large perfusion abnormality is seen. With peripartum cardiomyopathy, perfusion is normal, but LV cavity is dilated and the EF is poor. The LV features in tako-tsubo CM were described previously (see Case 12-10). The clinical presentation of dissection is more abrupt and the course is rapidly progressive unless emergency revascularization is done. The ECG often shows ST elevation but late presentation may make distinction difficult, and some patients develop LBBB.

Cases 12-12 and 12-13   MUGA Images of Patients With Systolic and Diastolic HF (Figures 12-12 and 12-13)

The woman in Figure 12-12 had no known CAD or risk factors but was scheduled to undergo chemotherapy for breast cancer, while the man in Figure 12-13 had hypertension and shortness of breath, thought to be due to HF.

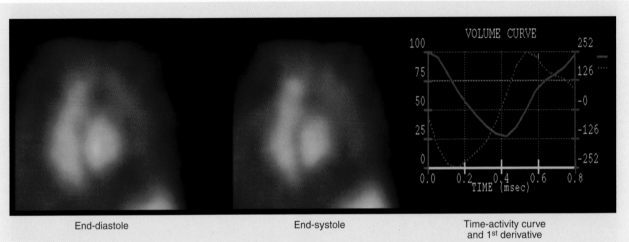

End-diastole   End-systole   Time-activity curve
and 1st derivative

■ **Figure 12-12** A gated equilibrium radionuclide angiogram in a modified left anterior oblique projection at end-diastole and end-systole. The time-activity curve and its first derivative are also shown. The EF, peak filling rate, time-to-peak filling rate, and atrial contribution to LV filling are normal. The dynamic images are shown in Video 12-7.

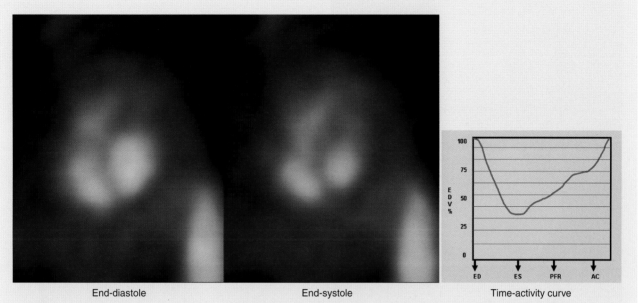

End-diastole   End-systole   Time-activity curve

■ **Figure 12-13** Same format as above. The LVEF is normal but the peak filling rate (PFR) is reduced and the atrial contribution (AC) to LV filling is increased, although the EF is normal, suggestive of diastolic LV dysfunction. ED and ES indicate end-diastole and end-systole, respectively. The dynamic images are shown in Video 12-8.

Comments

MUGA can evaluate not only systolic LV function, but also diastolic function. The diastolic indices include the peak filling rate (normalized to the end-diastolic volume), the time-to-peak filling rate, and the percent atrial contribution to LV filling. With diastolic dysfunction, the peak filling rate decreases (the slope is less steep), the time-to-peak rate lengthens, and the atrial contribution to LV filling increases. These are analogous to E/A ratio by Doppler echocardiography. In Figure 12-12, the EF and diastolic function are normal, while in Figure 12-13 the EF is normal, but the diastolic function is abnormal. The MUGA is still widely used to monitor patients undergoing chemotherapy and in patients with poor acoustic windows for 2DE.

Case 12-14   **Pacemaker-Induced LV Dysfunction (Figure 12-14)**

A 60-year-old man with sick sinus syndrome had a single-lead RV pacemaker inserted for symptomatic bradycardia. The LV function was normal before pacemaker insertion. After insertion, he started to have shortness of breath on exertion. He underwent exercise testing with imaging. The images are shown in Figure 12-14.

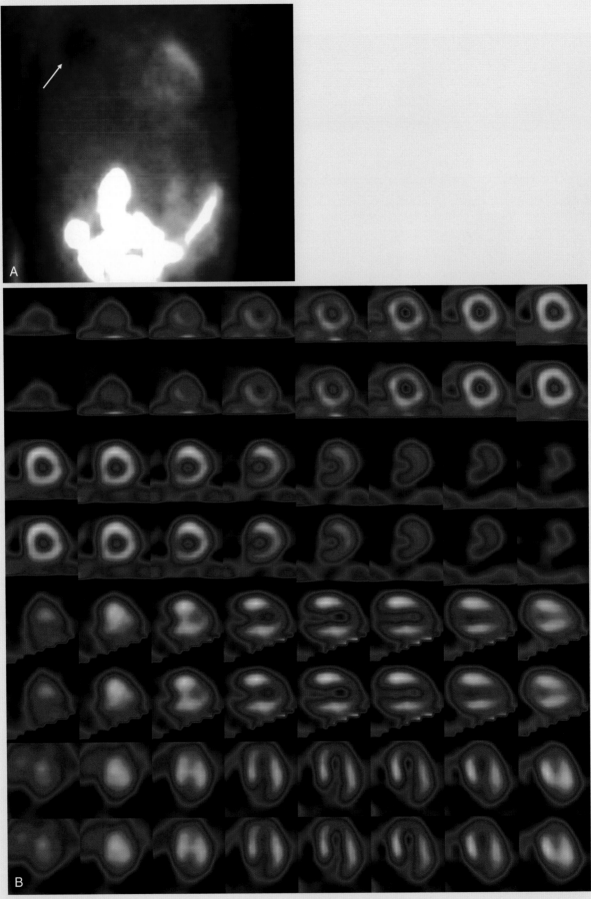

■ Figure 12-14 Gated SPECT sestamibi perfusion images in a patient with a pacemaker. The raw images show the pacemaker (**A,** *white arrow*). The perfusion pattern is normal except for apical thinning (**B**).

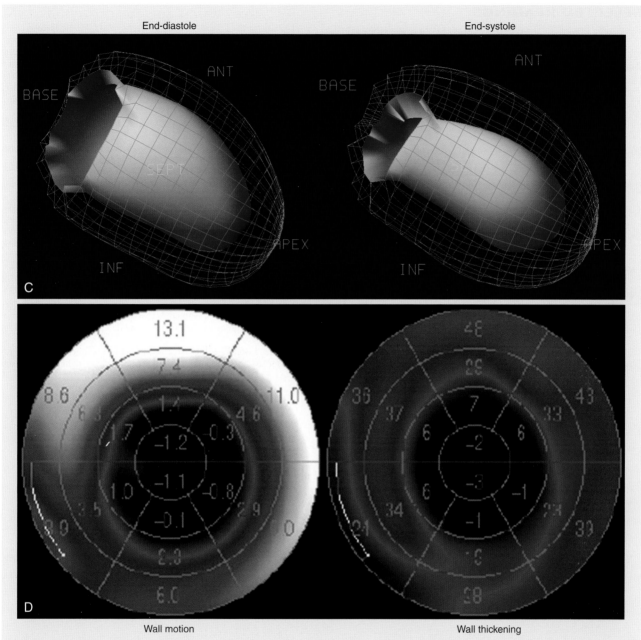

■ **Figure 12-14—Cont'd** The 3D images at end-diastole and end-systole show apical dyskinesia **(C)**. The quantitative analysis of motion and thickening in a 20-segment model is shown in **D**. The dynamic images are shown in Video 12-9.

Comments

Pacemaker syndrome occurs when dyssynchronous contraction results in a WMA and, potentially, a noticeable drop in EF. The images show dyskinesia of the apex even though there is no perfusion abnormality; the perfusion-function mismatch is characteristic. At times, because of the severe WMA, a mild perfusion defect due to partial volume effect can be seen. In some patients, biventricular pacing is needed to correct the problem.

SELECTED READINGS

Agarwal S, Tuzcu EM, Desai MY, et al: Updated meta-analysis of septal alcohol ablation versus myectomy for hypertrophic cardiomyopathy, *J Am Coll Cardiol* 55:823–834, 2010.

Aqel RA, Hage FG, Zohgbi GJ, et al: Serial evaluations of myocardial infarct size after alcohol septal ablation in hypertrophic cardiomyopathy and effects of the changes on clinical status and left ventricular outflow pressure gradients, *Am J Cardiol* 101:1328–1333, 2008.

Atchley AE, Kitzman DW, Whellan DJ, et al: Myocardial perfusion, function, and dyssynchrony in patients with HF: baseline results from the single-photon emission computed tomography imaging ancillary study of the heart failure and a controlled trial investigating outcomes of exercise training (HF-ACTION) trial, *Am Heart J* 158:S53–S63, 2009.

The BEST investigators: A trial of the beta-blocker bucindolol in patients with advanced chronic HF, *N Engl J Med* 344:1659–1667, 2001.

Carrió I, Cowie MR, Yamazaki J, et al: Cardiac sympathetic imaging with mIBG in HF, *JACC Cardiovasc Imaging* 3:92–100, 2010.

de Groote P, Millaire A, Foucher-Hossein C, et al: Right ventricular ejection fraction is an independent predictor of survival in patients with moderate HF, *J Am Coll Cardiol* 32:948–954, 1998.

Dorfman TA, Iskandrian AE: Takotsubo cardiomyopathy: state-of-the-art review, *J Nucl Cardiol* 16:122–134, 2009.

Fang J, Mensah GA, Croft JB, et al: Heart failure-related hospitalization in the U.S., 1979 to 2004, *J Am Coll Cardiol* 52:428–434, 2008.

Ghali JK, Krause-Steinrauf HJ, Adams KF, et al: Gender differences in advanced HF: insights from the BEST study, *J Am Coll Cardiol* 42:2128–2134, 2003.

Hogg K, Swedberg K, McMurray J: Heart failure with preserved left ventricular systolic function; epidemiology, clinical characteristics, and prognosis, *J Am Coll Cardiol* 43:317–327, 2004.

Hunt SA, Abraham WT, Chin MH, et al: ACC/AHA 2005 Guideline Update for the Diagnosis and Management of Chronic Heart Failure in the Adult: a report of the American College of Cardiology/American Heart Association Task Force on Practice Guidelines (Writing Committee to Update the 2001 Guidelines for the Evaluation and Management of Heart Failure): developed in collaboration with the American College of Chest Physicians and the International Society for Heart and Lung Transplantation: endorsed by the Heart Rhythm Society, *Circulation* 112(12):e154–e235, 2005.

Levy D, Kenchaiah S, Larson MG, et al: Long-term trends in the incidence of and survival with HF, *N Engl J Med* 347:1397–1402, 2002.

Iskandrian AE, Garcia EV: *Nuclear Cardiac Imaging: Principles and Applications*, ed 4, New York, 2008, Oxford University Press.

Manno BV, Iskandrian AS, Hakki AH: Right ventricular function: methodologic and clinical considerations in noninvasive scintigraphic assessment, *J Am Coll Cardiol* 3:1072–1081, 1984.

Maron BJ, Maron MS, Wigle ED, et al: The 50-year history, controversy, and clinical implications of left ventricular outflow tract obstruction in hypertrophic cardiomyopathy from idiopathic hypertrophic subaortic stenosis to hypertrophic cardiomyopathy: from idiopathic hypertrophic subaortic stenosis to hypertrophic cardiomyopathy, *J Am Coll Cardiol* 54:191–200, 2009.

Maron MS, Olivotto I, Maron BJ, et al: The case for myocardial ischemia in hypertrophic cardiomyopathy, *J Am Coll Cardiol* 54:866–875, 2009.

Meyer P, Filippatos GS, Ahmed MI, et al: Effects of RV ejection fraction on outcomes in chronic systolic HF, *Circulation* 121:252–258, 2010.

Persson H, Lonn E, Edner M, et al: Diastolic dysfunction in HF with preserved systolic function: need for objective evidence:results from the CHARM Echocardiographic Substudy-CHARMES, *J Am Coll Cardiol* 49:687–694, 2007.

Chapter 13

Other Forms of Heart Disease

Fadi G. Hage, Fahad M. Iqbal, and Ami E. Iskandrian

KEY POINTS

- Myocardial ischemia can be due to diseases other than coronary atherosclerosis. Examples include endothelial dysfunction, bridging of coronary arteries, coronary artery spasm, LV hypertrophy, and certain types of anomalous origins of the coronary arteries. The ischemia in these patients can be detected by stress MPI.

- Anomalous origin of the left main coronary artery from the pulmonary artery in children may produce severe LV dysfunction; this represents a nice example of hibernating myocardium (if treated early, before necrosis).

- First-pass RNA can be used to detect and quantify intracardiac shunts, a seldom used indication because of the wide availability of alternative methods.

- Dextrocardia can affect image interpretation if unrecognized. Attention to the position of the RV is a good clue to the diagnosis.

- Cardiac transplantation continues to pose a challenge because the vasculopathy can be diffuse or focal. A combination of rest and exercise RNA and MPI might be of special interest in these patients.

- Attention to RV size and uptake on MPI can be good clues to the presence of an alternative etiology for chest pain in patients with a normal LV perfusion pattern (such as unsuspected pulmonary thromboembolism).

- Incidental findings on MPI are not uncommon and are discussed in Chapter 16.

- As more children with congenital heart disease are surviving into adulthood, increasing numbers of them also are requiring evaluations for chest pain, heart failure, and arrhythmias. Kawasaki disease, anomalous origin of the coronary arteries, and LV/RV hypertrophy are some of the causes of chest pain in this age group. Knowledge of the anatomy is important for precise interpretation of the images, whether by RNA or MPI.

- Although other imaging methods are used in adults with valvular heart diseases, MPI and RNA are still used to assess LV/RV function, ischemia, and LV dysfunction etiology in those with concomitant CAD.

- Some forms of reversible cardiomyopathy, such as cardiotoxicity, peripartum, and tako-tsubo cardiomyopathy, are discussed in Chapter 12.

BACKGROUND

In this chapter, we discuss less common applications of MPI and RNA in unique or special forms of heart disease. Alternative imaging methods, such as echocardiography, MRI, and CT, are more widely and appropriately used in some of these patients, but nuclear imaging remains an important imaging modality for some of them. The list of these diseases is long and some of the principles were outlined in the introductory bullets to this chapter and, thus, only a few examples will be used.

Case 13-1   Dextrocardia (Figure 13-1)

A 71-year-old man with ESRD, peripheral vascular disease, severe three-vessel CAD by coronary angiography (Figure 13-1, *A*), and moderate aortic stenosis presented with heart failure symptoms. Right heart catheterization demonstrated severe elevation of pulmonary capillary wedge pressure, severe pulmonary hypertension, and depressed cardiac index. The LV function was poor. He underwent rest and 4-hour delayed thallium-201 imaging to assess the extent of viability. The raw images show dextrocardia and situs inversus (Figure 13-1, *B*, and Video 13-1). The MPI showed a large perfusion abnormality in the territories of the LAD and RCA, with partial redistribution. There was severe LV dilatation and LV dysfunction (Figure 13-1, *C*, for uncorrected images and *D* for corrected images). If the dextrocardia is unrecognized, the abnormality could have been attributed to the LCX and RCA disease. He was offered CABG plus aortic valve replacement, but he declined. He died shortly afterward from sudden cardiac death.

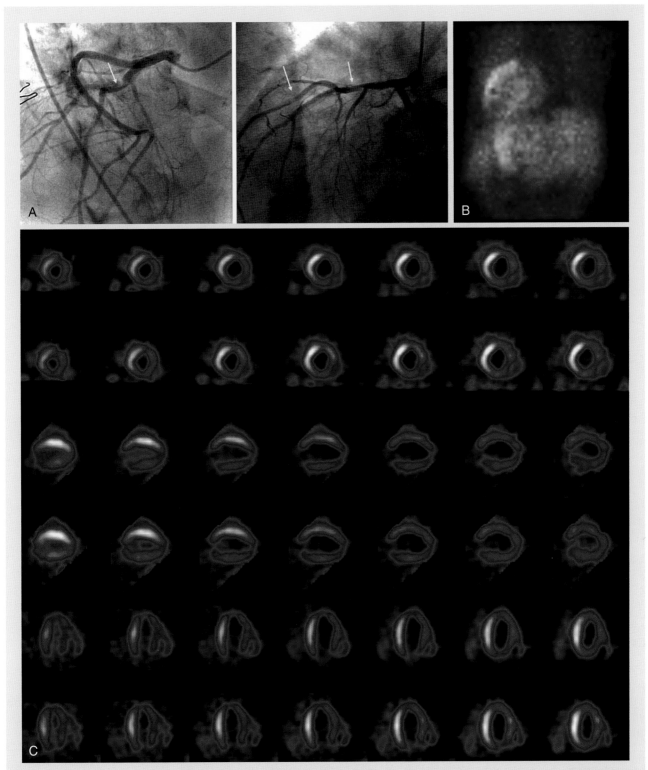

■ **Figure 13-1** Coronary angiogram show severe three-vessel CAD *(arrows)* **(A)**. The rotating images show the dextrocardia and situs inversus. Note that the liver is on the left side (**B** and Video 13-1). The rest and 4-hour delayed thallium-201 MPI scans show a large area of resting perfusion abnormality involving the septum and the inferior wall that improves partially on the delayed images (**C,** uncorrected).

(Continued)

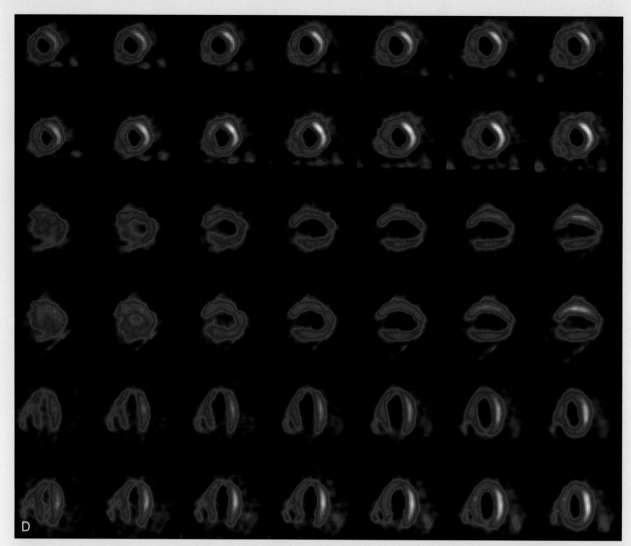

■ **Figure 13-1—Cont'd** The images are corrected post-acquisition to show the normal septal-lateral wall orientation **(D)**. In the uncorrected images, the abnormality could be attributed to LCX and RCA disease. The LV is severely dilated with an EF of 11%.

COMMENTS

Dextrocardia is a rare congenital heart disease, which can be either isolated or associated with other severe congenital abnormalities. Dextrocardia can be part of situs inversus (mirror-image dextrocardia), where the abdominal organs are also displaced in a mirror image. If unrecognized, an incorrect diagnosis could be made as the shortened septum is now in the usual position of the lateral wall. The images can be corrected after acquisition or the 180-degree acquisition arc can be changed from the standard RAO→LPO to LAO→RPO.

Case 13-2   Anomalous Origin of Coronary Arteries (Figure 13-2)

A 68-year-old woman underwent CT for suspected pulmonary embolism. The CT angiogram was negative, but the RCA was reported to have an anomalous origin. Subsequent coronary angiography confirmed that the RCA had an anomalous origin at the left coronary sinus of Valsalva (Figure 13-2, *A*). She underwent treadmill exercise testing and exercised for 7 minutes, achieving her target heart rate without angina or ST changes. The myocardial perfusion images were normal (Figure 13-2, *B*). She was managed conservatively.

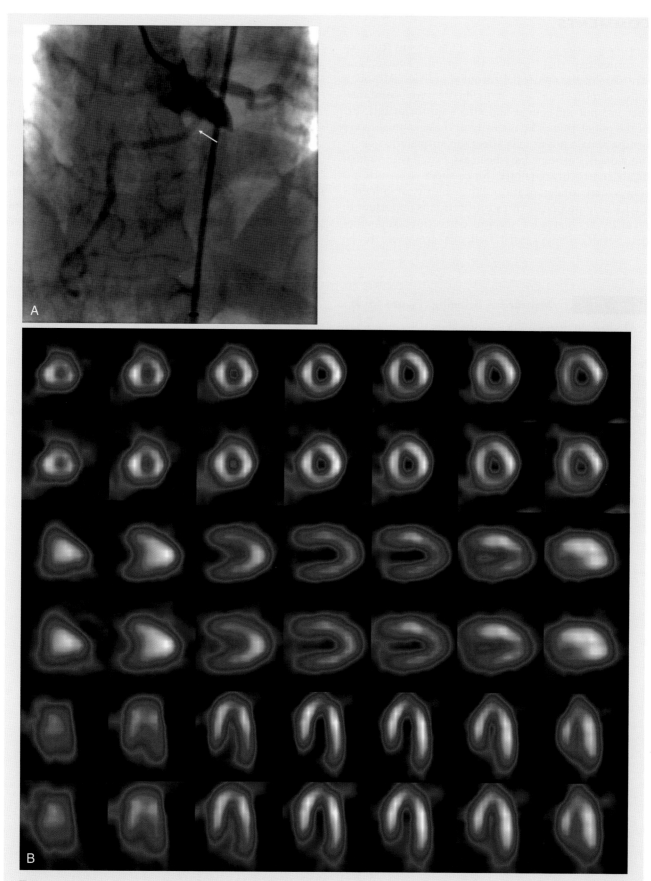

Figure 13-2 Coronary angiogram showing anomalous right coronary artery originating from the left coronary cusp (**A,** *white arrow*). Exercise MPI showed normal perfusion (**B**). The LVEF was normal.

COMMENTS

Coronary artery anomalies include a spectrum of abnormalities that involve the origin, course, and structure of the epicardial coronary arteries. Although these abnormalities are individually rare, combined they are not infrequent and affect approximately 1% of the population. The majority of these anomalies are benign and do not usually affect the normal life span of individuals, but some have been associated with sudden death and/or heart failure. Since the first manifestation is often sudden death and the majority of individuals are asymptomatic, risk stratification is important to identify candidates for surgical correction. Anomalies that result in myocardial ischemia are likely to be harbingers of poor outcome; in particular, anomalous left main coronary artery with a course between the major trunks (aorta and pulmonary artery), anomalous LAD with intraseptal course, a single coronary artery, and an anomalous coronary artery from the pulmonary artery are thought to be associated with ischemia. MPI offers an opportunity to determine the functional significance of these anomalies. MPI is preferably performed with exercise rather than with pharmacologic stress since ischemia is at least partially related to the increased demand associated with exercise, resulting in increased cardiac output, which stretches the arterial trunks and compresses or kinks the anomalous artery between the two trunks.

Case 13-3   **Myocardial Bridging (Figure 13-3)**

A 62-year-old man with dyslipidemia underwent left heart catheterization for the evaluation of chest pain. On coronary angiography, he had myocardial bridging of the LAD with severe LAD stenosis (Figure 13-3, *A*). Exercise MPI showed ischemia in the territory of the LAD, involving the anteroseptal area (Figure 13-3, *B*). He underwent stenting of the LAD, which resulted in symptom resolution and the resolution of ischemia on follow-up MPI (not shown).

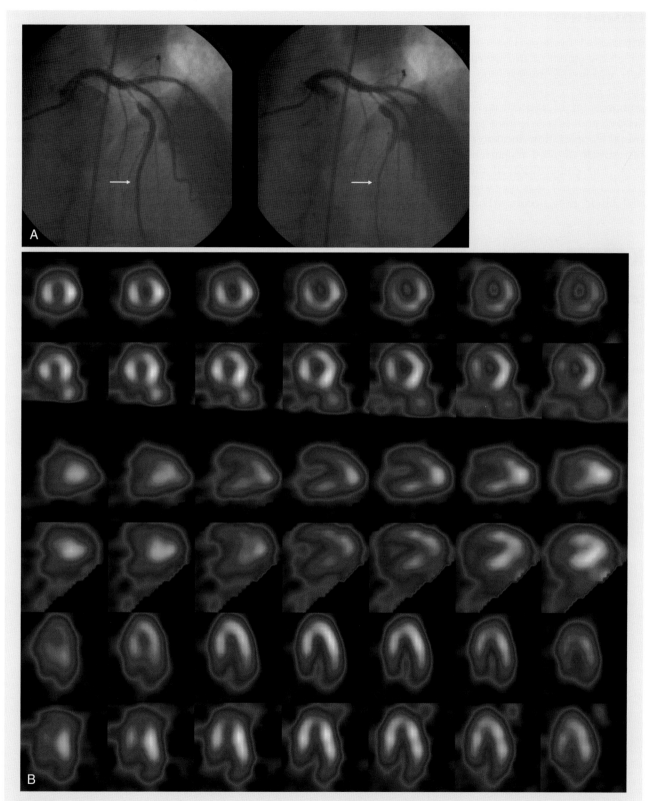

■ **Figure 13-3 A,** Coronary angiogram showing proximal LAD stenosis and LAD myocardial bridging over a long segment *(arrows)* in diastole *(left)* and systole *(right)*. **B,** Exercise MPI showing ischemia in the distribution of the LAD.

COMMENTS

Myocardial bridging is a congenital abnormality in which a segment of an epicardial coronary artery tunnels within the myocardium. When this intramural course is deep within the myocardium, systole causes compression of the coronary artery, which can be severe, and covers a long segment. Several studies, using Doppler flow measurements and intravascular ultrasound, showed impairment of myocardial blood flow. The compression of the coronary artery often extends to early diastole, when most of the myocardial blood flow occurs. Myocardial bridging usually involves the LAD or the septal perforator, but examples of bridging of the LCX and RCA have also been described. Bridging of the LAD and septal perforators are not uncommon in patients with hypertrophic cardiomyopathy and represents one of the mechanisms of ischemia in these patients. Tachycardia may be an important inducer of ischemia in these patients, as it decreases diastolic time and increases the time of compression. Treatments include medical therapy with beta-blockers and calcium channel blockers, stenting of the involved segment, CABG, and myotomy with unroofing of the coronary artery.

Case 13-4 Congenital Heart Diseases (Figure 13-4)

A 21-year-old woman presented with chest pain. She has a history of tetralogy of Fallot and pulmonary atresia, for which she had an RV to pulmonary artery homograft as a child, with subsequent stent placement and dilatations. She underwent regadenoson MPI, which showed normal perfusion and normal LV function. The RV is severely dilated and hypertrophied, indicating severe pulmonary hypertension (Figure 13-4). Right heart catheterization confirmed the presence of pulmonary hypertension. She underwent balloon dilatation of the conduit, with improvement in pressures and symptoms.

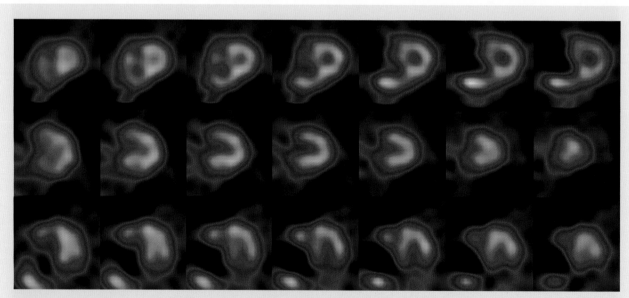

■ **Figure 13-4** Regadenoson MPI showing marked RV dilatation and hypertrophy. The LV perfusion pattern is normal.

COMMENTS

The geometrical shape and thinness of the RV myocardium are not as conducive to imaging as the LV using standard 2D imaging methodologies, such as echocardiography and SPECT. Techniques that can be helpful for the determination of RV function include MRI, first-pass radionuclide ventriculography, and tomographic gated blood pool imaging (gated blood pool SPECT is discussed in Chapter 4). Reliable assessment of RVEF is important in a number of diseases, such as cor pulmonale, pulmonary hypertension, valvular heart disease, RV dysplasia, and heart failure. The RV is also visualized during MPI studies and the RV function can be qualitatively assessed by the gated images. RV dilation, hypertrophy, or dysfunction on MPI performed for the assessment of chest pain can be the first clue to unsuspected pulmonary embolism and should not be ignored.

Case 13-5   Postcardiac Transplantation Vasculopathy (Figure 13-5)

This is the story of a patient with rapidly progressive coronary vasculopathy over a short time-frame requiring numerous imaging and coronary angiographic studies that were very helpful in monitoring deterioration and guiding the need for interventions. The only viable option for such a rapidly progressive case is retransplantation!

A 59-year-old man had cardiac transplantation in February 2009 for ischemic cardiomyopathy, doing well initially. The 2DE showed a normal LVEF of 70%. He had normal stress and rest MPIs (Figure 13-5, *A*, *B*). In February 2010, he had dyspnea on exertion and easy fatigability. The EF by 2DE was 65%. The SPECT images were abnormal (Figure 13-5, *C*). Coronary angiography showed a 60% LAD stenosis, occlusion of the diagonal branch, 75% stenosis of the LCX and obtuse marginal branch (OM-1), and occlusion of the distal RCA. The two lesions (in LCX and OM-1) were stented. In March 2010, he continued to have dyspnea on exertion. Imaging using PET/CT showed ischemia and scar in the LAD territory and ischemia in the RCA territory (Figure 13-5, *D*). Repeat coronary angiography showed proximal 70% LAD stenosis and was stented. In September 2010, he had heart failure symptoms, and a repeat PET study showed three-vessel ischemia (Figure 13-5, *E*). In October 2010, coronary angiography showed severe three-vessel disease and he received four more stents (one in the LAD and three in the LCX). He was listed for retransplantation because of continued symptoms and inability to revascularize diffuse CAD.

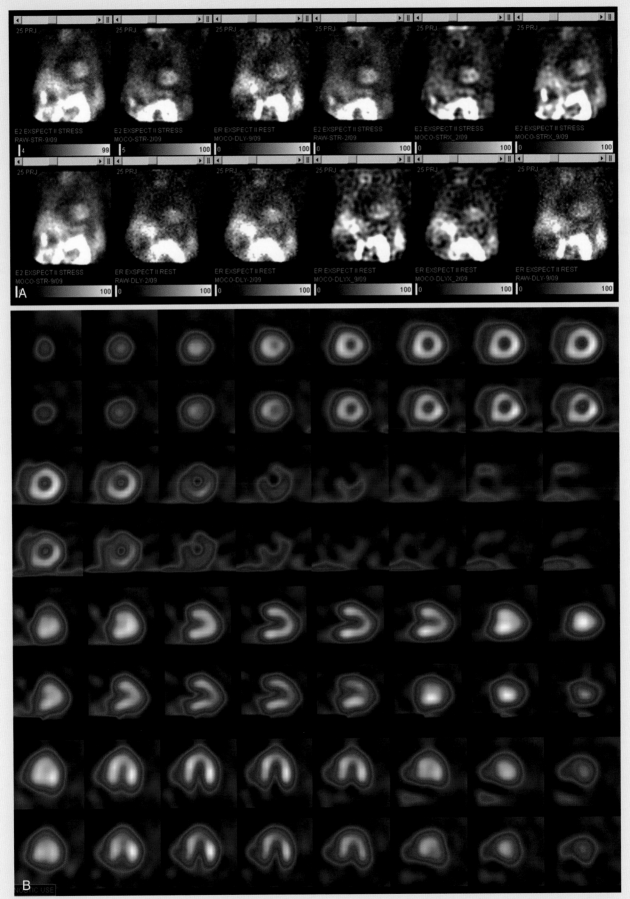

■ **Figure 13-5** Raw images showing classic findings with large region of photon-deficiency around the heart due to a markedly enlarged pericardium; virtually no cavity can be seen due to rocking of the heart in the large pericardium; enlarged RV **(A)**. Normal rest/stress sestamibi SPECT **(B)**.

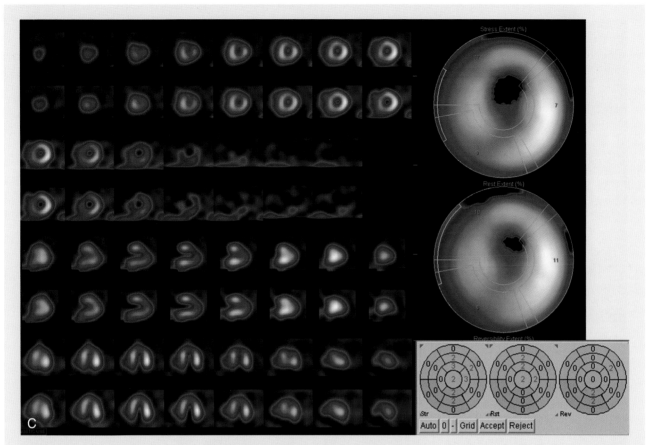

■**Figure 13-5—Cont'd** Abnormal rest/stress sestamibi SPECT obtained 1 year later, showing reversible defects in the distal anterior wall, apex, and distal anterolateral area **(C)**.

(Continued)

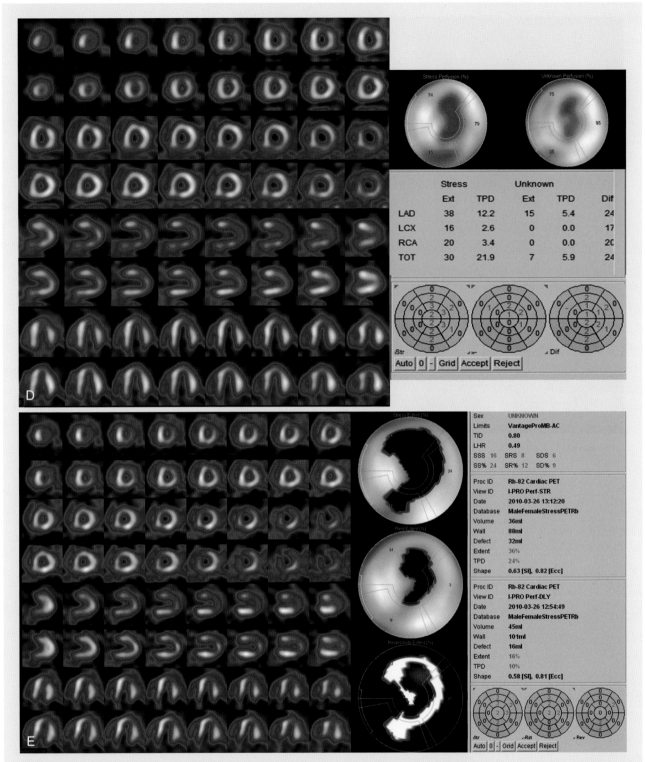

■ Figure 13-5—Cont'd Highly abnormal rest/stress Rb-82 PET obtained 1 month later, showing reversible defects in anterior, lateral, and inferior walls (**D**). Even more abnormal rest/stress Rb-82 PET obtained 6 months after initial PET scan (**E**). The stress images are in the *top rows* in each panel, while the rest images are in the *bottom rows*. The polar maps and segmental scores are shown in the *last two panels*.

COMMENTS

Coronary artery vasculopathy is a leading cause of mortality after heart transplantation. Most heart transplant centers utilize a screening program of routine invasive coronary angiograms in order to identify the presence and severity of the process. There is, therefore, of great interest in the development of noninvasive methods for this purpose. The vasculopathy can be focal or diffuse. The focal type is readily detected by stress MPI, if severe. The diffuse type is more difficult to detect and a combination of rest/exercise RNA using the first-pass method and MPI (see Chapter 4) is more helpful in these patients, but more data are needed. In this patient, MPI with sestamibi and PET with rubidium were very helpful in patient management.

(Case courtesy of Timothy M. Bateman, MD, Co-Director, Cardiovascular Radiologic Imaging, Mid-America Heart Institute, Professor of Medicine, University of Missouri-Kansas City School of Medicine.)

SELECTED READINGS

Avakian SD, Grinberg M, Meneguetti JC, et al: SPECT dipyridamole scintigraphy for detecting coronary artery disease in patients with isolated severe aortic stenosis, *Int J Cardiol* 81:21–27, 2001.

Bonow RO, Carabello BA, Chatterjee K, et al: 2008 Focused Update Incorporated into the ACC/AHA 2006 Guidelines for the Management of Patients With Valvular Heart Disease: A Report of the American College of Cardiology/American Heart Association Task Force on Practice Guidelines (Writing Committee to Revise the 1998 Guidelines for the Management of Patients With Valvular Heart Disease). Endorsed by the Society of Cardiovascular Anesthesiologists, Society for Cardiovascular Angiography and Interventions, and Society of Thoracic Surgeons, *J Am Coll Cardiol* 52:e1–142, 2008.

Chen M, Lo H, Chao I, et al: Dipyridamole Tl-201 myocardial single photon emission computed tomography in the functional assessment of anomalous left coronary artery from the pulmonary artery, *Clin Nucl Med* 32:940–943, 2007.

De Luca L, Bovenzi F, Rubini D, et al: Stress-rest myocardial perfusion SPECT for functional assessment of coronary arteries with anomalous origin or course, *J Nucl Med* 45:532–536, 2004.

Demirkol MO, Yaymaci B, Debeş H, et al: Dipyridamole myocardial perfusion tomography in patients with severe aortic stenosis, *Cardiology* 97:37–42, 2002.

Lee YS, Moon DH, Shin JW, et al: Dipyridamole TI-201 SPECT imaging in patients with myocardial bridging, *Clin Nucl Med* 24:759–764, 1999.

Tamás E, Broqvist M, Olsson E, et al: Exercise radionuclide ventriculography for predicting post-operative left ventricular function in chronic aortic regurgitation, *JACC Cardiovasc Imaging* 2:48–55, 2009.

Thomas GS, Kawanishi DT: Situs inversus with dextrocardia in the nuclear lab, *Am Heart Hosp J* 6:60–62, 2008.

Turgut B, Kitapci MT, Temiz NH, et al: Thallium-201 myocardial SPECT in a patient with mirror-image dextrocardia and left bundle branch block, *Ann Nucl Med* 17:503–506, 2003.

Vallejo E, Morales M, Sánchez I, et al: Myocardial perfusion SPECT imaging in patients with myocardial bridging, *J Nucl Cardiol* 12:318–323, 2005.

Wu Y, Yen R, Lee C, et al: Diagnostic and prognostic value of dobutamine thallium-201 single-photon emission computed tomography after heart transplantation, *J Heart Lung Transplant* 24:544–550, 2005.

Yasuda H, Taniguchi K, Takahashi T, et al: Thallium-201 single-photon emission computed tomography: quantitative assessment of left ventricular perfusion and structural change in patients with chronic aortic regurgitation, *Clin Cardiol* 28:564–568, 2005.

Zurick AO, Klein JL, Stouffer GA: Scintographic evidence of severe myocardial hypoperfusion in a patient with left anterior descending coronary artery bridging–case report and review of the literature, *Am J Med Sci* 336:498–502, 2008.

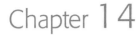

Chapter 14

Patients With Chest Pain in the Emergency Department

Fadi G. Hage, Eva V. Dubovsky, and Ami E. Iskandrian

KEY POINTS

- History, physical examination, 12-lead ECG, and serum markers are useful, but not sufficient, for diagnosing ACS and for risk stratification in the ED.

- MPI can be useful in the decision-making process in patients with suspected ACS in the ED and can be cost-effective if used in suitably selected patients.

- The logistics of ED imaging are not insurmountable but require coordination between ED staff and the nuclear laboratory and a good method of communication between the two. In most institutions, this is performed 8 to 12 hours daily and on weekdays only.

- Normal perfusion on rest MPI in a patient with chest pain in the ED predicts a low risk for cardiovascular events, especially if obtained during the episode or soon after resolution.

- A normal rest MPI in patients at intermediate or high clinical risk of ACS should be followed up with an outpatient stress MPI.

- An abnormal rest MPI in ED patients can occur in patients with ischemia (but no infarction) who have normal serum troponin levels and no acute ST/T changes.

- A stress rather than a rest MPI can be considered in patients suspected of having ACS in the ED if they are pain free and have two sets of negative cardiac markers and no acute ischemic ECG changes.

- A perfusion defect on rest MPI in patients with chest pain in the ED and with no history of prior MI should prompt admission to the hospital with plans for early coronary angiography. Such an abnormal perfusion pattern can represent myocardial ischemia or necrosis. The presence of a regional wall motion/thickening abnormality does not help in the differentiation but normal regional function favors ischemia.

- A normal rest MPI can be observed in patients with ischemia if the tracer injection is performed long after the resolution of chest pain. The precise window of opportunity is not well defined but some have suggested 2 hours. We believe that for better sensitivity, this window should be as narrow as possible, and preferably less than 1 hour.

- Rest-BMIPP (β-methyl-*p*-[^{123}I]iodophenyl-pentadecanoic acid) may be useful for imaging patients presenting to the ED after symptom resolution. This tracer however is not yet approved for clinical use in the United States.

BACKGROUND

Evaluating patients presenting to the ED with chest pain suspicious for ACS continues to be a challenge to both emergency physicians and consulting cardiologists. The initial questions posed are:

1. Is emergent treatment in the ED warranted?
2. What is the disposition of the patient: admit to the inpatient or observation unit or discharge home?

This is obviously not an idle question; millions of patients in the United States, and many more across the globe, have such a presentation. The decision-making in these situations has enormous personal, social, and economic implications. An overly conservative strategy of admitting all patients suspected of having ACS places an excessive economic burden on the health care system and stretches the availability of inpatient beds. On the other hand, ED physicians are acutely aware of the small but medicolegally significant proportion of patients who are inappropriately discharged home while having true ACS only to develop MI or sudden cardiac death shortly afterwards.

An ECG should be performed within 5 minutes of presentation and interpreted immediately to help stratify patients with ST elevation to immediate coronary angiography with PCI or, alternatively, fibrinolytic therapy. The ECG can also be helpful in confirming the diagnosis of ACS and in risk stratification in patients without ST elevation. However, a normal ECG (or one with nonspecific findings) is not uncommon in patients presenting to the ED with chest pain or pain-equivalent symptoms and should not be used to exclude the diagnosis of ACS. Similarly, an elevated cardiac troponin assay at presentation to the ED signifies a high-risk patient, but since several hours are required after symptom onset for cardiac troponins to become detectable in the serum, its absence is not reassuring. Furthermore, even patients with normal serial cardiac markers can be at high risk of future MI since rest (unstable) angina does not necessarily result in elevation of serum biomarkers.

In Figure 14-1, we show a suggested flowchart for the evaluation of patients presenting to the ED with chest

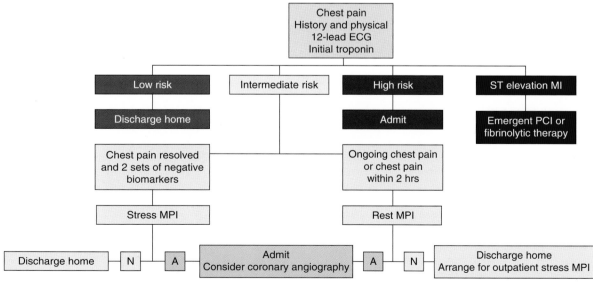

■ **Figure 14-1** Suggested flow diagram for patients presenting to the ED with chest pain and/or symptoms concerning for ACS. MPI is indicated in patients deemed at intermediate risk. *A,* Abnormal MPI; *N,* normal MPI.

pain and/or chest pain–equivalent symptoms such as dyspnea or jaw pain. In our experience, after the screening ECG is interpreted and STEMI is excluded, a detailed history is the most important factor that can help triage the patient. A clinical assessment is formed that incorporates findings on the history and physical examination, ECG, laboratory tests (including troponins), and other available pertinent results such as chest radiography. Patients judged to have an MI or determined to be at high risk for short-term adverse events are admitted to the hospital for further treatment and evaluation that may include coronary angiography. Alternatively, patients judged to have noncardiac chest pain or who are at low risk can be safely discharged home to follow-up with their primary care physicians who can consider further work-up as deemed appropriate.

For patients in the intermediate-risk group, MPI could help in the decision-making process. The following cases illustrate the usefulness of MPI in these patients and the pitfalls that should be avoided.

Case 14-1   **Chest Pain With Negative Biomarkers (Figure 14-2)**

A 43-year-old woman with hypertension developed chest pain radiating to the left arm, described as squeezing in nature, while driving to work. She does not smoke tobacco but has a significant family history for premature CAD. She was pain free when she arrived in the ED. The physical examination was benign. There were no acute ischemic changes on the ECG. Initial cardiac markers were negative.

A rest MPI was performed (Figure 14-2, *A*) and revealed normal perfusion and LV function. The tracer was injected 2 hours after onset of the pain. The patient was discharged home. She underwent regadenoson MPI 2 days later (she could not walk on a treadmill due to a recent history of lower extremity trauma). The stress images were also normal (Figure 14-2, *B*). She was treated with risk factor modifications.

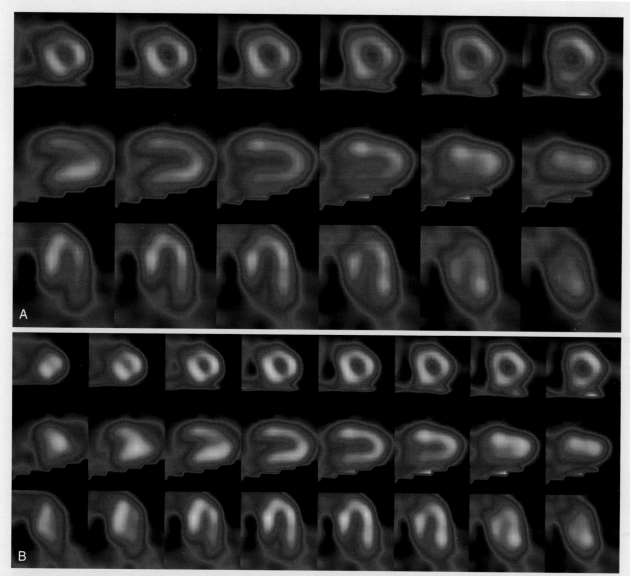

■ **Figure 14-2** Rest MPI performed with tracer injection in the ED revealing normal perfusion **(A)**. The LVEF was normal at 71%. The stress images were obtained 2 days later with regadenoson, again showing a normal perfusion pattern **(B)**.

COMMENTS

The majority of patients presenting to the ED with chest pain have a normal or nondiagnostic ECG. When management is directed by clinical examination, ECG, and initial cardiac markers, an important percentage of patients with ACS (including MI) are erroneously discharged home.

Approximately 50% are admitted to the hospital, but more than 50% of them will not have ACS as their final diagnosis. Multiple observational and randomized studies have demonstrated the usefulness of rest MPI in reducing unnecessary hospitalizations and cost in patients with suspected ACS, compared to routine care. The true value of a rest MPI is apparent when it is completely normal. In a patient with active chest pain presenting to the ED, a negative scan rules out the diagnosis of MI and has a very high negative predictive value for subsequent cardiac events over the next few months.

In the large Emergency Room Assessment of Sestamibi for the Evaluation of Chest Pain (ERASE chest pain) trial, which randomized 2475 patients with chest pain or other symptoms suggestive of ACS with a normal or nondiagnostic ECG to usual care versus care directed by Tc-99m sestamibi or tetrofosmin rest MPI, hospitalization in patients not having ACS was significantly decreased (42% vs. 52%, $p < .001$). There was no difference on triage of patients with ACS (including those having MI) and no difference in 30-day outcomes. In this study, a rest MPI added an average of 30 minutes to the evaluation but reduced unnecessary hospitalizations without adversely affecting outcomes or reducing indicated hospitalizations. A cost-effectiveness analysis of a multicenter study by Heller et al. suggested a mean cost savings per patient of $4,258; in a smaller randomized study, Stowers et al. found a median hospital cost saving per patient of $1,843 in the MPI group.

Case 14-2   **Abnormal Rest MPI After Subsidence of Chest Pain (Figure 14-3)**

A 34-year-old woman with no prior cardiac history or risk factors for CAD presented to the ED within 1 hour of onset of chest pain with associated nausea. She did not have a family history of premature CAD and was not on any medications. Her physical examination was unrevealing except for an elevated blood pressure of 153/92 mm Hg. The ECG showed nonspecific T-wave changes but no ST shifts and no Q waves. Initial troponin was negative. Rest MPI performed during the episode of chest pain revealed a moderate-sized perfusion defect in the distribution of the LCX with normal LVEF (Figure 14-3, *A*, *B*). The patient was admitted to the cardiac care unit and treated for ACS. Serial cardiac markers showed an increase in the troponin I and CK-MB levels. Coronary angiogram (Figure 14-3, *C*) showed an occlusion at the ostium of the second obtuse marginal branch of the LCX, which was successfully treated with a drug-eluting stent.

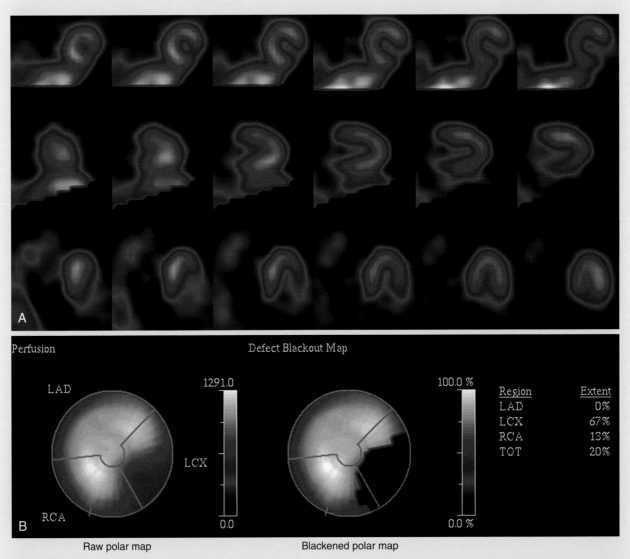

■ **Figure 14-3** Rest MPI performed after injection of tracer during active chest pain in the ED. There is an LCX abnormality **(A)**. The polar maps reveal the abnormality to be moderate sized **(B)**.

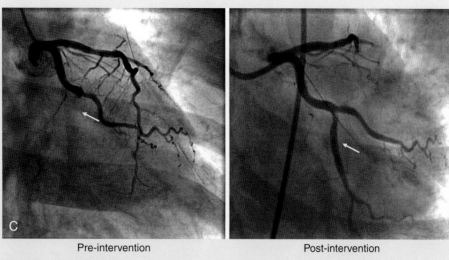

Pre-intervention   Post-intervention

■ **Figure 14-3—Cont'd** Coronary angiogram showing the culprit lesion in the second obtuse marginal *(arrows)* **(C)**.

COMMENTS

Rest MPI is more sensitive than ECG or initial cardiac markers for the detection of an acute non-STEMI. While cardiac troponins are a highly sensitive and specific marker of myocardial necrosis, detection in the serum can be delayed for several hours after the ischemic episode. The management of patients with ST elevation, ST depression, hemodynamic instability, or electric instability should be performed without the need for any imaging. Many patients, however, have baseline abnormalities on their ECG that preclude appropriate interpretation or present with nonspecific changes or normal ECG.

A rest MPI can show abnormalities in patients with ischemia but no infarction even though biomarkers are normal, especially if the tracer is injected while the pain is ongoing, as was performed in this patient. The posterior location of the MI in our patient may have masked the ECG findings. In the study by Varetto et al. of 64 patients suspected of having an ACS on presentation to the ED with nondiagnostic ECG, resting Tc-99m sestamibi MPI had a sensitivity of 100% for the detection of MI or significant CAD (13 patients with MI and 14 patients with significant CAD), a specificity of 92%, and a negative predictive value of 100% for subsequent cardiac events over an 18-month follow-up period.

Case 14-3   **Stress Testing After Rest MPI (Figure 14-4)**

A 49-year-old man with a history of type 2 DM, hyperlipidemia, and asthma presented to the ED with a several-day history of intermittent chest pain. At presentation, he had been pain free for 2 hours. His initial work-up, including ECG and cardiac markers, was negative. An initial normal rest MPI was followed by an exercise stress test. The test was stopped after he walked 4.5 minutes and achieved a peak heart rate of 124 bpm with the development of chest pain. The MPI revealed a reversible defect (Figure 14-4, *B*). Coronary angiography showed severe three-vessel CAD. He subsequently underwent CABG with no complications.

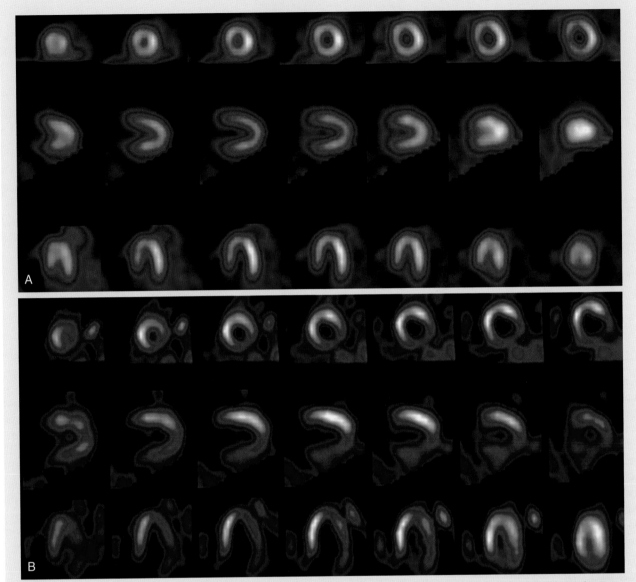

■ **Figure 14-4** Rest MPI showing a normal perfusion pattern **(A)**. The exercise MPI shows perfusion abnormalities in the RCA and LCX territories at a low level of exercise with transient ischemic dilatation **(B)**. The LVEF was 57%. Coronary angiography showed three-vessel disease (not shown).

COMMENTS

The sensitivity of rest MPI to detect perfusion abnormalities falls with increasing time from symptom resolution. MPI has an almost 100% sensitivity for the detection of ischemia if injection of the flow tracer is performed *during* active chest pain. Emphasis should be placed on the timing of the tracer (Tc-99m) injection rather than imaging (imaging is generally performed 1 hour after injection). On the other hand, LV function is representative of the function at the time of imaging rather than tracer injection, and therefore, regional wall motion abnormalities may not be apparent if imaging is delayed until after ischemia resolution, even though a perfusion abnormality will still be present. The presence of a wall motion abnormality, however, does not necessarily mean myocardial necrosis; it could simply be due to postischemic stunning. As this case illustrates, it is important to realize that a normal MPI performed *after* symptom resolution should be followed-up by a stress test in intermediate- to high-risk patients. Studies in which Tc-99m sestamibi was injected after balloon deflation during PCI have revealed that perfusion is normal in most patients when injection is delayed 90 to 120 minutes; abnormal in only 15% of those injected 30 to 60 minutes after balloon deflation; and abnormal in all patients when the tracer is injected during balloon occlusion. Obviously, balloon occlusion differs from unprovoked ischemia in its impact on the threshold of ischemia detection, but the principle remains the same.

Case 14-4 **Attenuation Artifact Versus True Perfusion Defect (Figure 14-5)**

A 78-year-old man presented to the ED with chest tightness and shortness of breath. A rest MPI showed decreased perfusion in the inferior myocardium with depressed LVEF and a diffuse wall motion abnormality (Figure 14-5, *A*). The patient was admitted to the hospital. An adenosine MPI was performed, showing a fixed abnormality in the inferior myocardium that is unchanged compared to the rest MPI. Attenuation-correction using gadolinium line sources corrected the inferior perfusion abnormality, which was thought to be due to diaphragmatic attenuation artifact superimposed on partial volume effect due to the wall motion abnormality (Figure 14-5, *B*). A prior MPI, performed 3 years earlier, showed a similar perfusion pattern but the left ventricular function was better preserved. The patient was managed for nonischemic heart failure and discharged without undergoing repeat coronary angiography. He had no vascular events during long-term follow-up and a left heart catheterization, performed at another institution, showed normal coronary angiography.

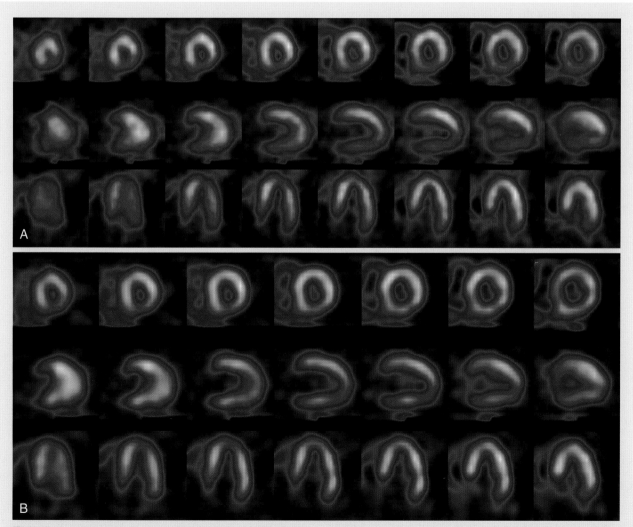

■ **Figure 14-5** Rest MPI showing mild inferior abnormality that is unchanged from a study conducted 3 years earlier **(A)**. With attenuation correction, the perfusion pattern is normal **(B)**. The LVEF was reduced. This patient is known to have a dilated cardiomyopathy.

COMMENTS

Rest MPI is useful in the ED in patients who have had no prior MI because both old and new MIs (as well as ischemia) can demonstrate a perfusion abnormality and it is difficult to differentiate between the two. The reality, however, is that patients with no CAD but other forms of cardiomyopathy can also present with chest pain. Obviously, patients with a depressed LVEF, especially if previously undiagnosed, require admission to the hospital and treatment.

The Achilles heel of MPI in the ED, especially in patients with enlarged hearts, is attenuation artifacts, namely diaphragmatic attenuation in men and breast attenuation in women. Unlike conventional stress/rest imaging, here the decision has to be made on a single set of images. The use of attenuation correction therefore becomes even more important in identifying artifacts. Needless to say, high-quality images are a prerequisite and imaging should be repeated if there is excessive motion or extracardiac activity interfering with image interpretation.

Case 14-5   Metabolic Imaging (Figure 14-6)

A 73-year-old woman known to have DM, hypertension, and hyperlipidemia for more than 20 years but with no known prior cardiac disease presented to the ED at noon after experiencing intermittent chest pains for a total of 4 hours during the previous night. The patient was chest pain free on presentation and had no ECG changes except for evidence of LV hypertrophy. Cardiac troponin was negative on serial testing. An I-123 BMIPP rest scan was performed as part of a research project in addition to thallium-201 imaging. The thallium images showed a mild lateral wall abnormality while the BMIPP images showed a more convincing moderate-sized defect in the lateral wall of the left ventricle (Figure 14-6). The patient was admitted to the cardiac care unit where subsequent coronary angiography confirmed a tight stenosis in the LCX that was treated with PCI.

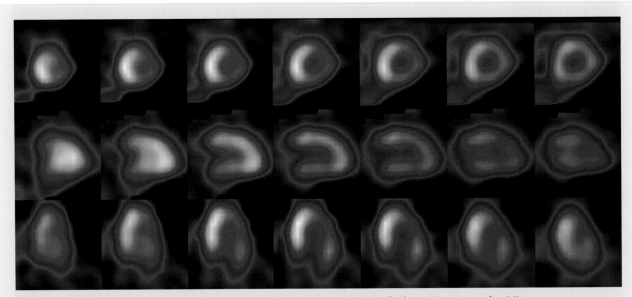

■ **Figure 14-6** Rest BIMPP SPECT images showing decreased uptake in the lateral wall. The LVEF was normal at 56%.

COMMENTS

As mentioned earlier, the sensitivity for detecting perfusion abnormalities drops when imaging patients using Tl-201 or Tc-99m–labeled perfusion tracers the longer one waits after symptom resolution. I-123 BMIPP, if approved, is ideally suited for the purpose of detecting remote ischemia. Long-chain fatty acids are the main source of energy for the normoxic heart. BMIPP is a methyl-branched modified fatty acid that does not undergo beta-oxidation and is therefore metabolically trapped in the myocardium with slow washout, allowing for excellent high-quality imaging. The delay in normalization of fatty acid metabolism after normalization of perfusion has facilitated the concept of ischemic memory. In essence, after an ischemic episode fatty acid metabolism may be abnormal for hours to days. Thus, in a patient presenting several hours after symptom resolution, rest BMIPP imaging may show an area of sustained metabolic abnormality despite a normal rest Tc-99m (or Tl-201) MPI. The diagnostic yield of a rest-BMIPP scan may be comparable to a stress-MPI and can be particularly attractive to perform in the ED setting in unstable patients not suitable to undergo stress. A recent study evaluated the efficacy and safety of BMIPP in patients who presented to an ED with symptoms suggestive of ACS. The BMIPP scanning added an incremental value to currently available clinical information for the early diagnosis of ACS and allowed for the determination to be made much earlier in the evaluation process.

Case 14-6   Abnormal Exercise MPI (Figure 14-7)

A 72-year-old woman with DM, hypertension, and continued tobacco use presented to the ED with episodic atypical chest pain of several weeks' duration. She was pain-free at the time of presentation. ECG and troponin levels were normal. Since the patient presented at night, she had two sets of negative cardiac markers before the morning and underwent exercise MPI. After 4 minutes on the treadmill, she had ST segment depression on the ECG and developed chest pain. MPI revealed decreased tracer uptake in the anterior, septal, and inferior myocardium (Figure 14-7, *A*). The LVEF was normal. Coronary angiography showed occlusion of the LAD and severe disease of the RCA (Figure 14-7, *B*). She underwent PCI with stent placement in the RCA. There was no evidence of MI on serial measurements of cardiac markers.

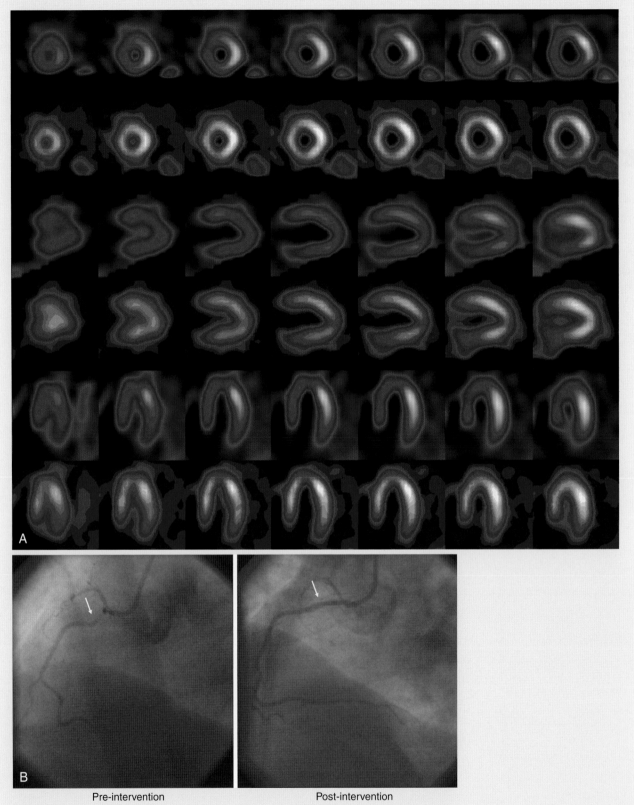

Pre-intervention   Post-intervention

■ **Figure 14-7** Exercise/rest MPI showing reversible perfusion abnormalities in the LAD and RCA territories **(A)**. The polar maps show the abnormality to be large, involving 30% of the myocardium (not shown). Coronary angiogram showing severe stenosis of the RCA *(arrows)*, which was stented **(B)**. The mid LAD was occluded and the distal vessel had a poor runoff (not shown).

COMMENTS

Although a normal rest MPI in the ED setting is reassuring, a small percentage of patients manifest ischemia only during stress testing and, therefore, a follow-up stress study should be performed shortly after discharge from the ED. In patients who are chest pain free on presentation, a resting MPI is less useful as detailed in Case 14-5. If myocardial necrosis is excluded through serial evaluation of cardiac biomarkers, an exercise or vasodilator stress imaging can be utilized to guide management. Such an approach is safe and can efficiently reduce unnecessary admissions while reliably identifying patients with evidence of stress-induced myocardial ischemia, thereby substantially shortening length of stay and decreasing cost. This approach is also very useful in patients who present at night or in the early morning to the ED when there is no 24-hour imaging service available. Stress testing early the next day is ideal, and optimally the results from two sets of biomarkers should be available. In this patient, exercise testing reproduced the pain and was associated with ST depression and multivessel reversible perfusion abnormality. Same-day coronary angiography showed three-vessel disease and the patient underwent an uneventful CABG.

Case 14-7 Stress Imaging Only (Figure 14-8)

A 60-year-old woman known to have hypertension and hyperlipidemia but with no known prior cardiac disease presented to the ED with chest pain for the previous 8 hours. The patient described the pain as aching to burning in quality with radiation to the left shoulder and the left side of the neck. She has a long history of gastroesophageal reflux disease that has caused her to have a burning sensation in her epigastric area and at times in the chest as well. The current pain is described as being different from her "usual" reflux pain and was resolved after taking a 325mg aspirin tablet at home more than 2 hours prior to presentation. The ECG and cardiac troponin levels were normal. The patient was exercised on a treadmill the same afternoon; she exercised for more than 10 minutes using the Bruce protocol without chest pain. The MPI showed normal perfusion and a normal LVEF (Figure 14-8). A rest study was not performed and the patient was discharged home to follow up with her primary care physician for further evaluation and management of her esophageal disease.

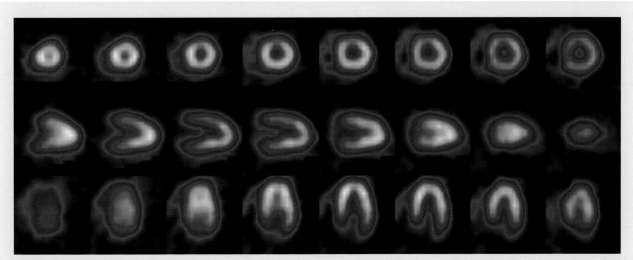

■ Figure 14-8 Exercise-only MPI after 10 minutes 10 seconds on a treadmill using a Bruce protocol showing a normal perfusion pattern. The LVEF was normal.

COMMENTS

Although there are multiple protocols for the performance and acquisition of MPI, stress-only MPI has many advantages. This protocol consists of performing stress imaging as the initial procedure, and if the images are entirely normal (as in this case), then there is no need to proceed to rest imaging and the study is complete. This protocol is more convenient to the patient, saves money and time, and importantly, decreases radiation exposure. There is now convincing evidence that patients with normal stress-only images have a similar low mortality rate compared to those who have a normal stress and rest MPI. Indeed, this has been the norm for performing stress MPIs at our institution for many years. In order to avoid missing significant abnormalities, it is important to realize that if there is any uncertainty as to whether there is a perfusion defect on the stress images, a rest study is obtained. This same paradigm can be used in the ED, as was performed here, in patients who are appropriate to undergo stress testing. Obviously, this protocol requires high-quality images and experience in interpreting these images. The use of quantitative analysis and attenuation correction is helpful but not mandatory.

SELECTED READINGS

Abbott BG, Abdel-Aziz I, Nagula S, et al: Selective use of single-photon emission computed tomography myocardial perfusion imaging in a chest pain center, *Am J Cardiol* 87:1351–1355, 2001.

Aqel RA, Hage FG, Ellipeddi P, et al: Usefulness of three posterior chest leads for the detection of posterior wall acute myocardial infarction, *Am J Cardiol* 103:159–164, 2009.

Aqel R, Zoghbi GJ, Bender LW, et al: Myocardial perfusion imaging after transient balloon occlusion during percutaneous coronary interventions, *J Nucl Cardiol* 14:221–228, 2007.

Barnett K, Feldman JA: Noninvasive imaging techniques to aid in the triage of patients with suspected acute coronary syndrome: a review, *Emerg Med Clin North Am* 23:977–998, 2005.

Chang SM, Nabi F, Xu J, et al: Normal stress-only versus standard stress/rest myocardial perfusion imaging: similar patient mortality with reduced radiation exposure, *J Am Coll Cardiol* 55:221–230, 2010.

Dilsizian V, Bateman TM, Bergmann SR, et al: Metabolic imaging with beta-methyl-p-[(123)I]-iodophenyl-pentadecanoic acid identifies ischemic memory after demand ischemia, *Circulation* 112:2169–2174, 2005.

Forberg JL, Hilmersson CE, Carlsson M, et al: Negative predictive value and potential cost savings of acute nuclear myocardial perfusion imaging in low risk patients with suspected acute coronary syndrome: a prospective single blinded study, *BMC Emerg Med* 9:12, 2009.

Fram DB, Azar RR, Ahlberg AW, et al: Duration of abnormal SPECT myocardial perfusion imaging following resolution of acute ischemia: an angioplasty model, *J Am Coll Cardiol* 41:452–459, 2003.

Heller GV, Stowers SA, Hendel RC, et al: Clinical value of acute rest technetium-99m tetrofosmin tomographic myocardial perfusion imaging in patients with acute chest pain and nondiagnostic electrocardiograms, *J Am Coll Cardiol* 31:1011–1017, 1998.

Iskandrian AE: Stress-only myocardial perfusion imaging a new paradigm. *J Am Coll Cardiol* 55:231–233, 2010.

Knott JC, Baldey AC, Grigg LE, et al: Impact of acute chest pain Tc-99m sestamibi myocardial perfusion imaging on clinical management, *J Nucl Cardiol* 9:257–262, 2002.

Kontos MC, Dilsizian V, Weiland F, et al: Iodofiltic acid I 123 (BMIPP) fatty acid imaging improves initial diagnosis in emergency department patients with suspected acute coronary syndromes: a multicenter trial, *J Am Coll Cardiol* 56:290–299, 2010.

Kontos MC, Jesse RL, Schmidt KL, et al: Value of acute rest sestamibi perfusion imaging for evaluation of patients admitted to the emergency department with chest pain, *J Am Coll Cardiol* 30:976–982, 1997.

Radensky PW, Hilton TC, Fulmer H, et al: Potential cost effectiveness of initial myocardial perfusion imaging for assessment of emergency department patients with chest pain, *Am J Cardiol* 79:595–599, 1997.

Stowers SA, Eisenstein EL, Th Wackers FJ, et al: An economic analysis of an aggressive diagnostic strategy with single photon emission computed tomography myocardial perfusion imaging and early exercise stress testing in emergency department patients who present with chest pain but nondiagnostic electrocardiograms: results from a randomized trial, *Ann Emerg Med* 35:17–25, 2000.

Swinburn JM, Stubbs P, Soman P, et al: A. Rapid assessment of patients with non-ST-segment elevation acute chest pain: troponins, inflammatory markers, or perfusion imaging? *J Nucl Cardiol* 9:491–499, 2002.

Tatum JL, Jesse RL, Kontos MC, et al: Comprehensive strategy for the evaluation and triage of the chest pain patient, *Ann Emerg Med* 29:116–125, 1997.

Udelson JE, Beshansky JR, Ballin DS, et al: Myocardial perfusion imaging for evaluation and triage of patients with suspected acute cardiac ischemia: a randomized controlled trial, *JAMA* 288:2693–2700, 2002.

Varetto T, Cantalupi D, Altieri A, et al: Emergency room technetium-99m sestamibi imaging to rule out acute myocardial ischemic events in patients with nondiagnostic electrocardiograms, *J Am Coll Cardiol* 22:1804–1808, 1993.

Wackers FJ: Chest pain in the emergency department: role of cardiac imaging, *Heart* 95:1023–1030, 2009.

Wackers FJ, Lie KI, Liem KL, et al: Potential value of thallium-201 scintigraphy as a means of selecting patients for the coronary care unit, *Br Heart J* 41:111–117, 1979.

Chapter 15

Viability Assessment

Ami E. Iskandrian and Jaekyeong Heo

KEY POINTS

- Assessment of myocardial viability is helpful in patients with severe CAD and severe LV dysfunction.

- Every living patient has viable myocardium; the question is not whether there is viable myocardium, but whether there is a sufficiently large area of viable myocardium to result in an improved outcome with coronary revascularization.

- The benefits of coronary revascularization include improvement of regional function, EF, quality of life, and survival.

- Viable but jeopardized myocardium is demonstrated on PET by a mismatch between myocardial flow and metabolism.

- Viable myocardium is demonstrated on SPECT by regional tracer concentration in the myocardium.

- Thallium-201, Tc-99m sestamibi, and Tc-99m tetrofosmin are sequestered within the cytoplasm and mitochondria, respectively; hence, their uptake requires an intact cell membrane, which indicates viable cells.

- LV dysfunction may be due to a combination of different pathophysiologic processes, such as hibernation, stunning, remodeling, and scar, either in a given patient or vascular territory. Additional factors, such as valvular heart disease and hypertensive cardiomyopathy, might also play a role in LV dysfunction.

- Appropriate patient selection, imaging protocol, and reporting can impact patient management and outcome.

- Patients with viable myocardium do better with coronary revascularization than medical therapy.

- Patients with extensive nonviable myocardium do not benefit from coronary revascularization; on the contrary, they do better with medical therapy.

BACKGROUND

The first description of myocardial stunning was by Heyndricks in 1975, subsequently modified by Braunwald and Kloner in 1982. The first description of hibernation was by Diamond in 1978, subsequently used by Rahimtoola in 1985. Since 1980, and with the advent of imaging, there has been an increasing interest in this topic with an ever-increasing number of publications (Figure 15-1). In 1989, Rahimtoola wrote, "hibernating myocardium is a relatively uncommon response to reduced myocardial blood flow (MBF) at rest whereby the heart down-regulates its function to the extent that the MBF and function are once again in equilibrium and, as a result, neither necrosis nor ischemic symptoms are present." That description is probably still true in some, but not all, patients.

There are several reasons why patients with CAD develop LV dysfunction. These include infarction (scar), hibernation, stunning, and remodeling, which refers to regional dysfunction in segments remote from culprit zones. Obviously, and not uncommonly, the dysfunction can be due to a coexisting problem, such as hypertension, valvular heart disease (either preexisting, such as aortic valve disease, or developing as a result of LV dysfunction, such as mitral regurgitation), or dilated cardiomyopathy, just to mention the most common causes.

Simply stated, the dysfunction can be described as either reversible, if the MBF is restored to normal (stunning and hibernation are prototypes of viable myocardium), or irreversible (scar); the fate of remodeled areas will depend on whether the initiating process was scar or hibernation/stunning (assuming there are no concomitant causes of dysfunction and coronary revascularization is feasible, complete, and maintained for a prolonged period of time).

Many PET studies validated Rahimtoola's observation and showed a reduction in resting MBF and increased glucose utilization (measured via F-18-fluorodeoxyglucose,

FDG), the flow-metabolism mismatch. The normal myocardium has several sources of energy production, but it uses glucose or fatty acids preferentially. Each mole of glucose produces 2 moles of ATP in the cytoplasm when metabolized anaerobically and 36 moles of ATP when metabolized aerobically in the mitochondria. Glycolysis generates 17% more ATP than fatty acids for an equal amount of oxygen used and is the reason why metabolism is shifted to glucose utilization in ischemic states.

Other studies, including those in animal models, however, challenged the temporal relationship between changes in MBF and LV dysfunction. What emerged is the following scenario: early after a severe stenosis develops, regional LV function decreases even though the resting MBF is normal. But because the hyperemic MBF is blunted (due to the severe stenosis), any increase in demand will produce an episode of stunning (regional dysfunction that persist after flow returns back to normal), which is a flow-function mismatch (reduced function but normal resting MBF). This stunning, however, is not isolated to a single episode; rather it keeps repeating itself with such frequency that the function never has a chance to return to normal. As function deteriorates, the MBF decreases because the demand is lower (setting the bar progressively lower). Unlike the original hypothesis, the reduction in MBF is a secondary phenomenon rather than the initiating element. Repetitive stunning, as this process is known, presents itself as chronic LV dysfunction. Adaptation results in structural changes in the myocardium that are collectively referred to as dedifferentiation, along with degeneration in the intracellular and extracellular structures. The intensity of these changes and the degree of LV dilatation will determine how completely and rapidly the function will normalize after coronary revascularization. Because of the tenuous relationship between supply and demand, these patients are at a higher risk for infarction and death. Finally, some studies have suggested that sudden death due to ventricular arrhythmias is due to functional dennervation involving segments even larger than those with flow or metabolic changes (so called perfusion–innervation mismatch).

Various imaging methods have relied on a number of different principles to elucidate what is viable and what is not. These studies have come to be known as viability testing. The implication being, that the techniques can identify patients with CAD and LV dysfunction who could benefit from coronary revascularization because the dysfunction is secondary to hibernation or stunning. As a caveat, there is no standard definition of what "benefit" means. "Benefit" has been previously defined as an improvement in regional function, EF, symptoms, quality of life, and/or survival. There are also no guidelines on when to assess for "benefit," because, as mentioned earlier, degenerative changes may take some time to recover, as long as 6 to 12 months!

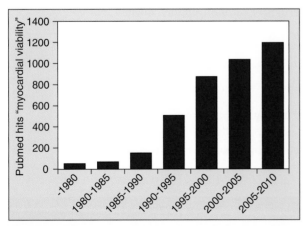

■ **Figure 15-1** The number of publications on myocardial viability over a 30-year period.

PATIENT SELECTION

Proper candidates for viability testing are patients with severe LV dysfunction (EF < 35%) and severe CAD. This is not a test for patients with a normal EF, diastolic heart failure, patients with mild CAD but with LV dysfunction, or patients with dilated cardiomyopathy. It may seem simple and straightforward, but we continue to be surprised by the nature of some of the requests!

This book will not discuss the role of other imaging modalities as they are discussed in the other companion books.

NUCLEAR IMAGING FOR VIABILITY ASSESSMENT

The use of PET is discussed in Chapter 18. What follows is a discussion on the use of single photon tracers, Tl-201– and Tc-99m–labeled tracers (sestamibi and tetrofosmin). Both Tl and Tc-tracers are considered flow tracers and their sequestration inside the cells (cytoplasm and mitochondria, respectively) require intact cell membrane (hence, the technique is sometimes described as testing cell membrane integrity). The uptake is proportional to regional MBF at rest, in fact, it may overestimate *resting* MBF. There is one difference, however, between the tracers and that is the process of redistribution; thallium redistributes and sestamibi/tetrofosmin do not (or do so minimally). That difference, therefore, dictates how imaging is done. With thallium, rest and 4-hour redistribution, stress and 4-hour delayed reinjection imaging, or stress, 4-hour delayed, and 24-hour delayed imaging can be performed. Tc tracers are used for rest, stress and rest, or rest and stress imaging. Many studies have found that thallium results are comparable to Tc tracers for viability testing, but we have used thallium in most of our studies (with or without sestamibi) using a protocol we have used for almost two decades. This is because we believe that a reduction in resting MBF does occur in some patients, or myocardial segments in a given patient, that can be missed by Tc tracers.

OUR VIABILITY PROTOCOL

We use rest and 4-hour delayed thallium imaging in patients with known severe CAD by coronary angiography or hemodynamically unstable patients. In these patients, we do not use stress testing as the question being asked is simple; is there sufficient viable myocardium that revascularization would benefit the patient? We continue to do these studies at the bedside in unstable patients using a mobile gamma camera and planar imaging.

In the remaining patients, we perform rest and 4-hour delayed thallium imaging followed by vasodilator sestamibi imaging. We compare the two thallium images to each other and compare the better of the two to the sestamibi images (all images are with gated SPECT). At one time, we gave a low dose of dobutamine after the first set of sestamibi images were acquired and acquired a second

set of sestamibi images (fourth set for the study) during the infusion to study contractile reserve. This is no longer done because the additional information was not helpful. We have, thus, limited the study to three sets of images.

On evaluating the images, we examine the L/H ratio and look for any evidence of redistribution on the delayed thallium images and stress-induced ischemia. One way of looking at the segments showing redistribution on the 4-hour delayed rest thallium images is that they are a poor man's PET perfusion–metabolism mismatch; the initial image is a flow image, but the delayed image is a metabolic image related to tracer exchange across metabolically active cell membranes. We use automated methods to quantify tracer uptake. If the two thallium images reveal severe and extensive fixed defects, we omit the stress portion. If the initial thallium images are normal, we omit the 4-hour delayed images.

CHARACTERIZATION OF DYSFUNCTIONAL MYOCARDIUM

When reviewing perfusion and regional function, we define segments (or more practically vascular territories or walls) as follows:

1. *Scar (nonviable):* Severe perfusion defect on initial thallium image (<50% tracer activity), no evidence of redistribution on the delayed thallium images, and no stress-induced ischemia (if a stress study was obtained). These segments have severe wall motion/thickening abnormalities at rest.
2. *Hibernating:* Reduced tracer activity on initial thallium images with evidence of redistribution on delayed thallium imaging. The stress images, if available, will show a more severe or extensive abnormality. These segments have severe wall motion/thickening abnormalities at rest.
3. *Stunning:* Reduced tracer activity on initial thallium images with no redistribution on delayed thallium images but with stress-induced ischemia (a stress study is needed to define stunning). These segments have severe wall motion/thickening abnormalities at rest.
4. *Remodeled:* These segments have reduced initial activity on thallium images with no redistribution on the delayed thallium images and no stress induced ischemia.

The entire protocol can be completed in 5 hours and provides comprehensive information on rest and stress perfusion and function. We do not routinely give nitroglycerin before thallium injection, but most of our patients are on long-acting nitrates. Further, we do not image at 24 hours as the image quality by then is poor and unreliable.

In some segments (walls or patients), there is slight redistribution on the thallium images or a slight stress-induced ischemia on the sestamibi images, but the activity level at its best is still very low. For example, the activity increases from 10% to 20% from the initial to the delayed thallium images. Twenty percent is still too low to have an impact on a positive outcome. Thus, not all reversible defects are created equal. Similarly, not all fixed defects are the same either. Fixed defects with greater than 50% activity have a sufficient amount of viable myocardium (subepicardial), which could be quite useful in preventing further remodeling, serious arrhythmias, and preserving diastolic function. They can even preserve the systolic function with exercise, which may produce symptomatic improvement, although it may not produce an improvement in the regional function at rest.

Tracer activity and recovery of function exist on a continuum. A good rule of thumb is that 80% tracer activity corresponds to an 80% chance for improvement and 40% represents a 40% chance for improvement with coronary revascularization. In general, the presence of ischemia is greater than 90% accurate in predicting functional recovery, if good target vessels are present. This is the reason for including a stress study in the protocol; reversibility is more commonly detected with stress than at rest.

REVERSIBILITY VERSUS VIABILITY

In conventional ischemia detection imaging, the terms *ischemia* and *scar* are used to reflect reversible and fixed defects, respectively. When it comes to viability assessment, these terms should be used more judiciously. For example, a mild fixed defect is a combination of scar and viable myocardium. Reporting it as scar is not really correct (is the glass half-full or half-empty?). With traditional reporting, the glass is half-empty. For the purpose of viability studies, we suggest a "glass half-full" approach to reporting. There is much more viability in the myocardium of patients with ischemic cardiomyopathy, in general, than our reports would suggest. This has been verified by several studies, as well as our own experience. In general, reversible defects (activity >50% on rest images), mild or moderate fixed defects (>70% and >50% activity, respectively), and normal segments are all viable. Thus, viable myocardium does not need to be *jeopardized*, a term often reserved for the presence of ischemia, and which we do not recommend. It is true, however, that the presence of ischemia makes it much more likely that these types of segments will recover after coronary revascularization, but improvement can occur in the other types of segments as well.

IMPLICATIONS OF THE VIABILITY STUDIES

Data from multiple single-center studies, taken collectively, shows that patients with viable myocardium tend to do better with coronary revascularization than with optimal medical management, while those with large areas of nonviable myocardium may actually do better with optimal medical management. Given the comorbid disease burden, patients who undergo coronary artery bypass surgery do better than those undergoing percutaneous coronary interventions. Our recent data are shown in Figure 15-2. Finally, segments are not the same as patients (they are useful for generating p values but have little clinical relevance). The presence of viability should be gauged for the entire LV myocardium, as well as each vascular territory. It is unlikely that a single segment abnormality will have a major impact on outcome whether or not a correct classification is completed. The presence of viable myocardium in at least 50% of two of the three vascular territories is a good threshold to start considering coronary revascularization. One final note, the location of viable myocardium is just as important as its extent. For example, patients with occlusion of the LAD after the first septal perforator branch and the first diagonal branch may have nonviable myocardium in the distal half of the anterior wall and septum (plus the apex) and viable myocardium in the basal half; coronary revascularization by implanting a mammary artery into the distal vessel will not be helpful to restore function even though half the vascular territory is viable!

ACUTE MYOCARDIAL INFARCTION

At times, it is important to determine the status of viability in a target vascular territory in patients who have regional dysfunction and an occluded artery in the setting of an acute MI. In general, the same principles should apply, including the need for stress testing, or the lack thereof. It should be remembered, however, that in acute occlusion, tracer injection before and after the vessel is opened has been used to assess the extent of the salvaged myocardium. The defect size, when the artery is occluded, defines the area at risk, while the defect size after recanalization defines the area of necrosis. The difference between the defect sizes defines the extent of myocardial salvage. In patients with an occluded artery, tracer delivery to the infarct zone is via collaterals, which often are underestimated by coronary angiography.

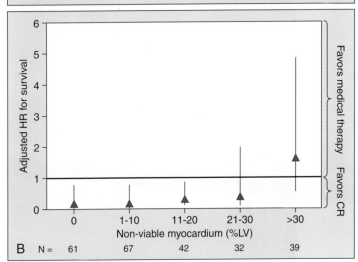

■ **Figure 15-2 A,** Kaplan-Meier survival curves of patients undergoing viability testing treated medically and with coronary revascularization. The survival is better with coronary revascularization. **B,** The hazard ratios for medical management versus revascularization in patients undergoing viability testing. Those with large nonviable myocardium do better with medical management, while those with small nonviable myocardium do better with coronary revascularization. *(From Hage FG, Venkataraman R, Aljaroudi W, et al. The impact of viability assessment using myocardial perfusion imaging on patient management and outcome,* J Nucl Cardiol *17:378-387, 2010.)*

Case 15-1   **Patient With Heart Failure (Figure 15-3)**

A 64-year-old man with known CAD presents with shortness of breath, nocturnal dyspnea, and occasional mild exertional angina. These symptoms have been increasing over a 9-month period. Risk factors include hypertension, hyperlipidemia, and smoking. Abnormal physical exam findings included sinus tachycardia, S_3 gallop, 1/6 systolic ejection murmur at the apex, and bilateral basilar rales. The ECG showed ST/T-wave changes. The 2DE showed an LVEF of 25% and mild mitral regurgitation. Coronary angiography showed severe three-vessel disease with an LV filling pressure of 25 mm Hg. The viability study is shown in Figure 15-3. The patient had an uneventful CABG and the EF normalized 3 months later.

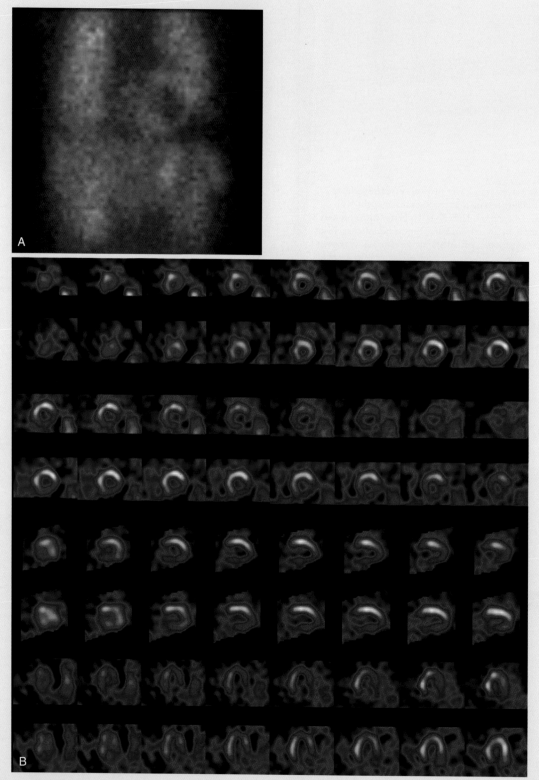

■ **Figure 15-3** Rest and 4-hour redistribution (delayed) thallium-201 gated SPECT images. The L/H ratio is markedly increased, consistent with an elevated LV filling pressure **(A)**. The perfusion images show a large abnormality on the initial images with considerable improvement (redistribution) on the delayed images consistent with hibernation **(B)**. Selected slices are shown. *Note:* It is important to be certain that the initial images are on the top and the delayed on the bottom because many computer programs may show the same set of images twice or in reverse order.

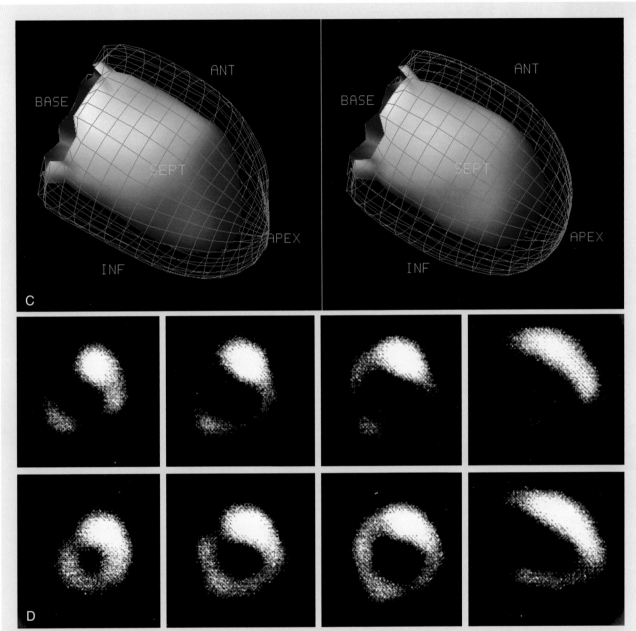

■ **Figure 15-3—Cont'd** The gated images in 3D show severe LV dysfunction (**C**). Another example of considerable redistribution, by rest/delayed thallium imaging, in a patient with severe LV dysfunction is shown in **D**.

Case 15-2   **Patient With Known CAD and Severe LV Dysfunction (Figure 15-4)**

A 66-year-old woman underwent stress testing because of chest pain and shortness of breath (Class IIB, NYHA). Her medications included an angiotensin-converting enzyme inhibitor, digoxin, a diuretic, a beta-blocker, aspirin, and a statin. The ECG showed LBBB. The 2DE showed severe LV dysfunction. The images are shown in Figure 15-4, *A* and *C* (top 2 rows). She subsequently underwent coronary angiography, which showed severe three-vessel disease and severe LV dysfunction. She then underwent rest-redistribution thallium imaging. The images are shown in Figure 15-4, *B* and *C* (bottom 2 rows). She underwent CABG and the EF normalized within 2 months of surgery.

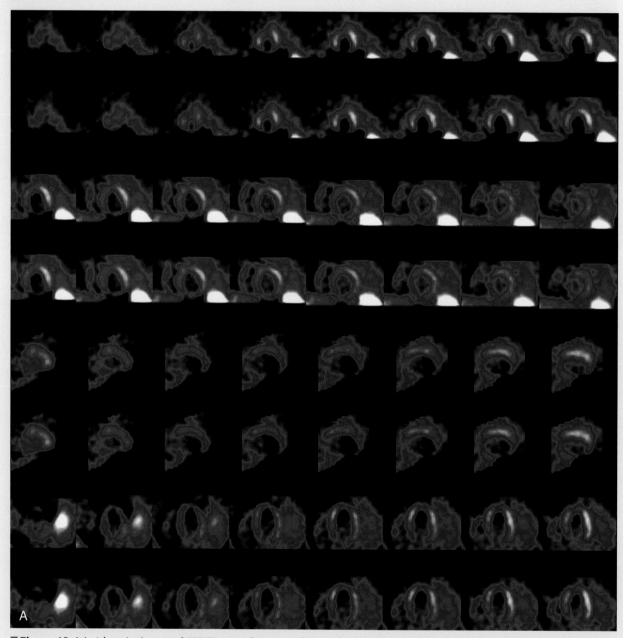

■ **Figure 15-4 A,** Adenosine/rest gated SPECT sestamibi images. There is a large perfusion abnormality on the sestamibi images.

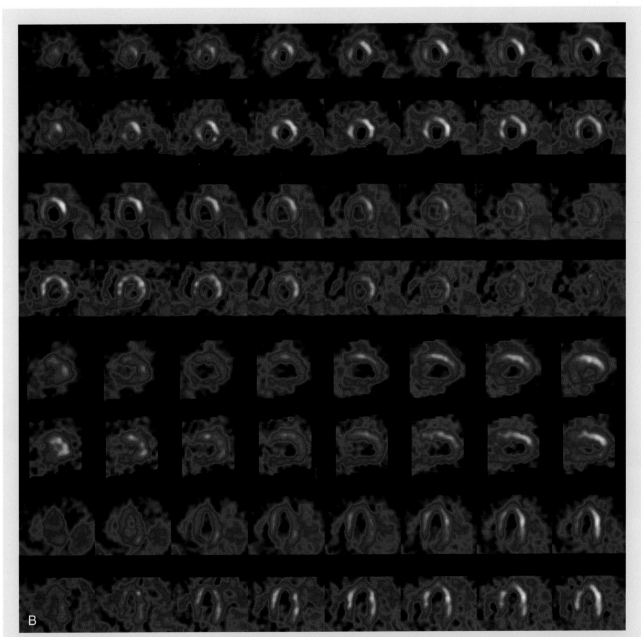

■ **Figure 15-4—Cont'd. B,** Rest-delayed thallium images. The initial thallium images show an abnormality similar to the one in the sestamibi images. However, the delayed thallium images show considerable redistribution.

(Continued)

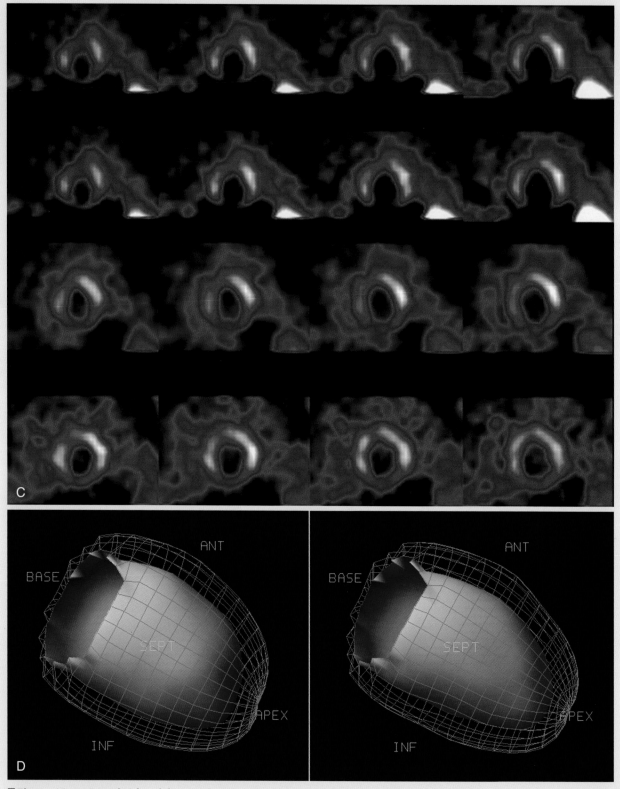

■ **Figure 15-4—Cont'd.** Selected slices are shown together for comparison **(C)**. The 3D gated images show severe LV dysfunction **(D)** . In this patient, the delayed thallium images were crucial for viability assessment.

Case 15-3   **Patient Listed for Cardiac Transplantation (Figure 15-5)**

A 49-year-old man with CAD and heart failure with low EF was transferred for cardiac transplantation consideration. He underwent viability testing. The results are shown in Figure 15-5. He subsequently underwent successful CABG and did well, with marked improvement in EF and symptoms.

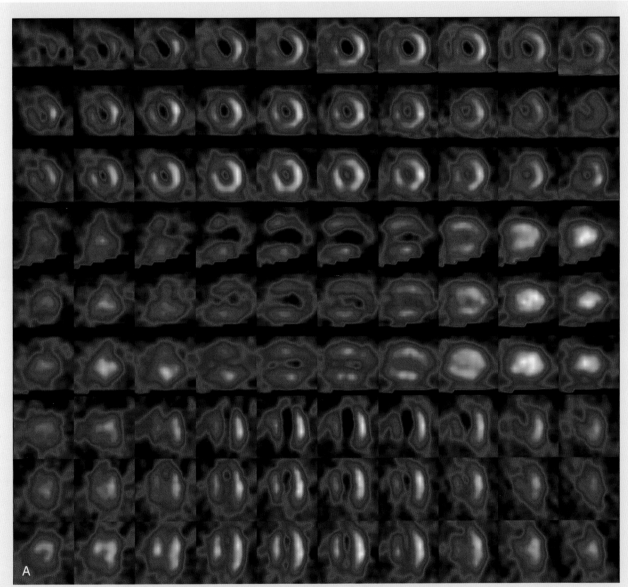

■ **Figure 15-5** The rest, 4-hour delayed thallium-201 images, and the regadenoson sestamibi images **(A)**. The initial thallium images reveal a large perfusion abnormality *(middle row)* with evidence of redistribution on the delayed images *(bottom row)*. The stress sestamibi images reveal a more severe and widespread ischemia *(top row)* with transient ischemic dilatation. The lung thallium uptake is increased (not shown) and the LV function is markedly decreased with an EF of 22%.

(Continued)

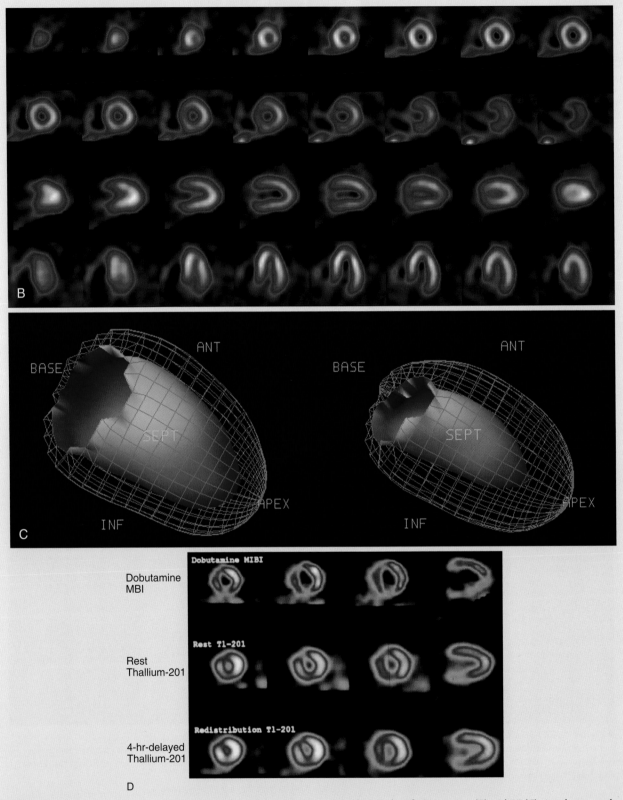

Dobutamine
MBI

Rest
Thallium-201

4-hr-delayed
Thallium-201

■ **Figure 15-5—Cont'd** The 1-year postoperative stress sestamibi images reveal normal perfusion pattern **(B)** and EF **(C)**. Another example using dobutamine as the stress agent in a patient with a history of bronchospasm is shown in **D**. The stress abnormality is more severe than the initial thallium abnormality.

Case 15-4 **Patient With Heart Failure and Not a Candidate for Coronary Revascularization (Figure 15-6)**

A 74-year-old woman underwent viability testing for heart failure symptoms. She had diabetes, hypertension, hyperlipidemia, and had previously undergone CABG and coronary interventions. The ECG showed RBBB. Significant physical findings included cardiomegaly, S$_3$ gallop, and the murmur of mitral regurgitation. Because of exercise limitations, she underwent adenosine stress testing. The images are shown in Figure 15-6. The coronary angiogram revealed severe CAD and poor run-off at the distal vessels. The 2DE showed moderate to severe mitral regurgitation and an enlarged, poorly functioning LV. She was not considered a good candidate for coronary revascularization and had ICD implantation.

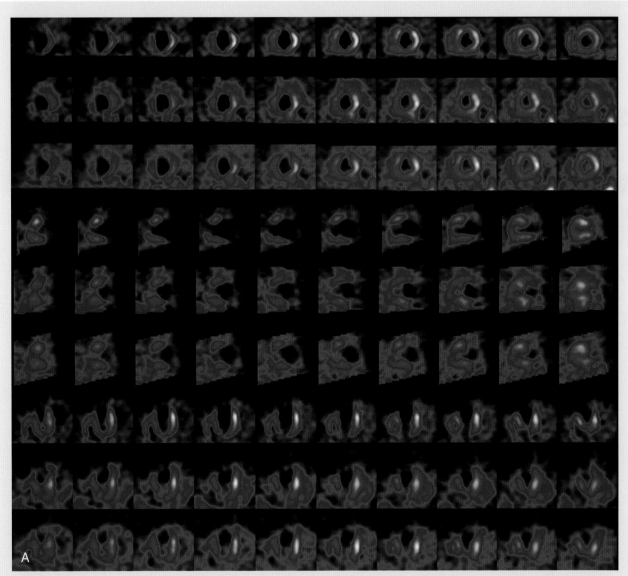

■ **Figure 15-6** Adenosine sestamibi and rest-redistribution thallium images are shown **(A)**. There are large and extensive perfusion defects on the initial thallium images *(middle row)*, which remain unchanged on the delayed thallium images *(bottom row)* or on the stress sestamibi images *(upper row)*.

(Continued)

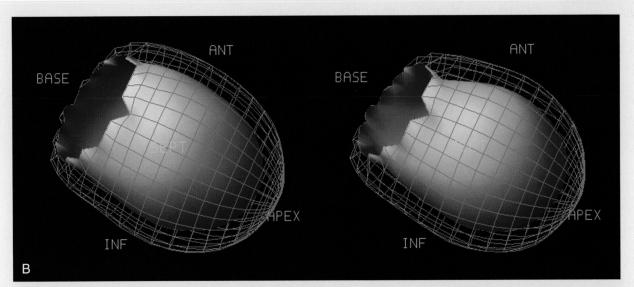

■**Figure 15-6—Cont'd.** The gated images reveal severe LV dysfunction with cavity dilatation **(B)**. In this patient, the same information was obtained from the thallium and sestamibi images.

Case 15-5   **Stress Testing in Patient With Heart Failure and Angina (Figure 15-7)**

A 67-year-old man underwent exercise testing for the evaluation of heart failure symptoms and chest pain. He had multiple coronary risk factors, including continued tobacco abuse. The physical examination was benign except for hypertension. The ECG showed LVH with ST-T changes. He exercised for 5 minutes on the treadmill and stopped because of shortness of breath. The exercise ECG was nondiagnostic for ischemia because of baseline ST changes. The images are shown in Figure 15-7. He did well following coronary angiography and revascularization. In this patient, the sestamibi images alone provided the needed information. The EF improved to 64% at 3 months after CABG, with the resolution of regional dysfunction.

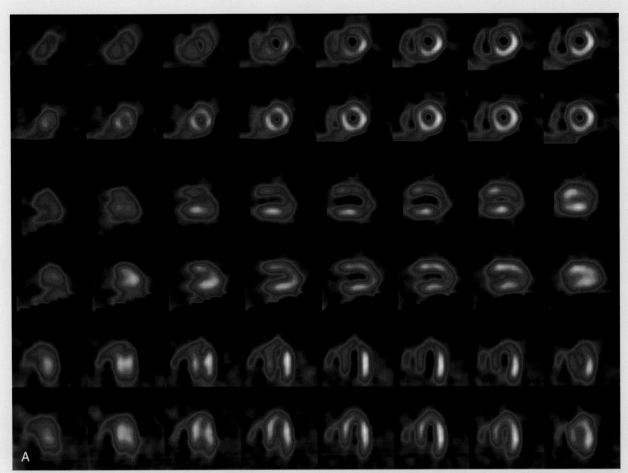

■ **Figure 15-7** Exercise and rest sestamibi images **(A)**. There are large perfusion defects with almost complete reversibility on the rest images.

(Continued)

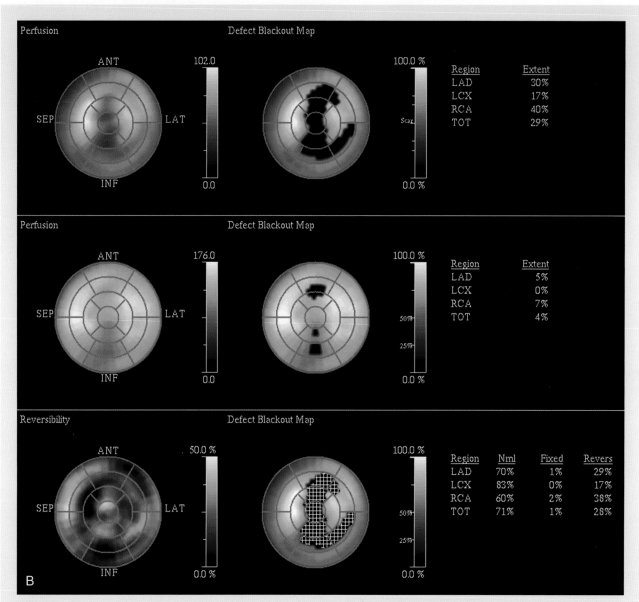

■ Figure 15-7—Cont'd The polar maps show the extent of the perfusion abnormality **(B)**. The regional LV function is depressed at rest (not shown), suggesting repetitive stunning as the cause of the LV dysfunction.

COMMENTS (Cases 15-1 through 15-5)

These five cases demonstrate a small spectrum of perfusion findings in patients with ischemic cardiomyopathy. In Case 1, the viable myocardium, based on the rest–delayed thallium imaging, in all likelihood represented hibernation, and stress-rest sestamibi images may have underestimated the degree of viability. This was evident in Case 2, where the stress and rest sestamibi images showed scar while the thallium images showed viable myocardium. In Case 3, the stress sestamibi images revealed a much greater degree of ischemia than the rest thallium images, which is expected because of the limited flow reserve in severe stenoses. The role of thallium imaging can best be appreciated by comparing the sestamibi images to the initial (top and middle rows) versus delayed thallium images (top and bottom rows). Hence, the thallium images added useful information. There was evidence of extensive nonviable myocardium regardless of which tracer or protocol was used in Case 4. In Case 5, on the other hand, the standard stress and rest sestamibi images revealed clear evidence of ischemia, which in this case meant viable myocardium. Thus, thallium imaging would not have added additional value in this patient. One final note: when using Tc-tracers, a rest-stress protocol may be superior to a stress-rest protocol because the rest study will not be affected by residual activity from the stress study.

These five cases also demonstrate the spectrums of regional dysfunction in relation to perfusion. Regional dysfunction was observed in segments with normal perfusion (remodeled), severe fixed defects (scar), rest reversible defects (hibernation), and stress-induced reversible defects (stunning).

SELECTED READINGS

Allman KC, Shaw LJ, Hachamovitch R, et al: Myocardial viability testing and impact of revascularization on prognosis in patients with coronary artery disease and left ventricular dysfunction: a meta-analysis, *J Am Coll Cardiol* 39:1151–1158, 2002.

Bax JJ, Schinkel AF, Boersma E, et al: Extensive left ventricular remodeling does not allow viable myocardium to improve in left ventricular ejection fraction after revascularization and is associated with worse long-term prognosis, *Circulation* 110:II18–II22, 2004.

Beanlands RS, Nichol G, Huszti E, et al: F-18-fluorodeoxyglucose positron emission tomography imaging-assisted management of patients with severe left ventricular dysfunction and suspected coronary disease: a randomized, controlled trial (PARR-2), *J Am Coll Cardiol* 50:2002–2012, 2007.

Beller GA, Budge LP: Viable: yes, no, or somewhere in the middle? *JACC Cardiovasc Imaging* 2:1069–1071, 2009.

Canty JM Jr., Fallavollita JA: Chronic hibernation and chronic stunning: a continuum, *J Nucl Cardiol* 7:509–527, 2000.

Chareonthaitawee P, Gersh BJ, Araoz PA, et al: Revascularization in severe left ventricular dysfunction: the role of viability testing, *J Am Coll Cardiol* 46:567–574, 2005.

Cleland JG, Pennell DJ, Ray SG, et al: Myocardial viability as a determinant of the ejection fraction response to carvedilol in patients with heart failure (CHRISTMAS trial): randomised controlled trial, *Lancet* 362:14–21, 2003.

Dilsizian V, Narula J: Qualitative and quantitative scrutiny by regulatory process: is the truth subjective or objective? *JACC Cardiovasc Imaging* 2:1037–1038, 2009.

Gioia G, Powers J, Heo J, et al: Prognostic value of rest-redistribution tomographic thallium-201 imaging in ischemic cardiomyopathy, *Am J Cardiol* 75:759–762, 1995.

Hage FG, Venkataraman R, Aljaroudi W, et al: The impact of viability assessment using myocardial perfusion imaging on patient management and outcome, *J Nucl Cardiol* 17:378–387, 2010.

Moore CA, Cannon J, Watson DD, et al: Thallium 201 kinetics in stunned myocardium characterized by severe postischemic systolic dysfunction, *Circulation* 81:1622–1632, 1990.

Narula J, Dawson MS, Singh BK, et al: Noninvasive characterization of stunned, hibernating, remodeled and nonviable myocardium in ischemic cardiomyopathy, *J Am Coll Cardiol* 36:1913–1919, 2000.

Rizzello V, Poldermans D, Biagini E, et al: Prognosis of patients with ischaemic cardiomyopathy after coronary revascularisation: relation to viability and improvement in left ventricular ejection fraction, *Heart* 95:1273–1277, 2009.

Schinkel AF, Bax JJ, Poldermans D, et al: Hibernating myocardium: diagnosis and patient outcomes, *Curr Probl Cardiol* 32:375–410, 2007.

Schinkel AF, Poldermans D, Elhendy A, et al: Assessment of myocardial viability in patients with heart failure, *J Nucl Med* 48:1135–1146, 2007.

Velazquez EJ, Lee KL, O'Connor CM, et al: The rationale and design of the Surgical Treatment for Ischemic Heart Failure (STICH) trial, *J Thorac Cardiovasc Surg* 134:1540–1547, 2007.

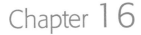

Chapter 16

Extracardiac Incidental Findings

Wael AlJaroudi, Eva V. Dubovsky, and Ami E. Iskandrian

KEY POINTS

- ECFs on nuclear SPECT MPI are not uncommon and can be easily missed.

- ECFs are seen in 1.7% (0-2.8%) of all cases, and 50% of these are unsuspected prior to the study.

- There is a large variability in the incidence of ECFs, depending on the reader's expertise.

- 27% of breast uptake lesions and 46% of focal lung uptake lesions are malignant.

- Patients with ECFs, such as a hiatal hernia, pericardial effusion, pulmonary embolism, aortic dissection, splenomegaly, gallbladder disease, and bone lesions, may have symptoms that can often mimic cardiac symptoms.

- Identifying and reporting ECFs can alert the treating physician to pursue a different diagnostic pathway.

- ECFs are best identified while viewing the raw (unprocessed planar) data in a cine format (cinematic projection).

- ECFs can be small or large and they can be single or multiple

- ECFs can be detected because of either increased (increased vascularity) or decreased (attenuation) tracer concentration in a region of interest.

- Tracer uptake is increased with inflammation, hypermetabolic activity, and malignancy (primary or metastatic).

BACKGROUND

"Perfusion" tracers such as Tl-201, Tc-99m sestamibi, and Tc-99m tetrofosmin are distributed to various organs according to regional MBF. Since resting MBF represents only ~4% of cardiac output, it is clear that most of the injected tracer dose is deposited outside the myocardium. These regions include the muscles, liver, kidneys, brain (in the case of Tl-201 only), bowel, salivary glands, and thyroid gland, to name just a few. There is also some activity in the lungs in the form of diffuse activity, which, in the case of Tl-201, has been used as a useful marker of elevated LV filling pressure. This type of activity should not be confused with the localized extracardiac activity being discussed in this chapter. At times, tracer activity is either detected at sites where it should not be or is not detected at sites where it should be. These constitute collectively incidental findings, which may in a given patient be more important than the cardiac perfusion study itself. If not detected and reported, a poor outcome might follow (e.g., from undiagnosed breast or lung cancer). Most of these incidental findings are detected by careful review of the rotating images; few, if any, are detected on tomographic slices or polar maps!

The most common ECFs are summarized in Table 16-1. We will present a series of case examples to illustrate the pertinent findings.

TABLE 16-1 Most Common Extracardiac Findings

DEFECT	LOCATION	CAUSES
Decreased uptake	Thorax	Permanent pacemaker/defibrillator
		Pleural effusion
		Pericardial effusion
		Widened mediastinum/aortic aneurysm/dissection
		Breast implants
	Abdomen	Liver (cyst, cirrhosis, ascites)
		Gallbladder stones/Cholecystitis
		Kidney (cyst, congenital absence)
Increased uptake	Head & neck	Thyroid (poor labeling, adenoma, malignancy, goiter)
		Parathyroid (adenoma, hyperplasia, malignancy)
	Thorax	Thymoma
		Hiatal hernia
		Elevated hemi-diaphragm
		Sarcoidosis (hilar/mediastinal/lung fibrosis)
		High lung to heart (L/H) Tl-201 uptake
		Lung nodules (primary or metastatic)
		Breast (carcinoma, nodules, lactating)
		Axillary (contamination, lymphangitic spread)
		Bone (multiple myeloma, severe anemia)
	Abdomen	Liver (hepatocellular cancer, metastasis)
		Stomach (poor labeling)
		Splenomegaly
	Cloth/skin	Contamination/residual activity at site of injection
	Miscellaneous	Dilated RV/pulmonary thromboembolism

Case 16-1　ICD/Pacemaker (Figure 16-1)

A 64-year-old man with ischemic cardiomyopathy (LVEF of 25%), status post placement of an ICD, underwent Tc-99m sestamibi stress/rest SPECT MPI to evaluate his recurrent chest pain. The rest raw image demonstrated a dilated heart with a photopenic area in the left upper chest at the site of the ICD.

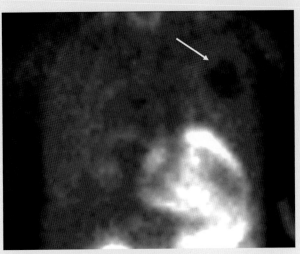

■ **Figure 16-1** Planar image showing a dilated heart and a significant photopenic area in the left upper chest wall *(white arrow)* consistent with an ICD.

COMMENTS

Permanent pacemakers and/or ICDs are commonly placed in the left or right subclavicular regions of the chest. On the raw images, they produce a significant photopenic area that can readily be identified unless a small field of view gamma camera is used and the position of the heart is at the bottom of the field of view, rather than at the center.

Case 16-2   Pleural Effusion (Figure 16-2)

A 58-year-old man underwent stress MPI prior to liver transplantation because of dyspnea on exertion. Significant physical exam findings included decreased breath sounds in the left lung field, hepatomegaly, positive fluid wave, and pedal edema. His laboratory values were significant for pancytopenia, acute kidney injury, mildly elevated bilirubin, and hypoalbuminemia. Stress SPECT MPI showed normal perfusion and an LVEF of 75%. The raw cine image (Figure 16-2, *A*) showed a large photopenic area shadowing almost the entire left lung field, consistent with a pleural effusion. The chest radiograph confirmed the diagnosis and showed a large pleural effusion (Figure 16-2, *B*). On the raw cine images, there was also a photopenic area around the liver, consistent with ascites (Figure 16-2, *C*). The field of view did not visualize the spleen, but the abdominal ultrasound did show significant ascites and splenomegaly.

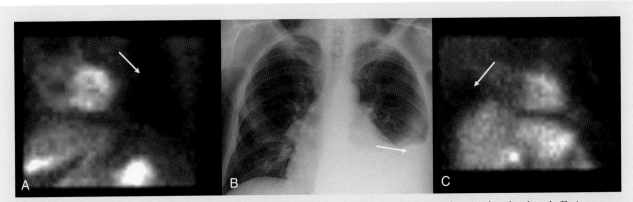

■ **Figure 16-2 A,** Planar image at rest showing a large photopenic area in the left lung field *(arrow)* that matches the pleural effusion seen on the chest radiograph (**B,** *arrow*). **C,** Same raw cine image in the right anterior projection showing a large photopenic area around the liver, consistent with ascites *(arrow).*

COMMENTS

Pleural effusions are common in patients with liver cirrhosis and hypoalbuminemia, but are also common in patients with congestive heart failure, lung cancer, and other conditions. Large effusions compress the lung and attenuate any lung activity, giving rise to a reverse pattern of lung activity (decreased rather than increased).

Case 16-3   **Pericardial Effusion (Figure 16-3)**

A 61-year-old woman with hypertrophic cardiomyopathy, no known coronary artery disease, class III-IV New York Heart Association heart failure symptoms, and symptomatic atrial fibrillation was initially referred for ablation therapy using pulmonary vein isolation. She was volume-overloaded on physical examination. After diuresis, she underwent stress SPECT MPI with Tc-99m sestamibi that showed normal perfusion and an LVEF of 57%. The raw cine image (Figure 16-3. *A*) showed a large photopenic area surrounding the heart, consistent with a pericardial effusion. Gated SPECT images (Figure 16-3. *B*) demonstrate swinging heart motion. 2D transthoracic echocardiogram confirmed the presence of a large (25 mm) pericardial effusion, but there were no echocardiographic signs of cardiac tamponade.

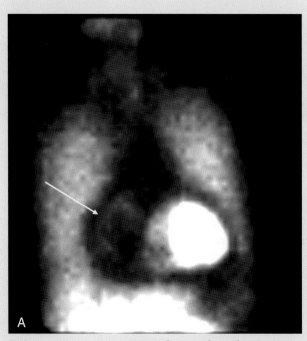

■ **Figure 16-3 A,** Raw cine image showing a large photopenic area surrounding the heart, suggestive of pericardial effusion *(arrow)*.

(Continued)

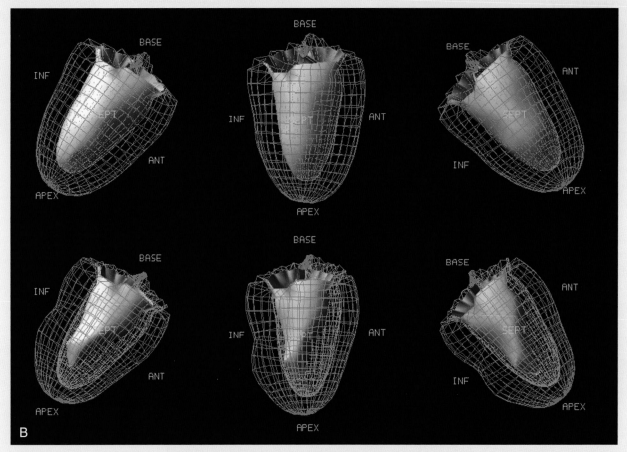

■ **Figure 16-3—Cont'd** The gated SPECT images **(B)** demonstrate swinging/translational motion of the heart (Video 16-1).

COMMENTS

The diagnosis of pericardial effusion by SPECT MPI is uncommon, but there are multiple published case reports. The raw cine images picked up a large photopenic area around the heart, suggestive of pericardial effusion that was not suspected by history or physical examination. The ECG showed atrial fibrillation but no electrical alternans, while the gated SPECT images demonstrated the swinging/translational motion of the heart (Figure 16-3, *B*, and Video 16-1).

Case 16-4   **Aortic Dissection (Figure 16-4)**

A 71-year-old woman presented to the ED with sudden onset of sharp chest pain, radiating to the neck and left shoulder. The pain was associated with nausea, diaphoresis, dyspnea, and dysphagia and was minimally relieved with sublingual nitroglycerin. Her past medical history was significant for hypertension, hyperlipidemia, and atrial fibrillation. Her medication list included warfarin, digoxin, lisinopril, HCTZ, and atenolol. She denied tobacco, alcohol, or illicit drug use. Her mother died of heart disease at age 40.

On physical exam, she appeared ill and in pain. Blood pressure was 152/68, pulse 81 irregular, and respirations were 24/min. She was afebrile, saturating 98% on a 2 L nasal cannula. Significant findings on exam included an increased jugular venous distention (10 cm) and a grade 2:6 systolic ejection murmur at the left lower sternal border.

Laboratory work-up was unremarkable except for a therapeutic international normalized ratio and intermediate troponin levels. The ECG (Figure 16-4, *A*) showed atrial fibrillation with non-specific T-wave changes. The chest radiograph (Figure 16-4, *B*) showed mediastinal enlargement, but was interpreted as having no significant change compared to one performed a year ago. She underwent a rest Tc-99m sestamibi SPECT MPI and was injected during active chest pains while in the ED. Rest SPECT MPI (Figure 16-4, *C*) revealed normal perfusion, the LVEF was 50% on gated images. She was admitted to the cardiac floor for monitoring. Shortly after, she had a cardiac arrest with pulseless electrical activity. She expired despite aggressive resuscitative efforts. Autopsy revealed a type A aortic dissection complicated by retrograde dissection with hemopericardium and hemothorax (Figures 16-4, *D*, *E*).The raw images showed a widened mediastinum and a photopenic area surrounding the heart, consistent with a pericardial effusion (Figure16-4F).

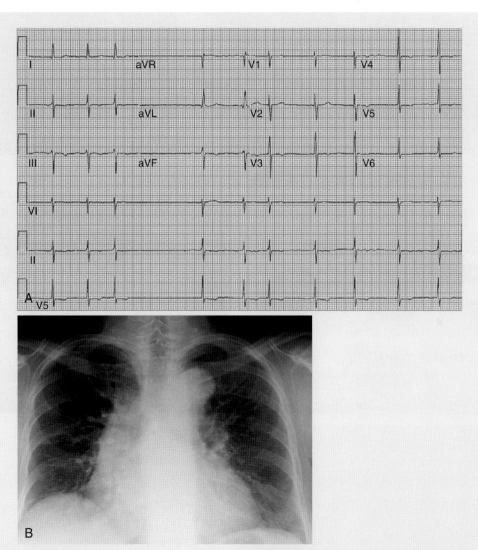

■**Figure 16-4 A,** 12-lead ECG obtained showing atrial fibrillation and nonspecific T-wave changes. The chest radiograph **(B)** demonstrates a widened mediastinum.

(Continued)

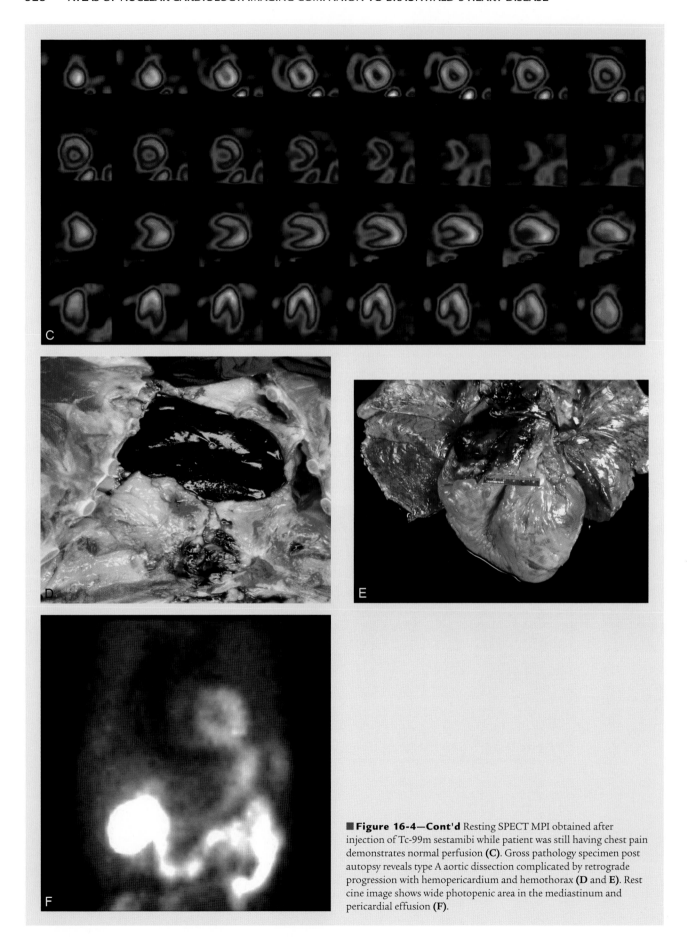

■ **Figure 16-4—Cont'd** Resting SPECT MPI obtained after injection of Tc-99m sestamibi while patient was still having chest pain demonstrates normal perfusion **(C)**. Gross pathology specimen post autopsy reveals type A aortic dissection complicated by retrograde progression with hemopericardium and hemothorax **(D and E)**. Rest cine image shows wide photopenic area in the mediastinum and pericardial effusion **(F)**.

COMMENTS

Ascending aortic dissection can mimic acute coronary syndrome and should always be on the differential diagnosis, especially with such a clinical presentation. When suspected, CT chest or transesophageal echocardiogram should be promptly performed followed by emergency surgery, if positive.

Case 16-5 Breast Implants (Figure 16-5)

A 55-year-old woman with alcoholic liver cirrhosis underwent stress SPECT MPI with Tc-99m sestamibi as part of the liver transplant work-up. Raw cine image demonstrated well-defined symmetrical breast shadows that are consistent with breast implants (Figure 16-5, *A*).

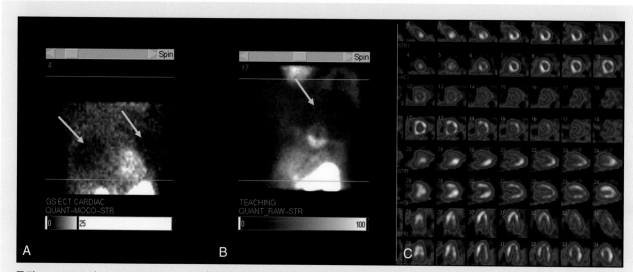

■**Figure 16-5** Planar image demonstrate bilateral photopenic areas in the breasts consistent with implants (**A,** *arrows*). **B** is a raw cine image demonstrating large breasts with significant attenuation artifact *(arrow)* in the anterior wall on the stress SPECT myocardial perfusion images (**C,** *top rows*) that corrects to normal perfusion after attenuation correction (**C,** *bottom rows*).

COMMENTS

Although breast implants are performed for cosmetic reasons, many are done after mastectomy for breast cancer. It is important to be diligent while looking at the raw images so as not to miss a recurrent breast cancer. Often a rim of breast tissue is seen overlying the implant anteriorly and can best be appreciated on cine images. The breast shadows appear symmetric and central in location. The attenuation by either natural breast or breast implant varies considerably and is not directly related to size. Breast tissue proper is more attenuating than fat tissue, which is abundant in redundant breasts (Figures 16-5, *B* and *C*).

Case 16-6 Liver Cyst (Figure 16-6)

A 91-year-old woman presented to the ED with nausea, vomiting, right-sided atypical chest pain, and upper abdominal pain. Stress/rest Tc-99m sestamibi SPECT MPI was normal. The raw cine image, however, showed photopenic areas in the liver suggestive of liver cysts (Figure 16-6, *A*). She underwent CT of the abdomen that showed multiple low attenuation lesions within the liver, predominantly medial segment left lobe, consistent with cysts, the largest 6.1 cm in size (Figure 16-6, *B*).

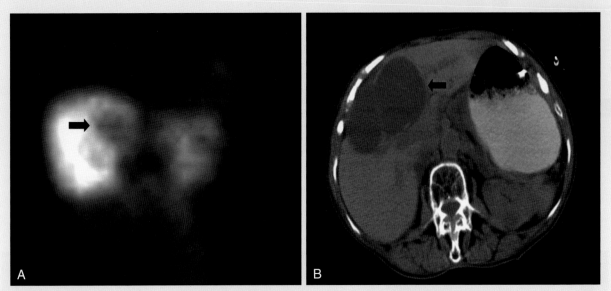

■ **Figure 16-6** Planar image demonstrating multiple photopenic areas in the liver (**A,** *arrow*), confirmed to be liver cysts on CT of the abdomen, shown as multiple low attenuation lesions within the liver, predominantly medial segment left lobe, up to 6.1 cm in size, without perceptible wall or septations (**B,** *arrow*) (*Reproduced from Venkatarman R, et al. J Nucl Cardiol 15:e23–e24, 2008.*)

COMMENTS

Hydatid cysts of the live are another type of cyst reported as an incidental finding by myocardial perfusion scintigraphy.

Case 16-7 | Ascitis (Figure 16-7)

A 51-year-old man with liver cirrhosis and portal hypertension secondary to chronic alcohol intake and hepatitis B and ESRD on hemodialysis was evaluated for liver and kidney transplantation. On examination, he was profoundly jaundiced and had spider angiomata, significant ascites with a fluid wave, and 3+ pitting edema. His labs were significantly abnormal, including thrombocytopenia, elevated creatinine, coagulopathy, hyperammonemia, severe hypoalbuminemia, and a profound hyperbilirubinemia. He underwent a stress MPI with Tc-99m sestamibi as part of the preoperative evaluation. The SPECT perfusion images were normal with an LVEF of 73%. The raw cine image showed a large photopenic area around the liver consistent with ascites (Figure 16-7, *A, arrow*) and splenomegaly (Figure 16-7, *B, star*). CT of the abdomen confirmed both findings (Figure 16-7, *C*).

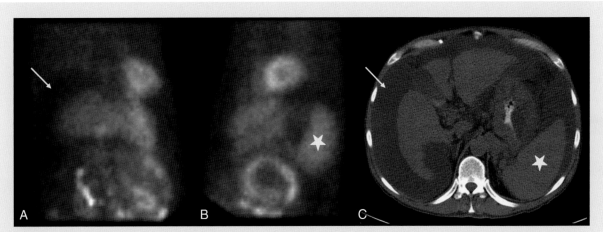

■ **Figure 16-7** Planar image showing ascites (**A,** *arrow*) and enhanced tracer uptake in the spleen with splenomegaly (**B,** *star*). The CT of the abdomen confirms the significant ascites (**C,** *arrow*) and enlarged spleen (**C,** *star*).

COMMENTS

Patients with liver cirrhosis often have ascites, which can cause diaphragmatic attenuation on perfusion imaging. In severe cases, pleural and pericardial effusions may also be seen. Splenomegaly also occurs commonly but is not specific to cirrhosis, it can be secondary to leukemia, lymphomas, and other conditions.

Case 16-8   **Liver Cirrhosis (Figure 16-8)**

A 61-year-old woman with liver cirrhosis secondary to hepatitis C was referred for transplant evaluation. Her physical examination was remarkable for spider angiomata and mild jaundice. She had no hepatomegaly or ascites. Adenosine gated SPECT sestamibi MPI was performed and showed normal perfusion and LVEF. Raw cine image showed absence of tracer uptake in the liver (Figure 16-8, *A*).

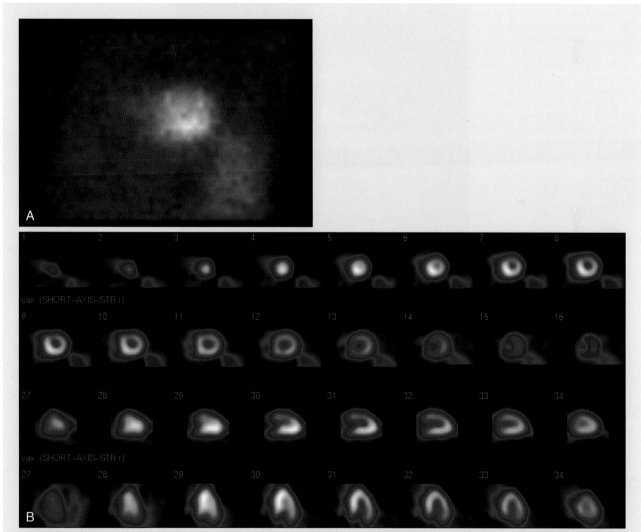

■ **Figure 16-8** Planar image showing lack of tracer uptake in the cirrhotic liver **(A)**. **B** is a SPECT myocardial perfusion image projection in short, vertical, and horizontal-long axes showing normal perfusion. Note the excellent image quality with good target to background contrast ratio.

COMMENTS

The liver has high tracer, activity, especially with vasodilator imaging. This is part of the reason for the 1-hour delay before image acquisition after tracer. Sestamibi is cleared through hepatobiliary excretion; as a result, liver and bowel activity may overlap cardiac activity. In this patient with severe liver disease, there was virtually no activity in the liver, which helped improve image quality by increasing target-to-background ratio (Figure 16-8, *B*).

Case 16-9   Thyroid Nodule (Figure 16-9)

A 78-year-old woman with multiple cardiac risk factors underwent stress MPI with Tc-99m sestamibi to evaluate left-sided chest pain. The stress test showed a large area of ischemia and the patient had three-vessel coronary artery disease by subsequent coronary angiography. The raw images showed focal tracer uptake in the thyroid gland consistent with a thyroid nodule (Figure 16-9). Unfortunately, the patient had a complicated postoperative course and expired.

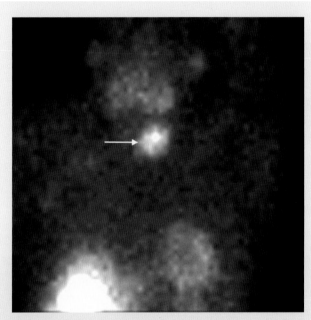

■ **Figure 16-9** Planar image showing focal uptake in the thyroid, consistent with a thyroid adenoma *(arrow)*.

COMMENTS

Tc-99m sestamibi uptake occurs in all vascular tumors, including thyroid and parathyroid gland adenomas or carcinomas.

Case 16-10   Thyroid Goiter (Figure 16-10)

A 58-year-old clinically euthyroid man with ESRD on hemodialysis underwent stress MPI prior to renal transplant. Significant exam findings included a left forearm AV fistula and an enlarged thyroid goiter. Thyroid stimulating hormone and free T_4 levels were normal. Stress MPI with Tc-99m sestamibi showed normal perfusion. Raw cine image showed enlarged goiter with tracer uptake and multiple complex nodules (Figure 16-10). Thyroid ultrasound confirmed the findings. Fine needle aspiration was recommended, but the patient was lost to follow-up.

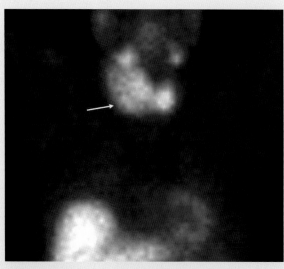

■ Figure 16-10 Planar image showing enlarged thyroid/goiter with enhanced tracer uptake and multiple complex nodules *(arrow).*

COMMENTS

Thyroid nodules, goiters, and malignancies demonstrate increased tracer uptake in pathologic cases. A "hot" thyroid nodule, however, does not necessarily imply malignancy, but needs to be further investigated. In a study of 339 patients with thyroid disease who underwent neck ultrasound and Tc-99m scintigraphy, the SPECT study increased the global accuracy of the diagnosis and altered management in two-thirds of cases. Anecdotally, there are many studies evaluating the role of Tc-99m sestamibi in diagnosing and staging thyroid cancer.

Case 16-11   Parathyroid Adenomas (Figure 16-11)

A 61-year-old woman with stage 5 CKD, and secondary parathyroid adenoma with elevated intact parathyroid hormone levels (2105 pg/ml, normal 12 to 65 pg/mL) underwent stress MPI before kidney transplantation. The raw cine image demonstrated increased tracer uptake in the parathyroid glands, consistent with parathyroid hyperplasia/adenoma.

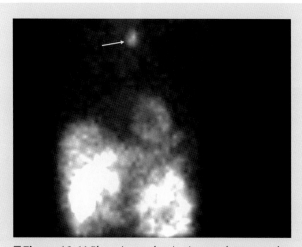

■ Figure 16-11 Planar image showing increased tracer uptake in the parathyroid *(arrow)* in a patient with ESRD and secondary hyperparathyroidism.

COMMENTS

Parathyroid hyperplasia and/or adenomas are commonly found in patients with ESRD. Tc-99m sestamibi SPECT has a high sensitivity for visualizing the parathyroid. It is routinely used for parathyroid scintigraphy in the preoperative setting to guide the surgeon; it is also useful in diagnosing a supernumerary parathyroid, which is the most common cause of relapse post-parathyroidectomy. In a case series of 44 patients, Tc-99m SPECT increased the diagnostic accuracy when compared to ultrasound and altered management in one-third of patients.

Case 16-12   Thymoma (Figure 16-12)

A 66-year-old woman with a history of DM, ESRD on hemodialysis, and hypertension, presented to the ED with substernal chest pain and dyspnea. Her physical examination was normal except for elevated blood pressure. The ECG showed normal sinus rhythm with LV hypertrophy. The laboratory work-up was unremarkable, including 3 sets of negative cardiac biomarkers.

She underwent a pharmacologic gated SPECT stress/rest MPI with T-99m sestamibi. The perfusion images showed mild ischemia in the left circumflex territory (Figure 16-12, *A*). Extracardiac activity was detected incidentally in the right hemithorax on the raw images (Figure 16-12, *B*) and prompted CT scan of the chest. The latter confirmed the presence of a smooth, uniformly enhancing mass in the right chest, adjacent but not infiltrating the ascending aorta (Figure 16-12, *C*). Also noted was a dissection of the thoracic aorta (Figure 16-12, *D*) extending from the aortic arch to the proximal descending part with moderate pericardial effusion (Figure 16-12, *E*). The patient underwent successful repair of the aortic dissection and resection of the 6-cm encapsulated mediastinal mass. The pericardial effusion was transudative, and the left circumflex coronary artery was diffusely diseased. The pathology report confirmed a well-encapsulated mass with a mixture of epithelial cells and lymphocytes, consistent with type B3 thymoma (Figures 16-12, *F* and *G*).

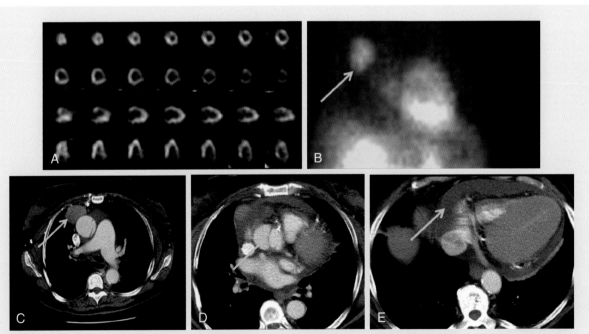

■ **Figure 16-12** Stress-rest SPECT MPI images (short, vertical, and long axes) demonstrate mild ischemia in the left circumflex coronary artery (**A**). **B** shows an extracardiac mass in the right hemithorax on the raw anterior planar images (*arrow*). Contrast-enhanced chest CT confirms the mass (**C**, *arrow*), dissection flap (**D**, *arrow*), and pericardial effusion (**E**, *arrow*).

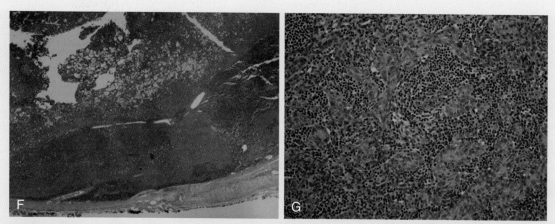

■**Figure 16-12—Cont'd** Low-power **(F)** and high-power **(G)** microscopy of the resected mass show well-encapsulated mass with a smooth surface and a mixture of epithelial cells and lymphocytes, consistent with type B3 thymoma. *(Reproduced from Bhambhvani PG, Dubousky E, Nath H, et al: Unusual incidental findings by SPECT myocardial perfusion imaging and CT in the same patient. J Nucl Cardiol 17;937–938, 2010.)*

COMMENTS

Thymomas are uncommon tumors in general, but can account for up to 20% of mediastinal neoplasms (the others include teratomas, thyroid cancers, and "terrible" lymphomas). Patients present with cardiac symptoms, such as chest discomfort or dyspnea. Almost half of patients can have myasthenia gravis symptoms, including weakness, diplopia, or dysphagia. Thymomas can progress to carcinoma, so surgical excision is the treatment of choice and is often curative. It can also help achieve remission of myasthenia gravis. The unique feature of this case is that neither the thymoma nor dissection were clinically suspected.

Case 16-13   Hiatal Hernia (Figure 16-13)

A 78-year-old man, with no known CAD, but with multiple cardiac risk factors, presented with burning epigastric pain and atypical chest pain. Stress MPI with Tc-99m sestamibi was performed and showed normal perfusion (Figure 16-13, *A*). Raw cine image (Figure 16-13, *B*) showed a large hiatal hernia.

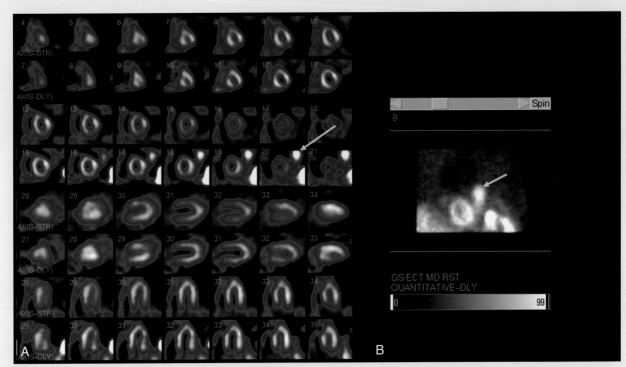

■ **Figure 16-13** Same-day stress/rest Tc-99m sestamibi SPECT images **(A)**. Note the increased tracer activity in the short- and horizontal-axis slices *(arrow)*. Also seen is the retrocardiac activity in the raw cine image **(B)**, consistent with a hiatal hernia.

COMMENTS

Tc-99m MPI agents are excreted by the hepatobiliary system. In patients with hiatal hernias, duodenogastric reflux can cause the tracer to reflux to the stomach and lower esophagus and appear as a hot spot behind the cardiac silhouette. The burning pain this patient experienced was probably due to gastroesophageal reflux and the hiatal hernia. He was treated with proton pump inhibitors and had no further chest pain at 2-year follow-up.

Case 16-14   **Sarcoidosis (Figure 16-14)**

A 57-year-old woman with hypertension and DM was scheduled for a stress MPI to evaluate atypical chest pain and dyspnea on exertion. The stress MPI showed normal perfusion and a preserved LVEF. The raw cine image, however, demonstrated multiple regions of localized tracer uptake in both lungs (Figure 16-14). Further work-up, including chest CT and pulmonary function testing, confirmed advanced pulmonary sarcoidosis with interstitial fibrosis and combined obstructive and restrictive lung physiology.

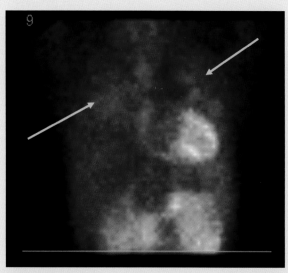

■ **Figure 16-14** Planar image showing patchy Tc-99m sestamibi uptake in both lungs *(arrows)* in a patient with known sarcoidosis.

COMMENTS

The typical pattern in sarcoid heart disease is pulmonary involvement with and without pulmonary hypertension and right ventricular dysfunction. Pulmonary nodules can be visualized, at least in some patients, but only before progressive fibrosis sets in. Sarcoidosis can also involve the myocardium, causing arrhythmias, myocardial scarring, and cardiomyopathy. Reversible perfusion defects are unusual despite the possibility that some of these granulomas might compress a coronary artery. If ischemia is detected, it is more likely due to microvascular disease.

Case 16-15   Increased Lung Thallium Uptake (Figure 16-15)

A 79-year-old man with CAD ischemic cardiomyopathy with an LVEF of 20%, and class III NYHA heart failure symptoms, was referred for a stress MPI because of recurrent chest pain. On physical examination, the patient was volume overloaded and had an S_3 gallop. The raw cine image showed diffuse increase in Tl-201 uptake in both lung fields with an elevated lung-to-heart ratio of 0.8 (upper normal is 0.5).

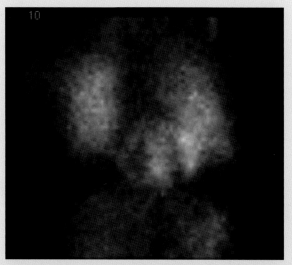

■ **Figure 16-15** Rest planar image showing increased diffuse Tl-201 uptake in bilateral lung fields, with increased lung-to-heart ratio.

COMMENTS

This type of increased lung activity is diffuse and not localized. The increased activity reflects elevation of LV filling pressures. As such it is not specific for CAD, but when seen in patients with CAD it is a marker of severe ischemia and poor outcome. We have seen examples of increased lung activity in patients with noncardiogenic pulmonary edema (i.e., a normal filling pressure); we believe it is due to capillary endothelial leakage.

Case 16-16   Lung Carcinoma (Figure 16-16)

A 78-year-old man was referred for stress MPI to evaluate dyspnea on exertion. The perfusion images were normal. However, the raw cine image showed focal increased uptake in the right lung. Chest CT confirmed a lung mass suspicious for cancer. The patient underwent resection and the mass was confirmed to be a squamous cell carcinoma.

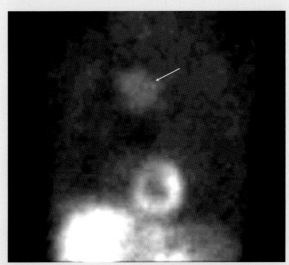

■ **Figure 16-16** Planar image showing focal tracer uptake in the right upper lung *(arrow)*. The biopsy was positive for squamous cell lung cancer.

COMMENTS

The sensitivity, specificity, and positive and negative predictive values of increased tracer uptake in a suspicious lung mass are 80%, 70%, 84%, and 64%, respectively. Data from a large retrospective study have shown that half of all lung masses found incidentally on raw cine images are malignant.

Tc-99m sestamibi is actively taken up intracellularly through the P-glycoprotein receptor. In recent studies, it was shown to be a noninvasive marker for the diagnosis of P-glycoprotein-related multidrug-resistant lung cancer and many other solid tumors. Tc-99m sestamibi had a 94% sensitivity to identify responders to chemotherapy, 90% specificity, and 92% accuracy.

Case 16-17   Breast Mass (Figure 16-17)

A 50-year-old man with DM and hypertension presented with right sided chest pain. Stress MPI with Tc-99m sestamibi showed normal perfusion. The raw cine image demonstrated a focal right breast mass. Biopsy was performed and pathologic examination was consistent with ductal carcinoma. He was referred for surgical resection and further management.

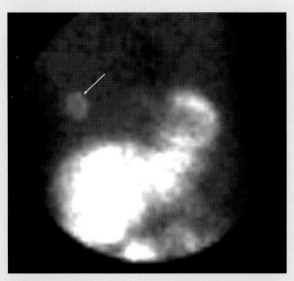

■**Figure 16-17** Planar image showed large left breast mass with increased tracer uptake *(arrow)* in a male with left-sided chest pain.

COMMENTS

Breast cancer in men accounts for 0.17% of all cancers, with 900 new cases per year. Risk factors include testicular abnormalities, including undescended testes, orchiectomy, elevated estrogen levels, chest radiation, and family history. Although gynecomastia is frequently seen with male breast cancer, there is no causal association, and is more likely secondary to elevated estrogen levels that are common in both conditions. Invasive ductal carcinoma is the most common type and frequently presents as a noncalcified mass. Tc-99m sestamibi can often visualize the tumor and this has been reported in a few cases.

Case 16-18   **Breast Mass (Figure 16-18)**

A 72-year-old woman with peripheral vascular disease, DM, and ESRD presented with chest pain and underwent stress MPI. The images were normal, but the raw images demonstrated focal tracer uptake in the breast.

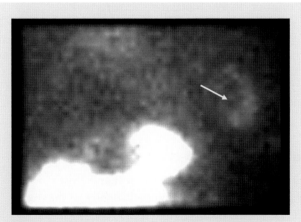

■**Figure 16-18** Planar image showed large focal Tc-99m uptake in the left breast *(arrow)*. Biopsy revealed intraductal adenocarcinoma.

COMMENTS

Breast cancer is the most common malignancy in women. Public awareness and screening have increased the detection rate and early therapy. Up to one-quarter of breast masses identified incidentally on Tc-99m SPECT are malignant. Recently, the Food and Drug Administration has approved the use of Tc-99m sestamibi for the diagnosis of primary, recurrent, or metastatic breast malignancy with or without lymphangitic spread. The tracer is also a noninvasive marker of P-glycoprotein mediated drug resistance and might help detect responders to chemotherapy.

| Case 16-19 | Lactating Breasts (Figure 16-19) |

A 36-year-old woman, recently postpartum and still lactating, underwent sestamibi stress MPI to evaluate chest discomfort and dyspnea. The perfusion images were normal and LVEF was 60%. The raw cine rotating images, however, revealed significant, homogenous/diffuse radioisotope tracer uptake in both breasts.

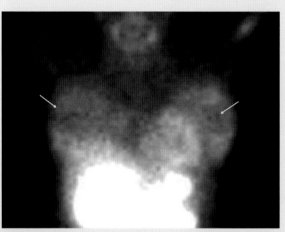

■ **Figure 16-19** Planar image demonstrating diffuse/ homogenous uptake of tracer in both breasts of a lactating woman (*arrows*).

COMMENTS

There have been two reported cases of Tc-99m uptake in bilateral breasts in lactating women and it is considered a physiologic finding. Tc-99m has a short halflife (6 hours) and less than 0.03% of the initial dose is excreted in breast milk. Withholding breast feeding for 12 to 24 hours is still recommended, as a conservative measure. Thus, although breasts often cause attenuation artifacts, they may in lactating women show the reverse finding of increased activity, which is not to be confused with lung activity.

Note: MPI might be helpful in new onset heart failure in the peripartum period where the differential diagnosis between peripartum cardiomyopathy and coronary artery dissection is not clear; these patients might also have a LBBB on the ECG, which makes the diagnosis more difficult.

| Case 16-20 | Axillary Lymph Node (Figure 16-20) |

A 50-year-old obese man underwent 2-day rest/stress Tc-99m sestamibi SPECT MPI. The rest raw cine image showed right axillary lymph node uptake of the tracer (Figure 16-20, *A, arrow*) and residual activity over the right arm at the site of the injection (*arrowhead*). The stress raw image did not show any tracer activity in the lymph node (Figure 16-20, *B*).

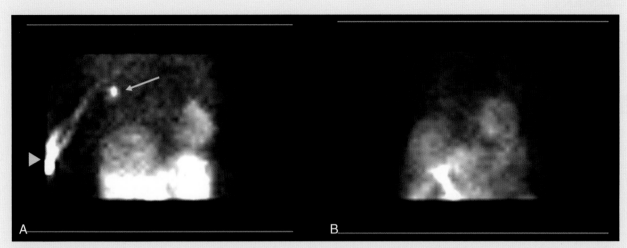

■ **Figure 16-20** Rest planar image showing right axillary lymph node *(arrow)* and skin infiltration *(arrowhead)* over the right arm **(A)**. **B** is the stress raw cine image performed the next day that showed resolution of the activity in the lymph node.

COMMENTS

Axillary lymph node uptake of the tracer can be secondary to inflammation or malignancy (such as lymphoma or lymphangitic spread), but it occurs most commonly from tracer infiltration during injection. It is very important to know in which arm the tracer was injected. Commonly, residual skin contamination or subdermal tracer infiltration are seen on the same side as the lymph node, confirming the diagnosis. Because of the short halflife of Tc-99m (6 hours), the stress raw images performed 24 hours later did not show any tracer uptake.

Case 16-21 Multiple Myeloma (Figure 16-21)

A 59-year-old man with CAD and bypass grafts underwent stress MPI to evaluate atypical left sided chest wall pain. Stress perfusion images showed mild ischemia, and subsequent left heart catheterization showed patent grafts but residual disease. The raw cine images (Figures 16-21, *A* and *B*) demonstrated increased uptake in bone (sternum and ribs). Chest CT showed lytic bony lesions. Further work-up, including bone marrow biopsy, confirmed the diagnosis of multiple myeloma.

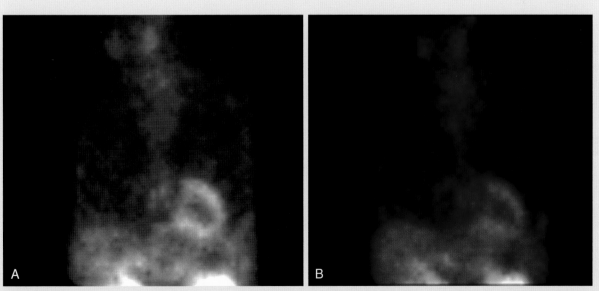

■ **Figure 16-21** Planar images showing increased tracer uptake in the rib cage and sternum as seen in gray scale **(A)** and thermal scale **(B)**.

COMMENTS

Tc-99m sestamibi has been used for more than a decade in the diagnosis, staging, management of multiple myeloma, and detecting recurrence post-chemotherapy. There have also been numerous case reports of bone marrow malignancies discovered incidentally on raw cine images. Focal tracer uptake is a better indicator of active disease than diffuse uptake.

Case 16-22 — Hepatocellular Carcinoma (Figure 16-22)

A 49-year-old man with advanced liver cirrhosis secondary to hepatitis C and worsening shortness of breath was referred for stress MPI prior to liver transplant surgery. The perfusion SPECT images and LVEF were normal. The raw cine image, however, demonstrated a mass with increased uptake in the right hepatic lobe (Figure 16-22, *A*). Abdominal CT with contrast revealed a 4.0 × 3.6 cm mass in the liver consistent with hepatocellular carcinoma (Figure 16-22, *B*).

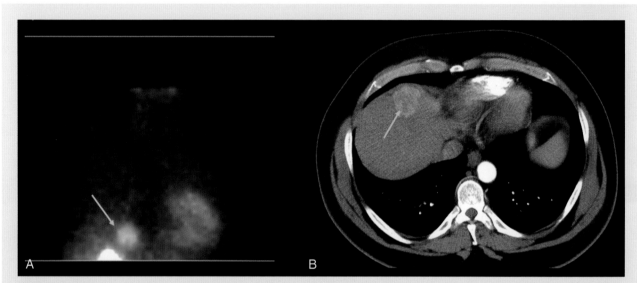

■ **Figure 16-22** Rest planar image showing a mass in the right hepatic lobe with increased tracer uptake (**A**, *arrow*). CT of the abdomen confirmed the mass (**B**, *arrow*).

COMMENTS

Tc-99m sestamibi is not a sensitive tracer for the diagnosis of hepatocellular carcinoma. In a small study of patients with confirmed diagnosis, SPECT perfusion imaging identified only 2 of 22 cases of hepatocellular cancer. However, other studies have shown that the lack of Tc-99m sestamibi uptake correlated with P-glycoprotein expression, a marker of multidrug resistance, and might have clinical implications in predicting patients' response to chemotherapy.

Case 16-23 — Contamination (Figure 16-23)

A 61-year-old woman with ischemic cardiomyopathy and heart failure underwent stress MPI with Tc-99m sestamibi for worsening shortness of breath and chest pain. The raw image shows a photopenic area in the right upper chest wall ICD and enhanced tracer uptake outside the body, consistent with spill contamination.

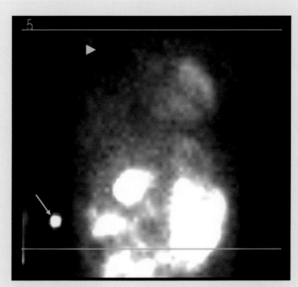

■ **Figure 16-23** Rest planar image showing tracer outside the body *(arrow)*, likely the result of cloth contamination. Another incidental finding is the ICD in the right upper chest wall *(arrowhead)*.

COMMENTS

Uncommonly, spill contamination can occur during tracer injection; the tracer falls on the patient's gown or skin. It is important to look at the rotating raw images to recognize that the tracer uptake is located outside the body.

Case 16-24   **Pulmonary Thromboembolism (Figure 16-24)**

A 61-year-old woman, who was recovering from pelvic surgery, became suddenly short of breath, diaphoretic, and had sharp chest pain on postoperative day 3. Significant exam findings included hypotension, tachypnea, and hypoxia. The lungs were clear bilaterally. The troponin level was elevated. The 12-lead ECG showed sinus tachycardia, and $S_1Q_3T_3$ pattern (Figure 16-24, *A*). Chest CT confirmed bilateral pulmonary emboli (Figure 16-24, *B*, *arrows*). The patient was initiated on anticoagulation and did well.

A stress MPI was performed prior to discharge and showed normal perfusion and LVEF. The gated images (in slices) showed a flattened interventricular septum and an enlarged and hypokinetic right ventricle (minimum thickening and volume changes from diastole to systole) (Figure 16-24, *C*).

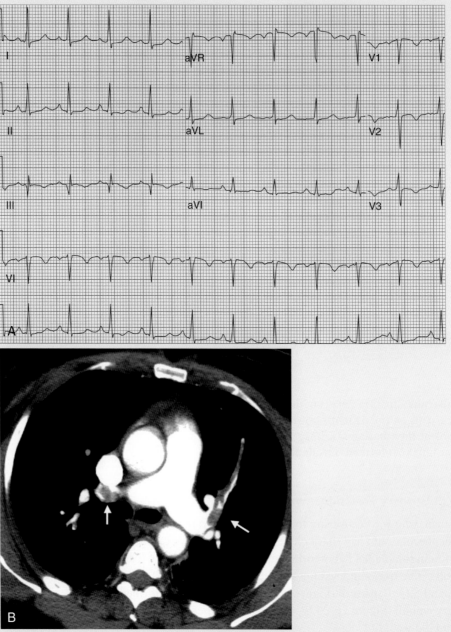

■**Figure 16-24** 12-lead ECG **(A)** showing sinus tachycardia and $S_1Q_3T_3$ (suggestive of pulmonary embolism). CT angiogram of the chest with contrast **(B)** demonstrates filling defects in bilateral pulmonary arteries (arrows) consistent with emboli.

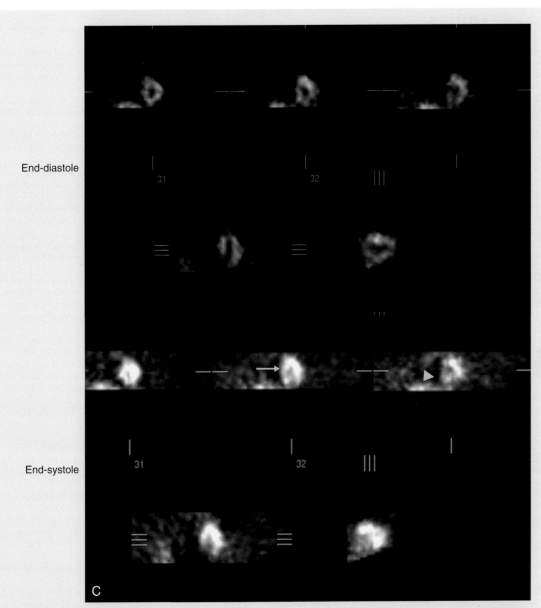

End-diastole

End-systole

C

■**Figure 16-24—Cont'd C,** Gated SPECT images in slices at end-diastole and end-systole demonstrate flattening of the interventricular septum (**D**-shape, *arrow*) throughout diastole and systole, dilated right ventricle *(arrowhead)* that is larger than the left ventricle, with minimal thickening and volume change through the cardiac cycle.

COMMENTS

Tc-99m sestamibi gated SPECT studies can assess the RV size and function when the images are displayed as slice projections. In many cases, the diagnosis of acute RV dysfunction was initially made from the gated SPECT studies, which led to the diagnosis of pulmonary embolism. The assessment of RV function with Tc-99m sestamibi has been shown to correlate well with contrast ventriculography, echocardiography, and equilibrium gated blood pool imaging. In the case we presented, the Tc-99m sestamibi gated SPECT images showed a flattened interventricular septum that suggests volume and pressure overload, and a dilated, hypocontractile right ventricle, which is a poor prognostic indicator.

SELECTED READINGS

Austin BA, Kwon DH, Jaber WA: Pericardial effusion on Tc-99m SPECT perfusion study, *J Nucl Cardiol* 15:e35–36, 2008.

Bhambhavani P, Dubousky E, Nath H, et al: Unusual incidental findings by SPECT myocardial perfusion imaging and CT the same patient, *J Nucl Cardiol* 17:937–938, 2010.

Chadika S, Kokkirala AR, Giedd KN, et al: Focal uptake of radioactive tracer in the mediastinum during SPECT myocardial perfusion imaging, *J Nucl Cardiol* 12:359–361, 2005.

Duarte PS, Zhuang H, Blasbalg R, et al: Hepatic cysts detected on myocardial perfusion scintigraphy, *Clin Nucl Med* 26:468–469, 2001.

Dunnwald LK, Gralow JR, Ellis GK, et al: Residual tumor uptake of [99mTc]-sestamibi after neoadjuvant chemotherapy for locally advanced breast carcinoma predicts survival, *Cancer* 103:680–688, 2005.

Eguchi M, Tsuchihashi K, Hotta D, et al: Technetium-99m sestamibi/tetrofosmin myocardial perfusion scanning in cardiac and noncardiac sarcoidosis, *Cardiology* 94:193–199, 2000.

Gedik GK, Bozkurt FM, Ugur O, et al: The additional diagnostic value of a single-session combined scintigraphic and ultrasonographic examination in patients with thyroid and parathyroid diseases, *Panminerva Med* 50:199–205, 2008.

Gedik GK, Ergün EL, Aslan M, et al: Unusual extracardiac findings detected on myocardial perfusion single photon emission computed tomography studies with Tc-99m sestamibi, *Clin Nucl Med* 32:920–926, 2007.

Hawkins M, Scarsbrook AF, Pavlitchouk S, et al: Detection of an occult thymoma on 99Tcm-Tetrofosmin myocardial scintigraphy, *Br J Radiol* 80:e72–e74, 2007.

Herzog E, Krasnow N, DePuey G: Diagnosis of pericardial effusion and its effects on ventricular function using gated Tc-99m sestamibi perfusion SPECT, *Clin Nucl Med* 23:361–364, 1998.

Hindié E, Zanotti-Fregonara P, Just P, et al: Parathyroid scintigraphy findings in chronic kidney disease patients with recurrent hyperparathyroidism, *Eur J Nucl Med Mol Imaging* 37:623–634, 2010.

Ho YJ, Jen LB, Yang MD, et al: Usefulness of technetium-99m methoxyisobutylisonitrile liver single photon emission computed tomography to detect hepatocellular carcinoma, *Neoplasma* 50:117–119, 2003.

Kalaga RV, Kudagi V, Heller GV: Role of Tc-99m sestamibi myocardial perfusion imaging in identifying multiple myeloma, *J Nucl Cardiol* 16:835–837, 2009.

Kamínek M, Myslivecek M, Skvarilová M, et al: Increased prognostic value of combined myocardial perfusion SPECT imaging and the quantification of lung Tl-201 uptake, *Clin Nucl Med* 27:255–260, 2002.

Karkavitsas N, Damilakis J, Tzanakis N, et al: Effectiveness of Tc-99m sestamibi compared to Ga-67 in patients with pulmonary sarcoidosis, *Clin Nucl Med* 22:749–751, 1997.

Kim YS, Cho SW, Lee KJ, et al: Tc-99m MIBI SPECT is useful for noninvasively predicting the presence of MDR1 gene-encoded P-glycoprotein in patients with hepatocellular carcinoma, *Clin Nucl Med* 24:874–879, 1999.

Langah R, Spicer K, Gebregziabher M, et al: Effectiveness of prolonged fasting 18f-FDG PET-CT in the detection of cardiac sarcoidosis, *J Nucl Cardiol* 16:801–810, 2009.

Liu M, Husain SS, Hameer HR, et al: Detection of male breast cancer with Tc-99m methoxyisobutyl isonitrile, *Clin Nucl Med* 24:882–883, 1999.

Mathew J, Perkins GH, Stephens T, et al: Primary breast cancer in men: clinical, imaging, and pathologic findings in 57 patients, *AJR Am J Roentgenol* 191:1631–1639, 2008.

Mohan HK, Miles KA: Cost-effectiveness of 99mTc-sestamibi in predicting response to chemotherapy in patients with lung cancer: systematic review and meta-analysis, *J Nucl Med* 50:376–381, 2009.

Moreno AJ, Carpenter AL, Pacheco EJ, et al: Large thoracic aortic aneurysm seen on equilibrium blood pool imaging, *Clin Nucl Med* 19:1113–1114, 1994.

Oskoei SD, Mahmoudian B: A comparative study of lung masses with 99mTechnetium Sestamibi and pathology results, *Pak J Biol Sci* 10:225–229, 2007.

Papantoniou V, Tsiouris S, Koutsikos J, et al: Scintimammographic detection of usual ductal breast hyperplasia with increased proliferation rate at risk for malignancy, *Nucl Med Commun* 27:911–917, 2006.

Pereira N, Klutz WS, Fox RE, et al: Identification of severe right ventricular dysfunction by technetium-99m-sestamibi gated SPECT imaging, *J Nucl Med* 38:254–256, 1997.

Ramakrishna G, Miller TD: Significant breast uptake of Tc-99m sestamibi in an actively lactating woman during SPECT myocardial perfusion imaging, *J Nucl Cardiol* 11:222–223, 2004.

Sanders GP, Pinto DS, Parker JA, et al: Increased resting Tl-201 lung-to-heart ratio is associated with invasively determined measures of left ventricular dysfunction, extent of coronary artery disease, and resting myocardial perfusion abnormalities, *J Nucl Cardiol* 10:140–147, 2003.

Shih W, Justice T: Massive left pleural effusion resulting in false-positive myocardial perfusion, *J Nucl Cardiol* 12:476–479, 2005.

Shih W, Kiefer V, Gross K, et al: Intrathoracic and intra-abdominal Tl-201 abnormalities seen on rotating raw cine data on dual radionuclide myocardial perfusion and gated SPECT, *Clin Nucl Med* 27:40–44, 2002.

Shih W, McFarland KA, Kiefer V, et al: Illustrations of abdominal abnormalities on 99mTc tetrofosmin gated cardiac SPECT, *Nucl Med Commun* 26:119–127, 2005.

Shih W, Shih GL, Huang W, et al: Duodenogastric reflux in a hiatal hernia seen as retrocardiac activity on 99mTc-tetrofosmin cardiac SPECT raw-data images, *J Nucl Med Technol* 35:252–254, 2007.

Shih WJ, Collins J, Kiefer V: Visualization in the ipsilateral lymph nodes secondary to extravasation of a bone-imaging agent in the left hand: a case report, *J Nucl Med Technol* 29:154–155, 2001.

Tallaj JA, Kovar D, Iskandrian AE: The use of technetium-99m sestamibi in a patient with liver cirrhosis, *J Nucl Cardiol* 7:722–723, 2000.

Teirstein AT, Morgenthau AS: "End-stage" pulmonary fibrosis in sarcoidosis, *Mt Sinai J Med* 76:30–36, 2009.

Thet-Thet-Lwin, Takeda T, Wu J, et al: Diffuse and marked breast uptake of both 123I-BMIPP and 99mTc-TF by myocardial scintigraphy, *Ann Nucl Med* 14:315–318, 2000.

Venkataraman R, Heo J, Iskandrian AE: Hepatic cysts detected on Tc-99m sestamibi gated cardiac SPECT images, *J Nucl Cardiol* 15:e23, 2008.

Chapter 17

Newer Tools for Assessment of Heart Failure

Ji Chen

KEY POINTS

- I-123 mIBG can be used to image adrenergic receptors in the heart using conventional planar or SPECT imaging.

- I-123 mIBG H/M measured from planar or SPECT images can provide important information on prognosis in HF patients. It is a more powerful predictor for SCD than LVEF.

- I-123 mIBG H/M measured from planar or SPECT images has been shown to be related to appropriate ICD discharges and the effect of CRT in HF patients, suggesting that mIBG imaging may aid in selection of HF patients who could benefit from ICD and/or CRT therapies.

- Viable but denervated myocardium is very sensitive to sympathetic stimulation and has been suggested to play a role in arrhythmogenesis in IHD.

- Mismatch between mIBG and SPECT perfusion imaging has been shown to be related to ventricular arrhythmias, suggesting that mIBG and MPI SPECT may aid in selection of IHD patients who could benefit from ICD therapy.

- Phase analysis has been developed and validated for measuring LV systolic dyssynchrony from gated SPECT MPI.

- Systolic dyssynchrony measured by phase analysis of gated SPECT MPI has been shown to correlate with systolic dyssynchrony measured by tissue Doppler imaging, and predicts response to CRT in HF patients.

- Phase analysis of gated SPECT MPI has been shown to assess regional activation and localize the site of latest mechanical activation.

- It has been shown that HF patients who undergo CRT with concordant LV pacing lead positioning (leads positioned at the site of latest mechanical activation as assessed by phase analysis) are more likely to have improved response to CRT than HF patients with discordant LV pacing lead positions.

- Phase analysis with multi-harmonic approximation has been shown to measure LV diastolic dyssynchrony from gated SPECT MPI. It has been shown that diastolic dyssynchrony is significantly more prevalent than systolic dyssynchrony and is related to cardiac risk factors and diastolic dysfunction in patients with ESRD and normal LVEF.

BACKGROUND

Two major tools of nuclear cardiac imaging have recently been developed for assessment of patients with HF. One is I-123 mIBG that can be used to image adrenergic receptors in the heart using conventional planar or SPECT imaging. I-123 mIBG imaging produces a quantitative index, heart-to-mediastinum ratio (H/M), which can evaluate receptor density and sympathetic tone. It has been shown that an abnormal H/M is an independent and more powerful predictor than LVEF for SCD in HF patients. Furthermore, H/M has been shown to be related to appropriate ICD discharges and the effectiveness of CRT in HF patients, suggesting that mIBG imaging may aid in selection of HF patients who could benefit from ICD and/or CRT therapies. In addition, mIBG defect score and mIBG-perfusion mismatch score have

been shown to relate to ventricular arrhythmias in IHD patients, further suggesting that mIBG and MPI SPECT may aid in selection of IHD patients who could benefit from ICD therapy.

Another major tool in the assessment of HF is phase analysis of gated SPECT MPI that can measure LV systolic and diastolic dyssynchrony. LV systolic dyssynchrony, measured by phase analysis of gated SPECT MPI, has been shown to correlate with that measured by tissue Doppler imaging. In addition, phase analysis has been shown to identify optimal LV pacing lead position for CRT and to predict response to CRT in HF patients. Recently, phase analysis with multi-harmonic approximation has been shown to assess LV diastolic dyssynchrony—a new LV parameter detected by MPI. In this chapter, both cutting-edge tools of nuclear cardiac imaging for assessment of HF are demonstrated using patient examples.

Case 17-1   **Patients With Normal and Abnormal mIBG Uptake Measured by I-123 mIBG Planar Imaging (Figure 17-1)**

The patient in Figure 17-1, *A*, is a 68-year-old man with NYHA class II, ischemic cardiomyopathy, and LVEF of 35%. The H/M by mIBG imaging was 1.69. He was under optimal medical therapy, but without ICD. He had no cardiac event during a 2-year follow-up. The patient in Figure 17-1, *B*, is a 51-year-old man with NYHA class II, ischemic cardiomyopathy, and LVEF of 33%. The H/M was 1.38. He was also under optimal medical therapy, but without ICD. He experienced cardiac death 8 months after the mIBG scan.

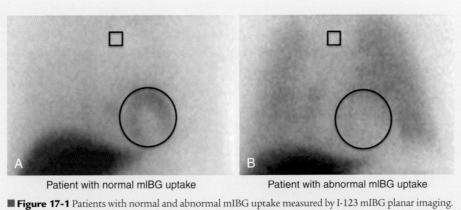

■ **Figure 17-1** Patients with normal and abnormal mIBG uptake measured by I-123 mIBG planar imaging. Two patient examples are shown in this figure. **A** shows a patient with normal mIBG uptake, whereas **B** shows a patient with abnormal mIBG uptake. Two ROIs are drawn on each planar image for calculating H/M (the mean counts in the heart ROI divided by the mean counts in the mediastinum ROI).

COMMENTS

H/M measured from I-123 mIBG planar imaging has been shown to predict adverse cardiac events in HF patients with an optimal cutoff value of 1.60. The two patients had similar baseline characteristics, but one with H/M > 1.60 and the other with H/M < 1.60. The two cases demonstrate that H/M measured from I-123 mIBG planar imaging can provide independent and incremental prognostic value in HF patients over baseline characteristics, such as NYHA class, HF etiology, and LVEF.

Case 17-2	Patients With Normal and Abnormal mIBG Uptake Measured by I-123 mIBG SPECT Imaging (Figure 17-2)

Control subject in a multicenter trial of mIBG (Figure 17-2, *A*). This subject had normal mIBG uptake. The H/M measured by I-123 mIBG SPECT was 3.56.
An HF patient in the same multicenter trial, but with an abnormal mIBG uptake (Figure 17-2, *B*). The H/M measured by I-123 mIBG SPECT was 0.93.

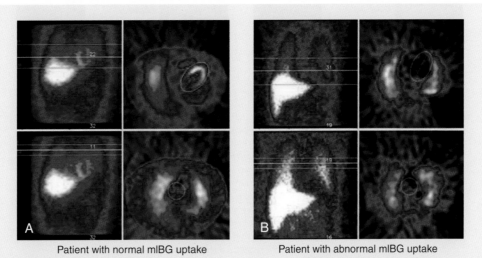

■ **Figure 17-2** Patients with normal and abnormal mIBG uptake measured by I-123 mIBG SPECT imaging. Two patient examples are shown in this figure. **A** shows a patient with normal mIBG uptake, whereas **B** shows a patient with abnormal mIBG uptake. In each panel, the heart and mediastinum ROIs are drawn on the heart and mediastinum transaxial images (reconstructed using FBP), which correspond to the *red lines* on the planar images next to them, respectively. The heart and mediastinum VOIs are then constructed to include the pixels within the heart and mediastinum ROIs in between the corresponding *green lines*, respectively. SPECT H/M is calculated by dividing the mean counts in the heart VOI by the mean counts in the mediastinum VOI.

COMMENTS

H/M measured from I-123 mIBG SPECT has shown to distinguish between abnormal and normal cardiac mIBG uptake. The optimal cutoff value of H/M for distinguishing normal from abnormal cardiac mIBG uptake depends on the image reconstruction method. For FBP, OSEM, and OSEM with DSP, the optimal cutoff values are 2.7, 2.6 and 4.0, respectively. The DSP H/M is larger than the FBP and OSEM H/M because DSP reduces background count level due to septal penetration, resulting in lower mediastinum VOI counts with DSP than with the other two reconstruction methods. H/M measured from I-123 mIBG SPECT, regardless of the reconstruction method used, has been shown to distinguish between normal and abnormal mIBG uptake with comparable sensitivity and specificity to the established H/M measured from I-123 mIBG planar imaging. This case demonstrates I-123 mIBG SPECT images with different mIBG uptakes in a normal subject and a HF patient and the effect of reconstruction method on the absolute values.

| Case 17-3 | Patients With Mismatched and Matched Defects on mIBG and MPI SPECT Images (Figure 17-3) |

A patient with IHD who had mismatched defects when comparing images from mIBG and perfusion (Figure 17-3, *A*). This patient had a large defect on the mIBG SPECT polar map. The mIBG defect region was well perfused, as shown on the MPI SPECT polar map. A second patient with IHD who had matched mIBG and perfusion defects (Figure 17-3, *B*). This patient had a large defect at approximately the same location with approximately the same extent on both mIBG and MPI SPECT polar maps.

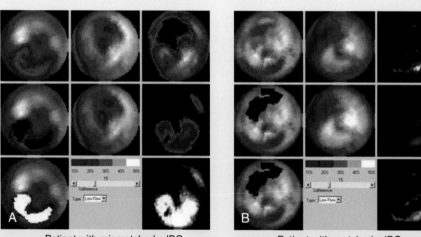

Patient with mismatched mIBG
and perfusion defects

Patient with matched mIBG
and perfusion defects

■ **Figure 17-3** Patients with mismatched and matched defects on mIBG and MPI SPECT images. Two patient examples are shown in this figure. **A** shows a patient with mismatched defects on the mIBG and MPI SPECT images, whereas **B** shows a patient with matched defects on the mIBG and MPI SPECT images. **A,** Shown on the *first row* from *left* to *right* are mIBG, perfusion, and their differential polar maps, respectively. Shown on the *left* in the *second row* is the mIBG blackout polar map, where the mIBG defect is identified *(blackened)* by use of an mIBG normal database, and the remaining normal areas are then used for normalization. The average count value in the entire region with normal mIBG uptake is computed for both the mIBG and perfusion images, and then the perfusion image is scaled so that its average value in the normal region is equal to that in the mIBG study (shown in the *middle* on the *second row*). The normalized mIBG distribution is subtracted from the normalized perfusion distribution (shown in the *right* on the *second row*). The difference between the two distributions is expressed as a percentage of the normalized perfusion distribution (shown in the *right* on the *third row*). A threshold for this percent difference can be set at any level. Regions in the normalized perfusion distribution that are above the threshold, and that also have abnormal mIBG uptake, are those that have relatively increased myocardial perfusion coexistent with relatively decreased mIBG uptake (i.e., a mismatch shown as the *white region* on the *left* on the *third row*). **B,** This patient has a large defect at approximately the same region on both mIBG and perfusion polar maps (i.e., a match).

COMMENTS

These cases demonstrate that IHD patients can have mIBG and perfusion defects, with either a mismatched or matched pattern. Data have shown that the extent of mIBG–perfusion mismatch, which represents the extent of viable but denervated myocardium, is related to future ventricular arrhythmias. Note that the tool demonstrated in this case has not yet been validated, and the optimal threshold for match-mismatch remains to be determined.

Case 17-4   Patient With Normal LV Systolic Synchrony (Figure 17-4)

This 55-year-old man with normal LVEF and normal QRS duration has normal LV synchrony. All LV regions start contraction at almost the same time; therefore, the phase polar map shows a uniform phase distribution and the phase band histogram is narrow and highly peaked.

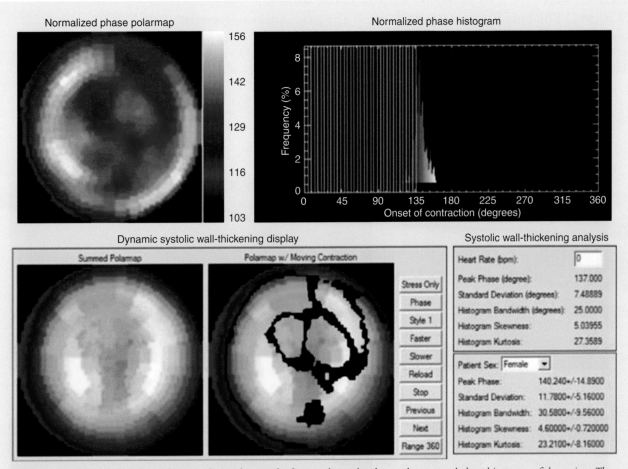

■ **Figure 17-4** Patient with normal LV systolic synchrony. The *first row* shows the phase polar map and phase histogram of the patient. The *second row* shows two perfusion polar maps and quantitative results. A cursor is placed on the phase histogram to represent a particular time bin during the cardiac cycle. The pixels in the second perfusion map, whose phases are within the time bin of the cursor, are blackened out. By continuously displaying the cursor, a dynamic display (Video 17-1) is created on the second perfusion map and represents the wave of onset of mechanical contraction of the ventricle.

COMMENTS

This example demonstrates the user interface of the software used to conduct phase analysis of gated SPECT MPI. The phase distribution array of a patient is displayed as a polar map. A phase histogram is displayed next to the phase polar map. The phase ranges from 0 to 360 degrees in the histogram, representing one cardiac cycle. If the patient's heart rate is known, the x-axis scale in the histogram can be converted to time. The y-axis of the histogram is frequency in percentage, representing the portion of the myocardium that starts contraction at a time bin during the cardiac cycle. A cursor is placed on the histogram to indicate a particular time bin during the cardiac cycle. As the cursor is sequentially displayed from the left to the right, a dynamic display is generated and shown next to the LV perfusion polar map. Users can stop and reload the cursor sequence, adjust its speed, and move a cursor to any particular time bin. Five quantitative indices (peak phase, phase standard deviation, histogram bandwidth, skewness, and kurtosis) describing the phase distribution are displayed and compared to the normal database.

Case 17-5   Nonresponder and a Responder to CRT (Figure 17-5)

At baseline, no LV dyssynchrony was present in this 67-year-old man with class III HF and LBBB. The phase distribution was relatively uniform and the corresponding phase histogram was a highly peaked, narrow distribution (Figure 17-5, *A*).
After 6-months of follow-up, no response to CRT was observed, as reflected by deterioration in NYHA functional class from III to IV. In addition, LVEF remained unchanged (32% at baseline vs. 33% at 6-month follow-up). On the other hand, the patient in Figure 17-5, *B*, responded to CRT. This 58-year-old woman with class III HF and LBBB had LV dyssynchrony at baseline. The phase distribution showed substantial nonuniformity, whereas the corresponding phase histogram had a widely spread distribution. After 6-month follow-up, she improved from NYHA functional class III to II, and her LVEF increased from 27% at baseline to 33% at 6 months.

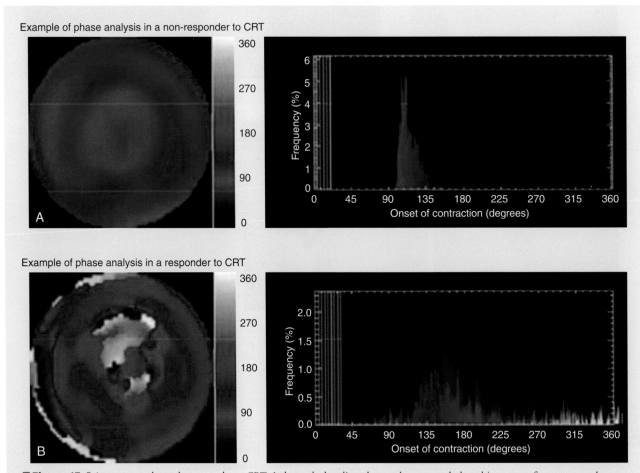

■ **Figure 17-5** A nonresponder and a responder to CRT. **A** shows the baseline phase polar map and phase histogram of a nonresponder to CRT. **B** shows the baseline phase polar map and phase histogram of a responder to CRT. *(Courtesy of Ami Iskandrian, MD).*

COMMENTS

The presence of LV dyssynchrony at baseline is an important predictor for CRT response. It has been shown that about one third of patients with narrow QRS durations had substantial LV dyssynchrony, and about one third of patients with wide QRS durations did not have LV dyssynchrony. These findings may explain why 30% to 40% of the patients who receive CRT do not respond to the therapy. The current standard criteria for CRT are NYHA class III or IV, LVEF ≤ 35% and QRS ≥ 120 msec), and to date do not include LV dyssynchrony by imaging.

| Case 17-6 | Patient With Favorable Response in LV Synchrony Immediately Post-CRT (Figure 17-6) |

A 72-year-old man with ischemic cardiomyopathy had NYHA class III symptoms. This patient had substantial LV dyssynchrony pre-CRT, as reflected by a nonuniform phase polar map and a wide phase histogram. He had a large myocardial scar. Regional scar extent analysis using a seven-segment model showed that 51%, 100%, and 58% of the septal, inferior, and lateral walls had myocardial scar. Regional phase analysis showed that the inferior wall had the latest activation, whereas the lateral wall had the latest activation without substantial myocardial scar (white arrow). The LV pacing lead was positioned at the lateral wall (red arrow), pacing the site of latest activation with viable myocardium. Comparing the pre-CRT phase polar map and phase histogram to those immediately post-CRT, this patient had a favorable acute response to CRT (phase standard deviation decreased from 28.9 to 15.4 degrees and phase bandwidth decreased from 88 to 50 degrees). His QRS duration also decreased from 142 to 132 msec. This patient did well at 1 year of follow-up and had no events (cardiac death, HF hospitalization, ICD shocks, CRT deactivation).

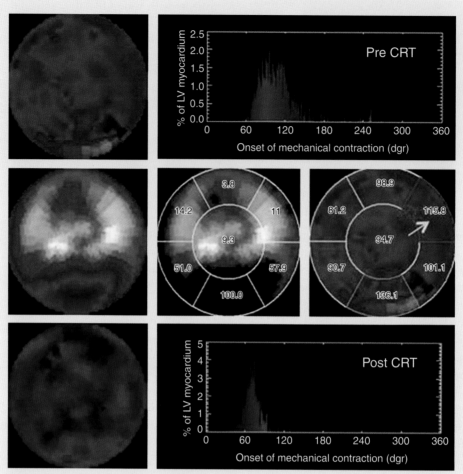

■ **Figure 17-6** A patient with a favorable response in LV synchrony immediately post-CRT. The *first row* shows the phase polar map and phase histogram of the patient pre-CRT. The *left* image in the *second row* shows the perfusion polar map of the patient. The *middle* image in the *second row* shows the myocardial scar analysis. The pixels in the perfusion polar map, whose counts are less than 50% of the maximum counts in the perfusion polar map, are blackened out. The perfusion polar map is divided into seven segments, and the scar extents are calculated and displayed for the seven segments. The *right* image in the *second row* shows the regional mean phases of the seven segments. The *white arrow* indicates the segment with the latest mechanical activation (having the largest mean phases) and no scar. The *red arrow* indicates the actual LV pacing lead position. The *third row* shows the phase polar map and phase histogram of the patient immediately post-CRT. *(Courtesy of Prem Soman, MD, PhD.)*

COMMENTS

In addition to baseline LV dyssynchrony, LV pacing lead position and myocardial scar burden are two important predictors for CRT response. It has been shown that the optimal LV pacing lead position for favorable CRT response is the site of latest mechanical activation with viable myocardium.

Case 17-7   **Patient With Deteriorative Response in LV Synchrony Immediately Post-CRT Due to Inappropriate LV Pacing Lead Position (Figure 17-7)**

A 65-year-old woman with nonischemic cardiomyopathy had NYHA class III symptoms. She had substantial LV dyssynchrony pre-CRT, as reflected by a nonuniform phase polar map and a wide phase histogram. She had no myocardial scar. Regional phase analysis showed that the inferolateral wall had the latest activation (white arrow); however, the LV pacing lead was positioned at the anteroseptal wall (red arrow). Comparing the pre-CRT phase polar map and phase histogram to those immediately post-CRT, this patient had acute deterioratiation after CRT (phase standard deviation increased from 19.8 to 37.4 degrees and phase bandwidth increased from 59 to 113 degrees). This patient had CRT deactivation due to worsened symptoms 15 days post-CRT.

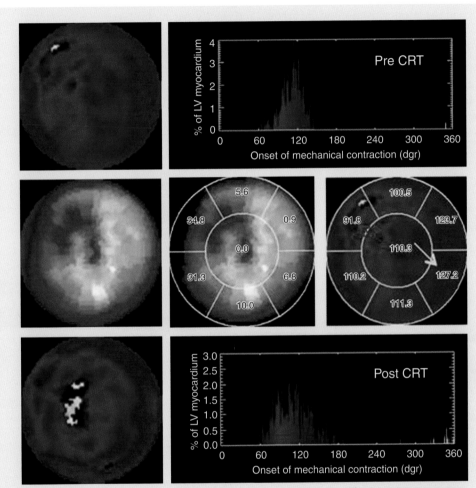

■ **Figure 17-7** A patient with deteriorative response in LV synchrony immediately post-CRT due to inappropriate LV pacing lead position. The *first row* shows the phase polar map and phase histogram of the patient pre-CRT. The *left* image in the *second row* shows the perfusion polar map of the patient. The *middle* image in the *second row* shows the myocardial scar analysis. The pixels in the perfusion polar map, whose counts are less than 50% of the maximum counts in the perfusion polar map, are blackened out. The perfusion polar map is divided into seven segments, and the scar extents are calculated and displayed for the seven segments. The *right* image in the *second row* shows the regional mean phases of the seven segments. The *white arrow* indicates the segment with the latest mechanical activation (having the largest mean phase). The *red arrow* indicates the actual LV pacing lead position. The *third row* shows the phase polar map and phase histogram of the patient immediately post-CRT. *(Courtesy of Prem Soman, MD, PhD.)*

COMMENTS

This example demonstrates that inappropriate LV pacing lead position can deteriorate LV synchrony. It has been shown that the optimal LV pacing lead position for favorable CRT response is the site of latest mechanical activation with viable myocardium.

Case 17-8   **Patient With Deteriorative Response in LV Synchrony Immediately Post-CRT due to Large Myocardial Scar Burden (Figure 17-8)**

A 61-year-old woman with ischemic cardiomyopathy had NYHA class III symptoms. She had substantial LV dyssynchrony pre-CRT, as reflected by a non-uniform phase polar map and a wide phase histogram. She had a very large myocardial scar. The scar extent was 52% of the ventricle. Regional phase analysis showed that the inferolateral wall had the latest activation (white arrow), and the LV pacing lead was positioned at the inferolateral wall (red arrow). Although there was concordant LV pacing lead position, there was a large myocardial scar in this region. Comparing the pre-CRT phase polar map and phase histogram to those immediately post-CRT, this patient had acute deterioration (phase standard deviation increased from 33.4 to 229 degrees and the bandwidth increased from 49.1 to 259 degrees). This patient had HF hospitalization 4 months post-CRT.

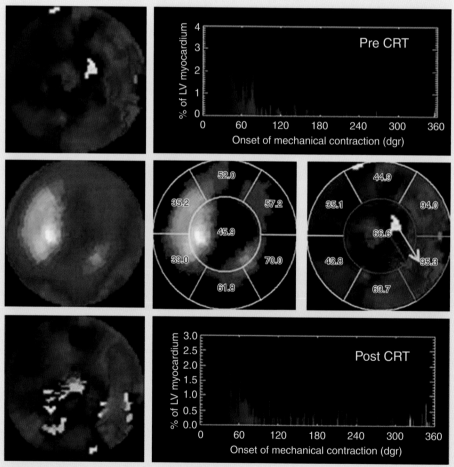

■ **Figure 17-8** A patient with deteriorative response in LV synchrony immediately post-CRT due to large myocardial scar. The *first row* shows the phase polar map and phase histogram of the patient pre-CRT. The *left* image in the *second row* shows the perfusion polar map of the patient. The *middle* image in the *second row* shows the myocardial scar analysis. The pixels in the perfusion polar map, whose counts are less than 50% of the maximum counts in the perfusion polar map, are blackened out. The perfusion polar map is divided into seven segments, and the scar extents are calculated and displayed for the seven segments. The *right* image in the *second row* shows the regional mean phases of the seven segments. The *white arrow* indicates the segment with the latest mechanical activation (having the largest mean phases). The *red arrow* indicates the actual LV pacing lead position. The *third row* shows the phase polar map and phase histogram of the patient immediately post-CRT. (*Courtesy of Prem Soman, MD, PhD.*)

COMMENTS

This example demonstrates that patients with large scar burden may not respond to CRT and may, in fact, have worsening of LV function, synchrony, and symptoms. It has been shown that a favorable response to CRT in patients with large myocardial scar burden is significantly lower than that in patients without or with small myocardial scar burden.

SELECTED READINGS

Arora R, Ferrick KJ, Nakata T, et al: I-123 MIBG imaging and heart rate variability analysis to predict the need for an implantable cardioverter defibrillator, *J Nucl Cardiol* 10:121–131, 2003.

Boogers MJ, Chen J, van Bommel RJ, et al: Optimal left ventricular lead position assessed with phase analysis on gated myocardial perfusion SPECT, *Eur J Nucl Med Mol Imaging*, 38: 230-238, 2011.

Chen J, Bax JJ, Henneman MM, et al: Is nuclear imaging a viable alternative technique to assess dyssynchrony? *Europace* 10(Suppl 3): III101–III105, 2008.

Chen J, Faber TL, Cooke CD, et al: Temporal resolution of multi-harmonic phase analysis of ECG-gated myocardial perfusion SPECT studies, *J Nucl Cardiol* 15:383–391, 2008.

Chen J, Garcia EV, Folks RD, et al: Onset of left ventricular mechanical contraction as determined by phase analysis of ECG-gated myocardial perfusion SPECT imaging: development of a diagnostic tool for assessment of cardiac mechanical dyssynchrony, *J Nucl Cardiol* 12:687–695, 2005.

Chen J, Garcia EV, Galt JR, et al: Optimized acquisition and processing protocols for I-123 cardiac SPECT imaging, *J Nucl Cardiol* 13:251–260, 2006.

Gould PA, Kong G, Kalff V, et al: Improvement in cardiac adrenergic function post biventricular pacing for heart failure, *Europace* 9:751–756, 2007.

Henneman MM, Bengel FM, van der Wall EE, et al: Cardiac neuronal imaging: application in the evaluation of cardiac disease, *J Nucl Cardiol* 15:442–455, 2008.

Henneman MM, Chen J, Dibbets P, et al: Can LV dyssynchrony as assessed with phase analysis on gated myocardial perfusion SPECT predict response to CRT? *J Nucl Med* 48:1104–1111, 2007.

Henneman MM, Chen J, Ypenburg C, et al: Phase analysis of gated myocardial perfusion SPECT compared to tissue Doppler imaging for the assessment of left ventricular dyssynchrony, *J Am Coll Cardiol* 49:1708–1714, 2007.

Jacobson AF, Senior R, Cerqueira MD, et al, for the ADMIRE-HF Investigators: Myocardial iodine-123 meta-iodobenzylguanidine imaging and cardiac events in heart failure. Results of the prospective ADMIRE-HF (AdreView Myocardial Imaging for Risk Evaluation in Heart Failure) study, *J Am Coll Cardiol* 55:2212–2221, 2010.

Kioka H, Yamada T, Mine T, et al: Prediction of sudden death by using cardiac iodine-123 metaiodobenzylguanidine imaging in patients with mild to moderate chronic heart failure, *Heart* 93:1213–1218, 2007.

Lin X, Xu H, Zhao X, et al: Repeatability of left ventricular dyssynchrony and function parameters in serial gated myocardial perfusion SPECT studies, *J Nucl Cardiol* 17:811–816, 2010.

Patel AD, Iskandrian AE: MIBG imaging, *J Nucl Cardiol* 9:75–94, 2002.

Simoes MV, Barthel P, Matsunari I, et al: Presence of sympathetically denervated but viable myocardium and its electrophysiologic correlates after early revascularised, acute myocardial infarction, *Eur Heart J* 25:551–557, 2004.

Trimble MA, Smalheiser S, Borges-Neto S, et al: Evaluation of left ventricular mechanical dyssynchrony as determined by phase analysis of ECG-gated myocardial perfusion SPECT imaging in patients with left ventricular dysfunction and conduction disturbances, *J Nucl Cardiol* 14:298–307, 2007.

Trimble MA, Velazquez EJ, Adams GL, et al: Repeatability and reproducibility of phase analysis of gated SPECT myocardial perfusion imaging used to quantify cardiac dyssynchrony, *Nucl Med Commun* 29:374–381, 2008.

Udelson JE, Shafer CD, Carrio I: Radionuclide imaging in heart failure: assessing etiology and outcomes and implications for management, *J Nucl Cardiol* 9:S40–S52, 2002.

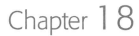

Chapter 18

Improving SPECT MPI Efficiency and Reducing Radiation

Ernest V. Garcia, Tracy L. Faber, and Fabio P. Esteves

KEY POINTS

- Improvements in reconstruction software and dedicated cardiac camera design now allow for efficient ultrafast MPI acquisition. Some of the acquisition time reduction may be traded off for a reduction in the injected radiopharmaceutical dose without loss of image quality.

- The tradeoff between acquisition time and dose reduction is approximately linear. Thus, an ultrafast MPI protocol using a 30-mCi dose and a 2-minute acquisition could be replaced with a 15-mCi dose and a 4-minute acquisition and receive very similar image quality and diagnostic accuracy with either protocol.

- New reconstruction algorithms use RRNR techniques that yield MPI images acquired in half the standard imaging times with superior image contrast and resolution and similar perfusion and function diagnostic performance, compared to standard SPECT.

- These RRNR reconstruction algorithms have been shown to provide LV volumes that correlate to standard SPECT, but are significantly smaller, and LVEFs that also correlate, but are lower due to smaller end-diastolic volumes.

- Innovative design of dedicated cardiac-centric cameras have in common that many detectors are constrained to simultaneously imaging the heart and use either conventional NaI crystals and PMT or the more beneficial solid-state detectors, such as CZT or CSI.

- Compared to standard SPECT devices, solid-state detectors are more efficient in how they convert the energy and location of the radiation absorbed by the detector to an electronic pulse, thus giving rise to significant improvements in energy and spatial resolution.

- Compared to standard SPECT, these new ultrafast cameras have potential for a 5- to 10-fold count sensitivity gain at no loss or even a gain in contrast and spatial resolution.

- These new ultrafast cameras with solid-state detectors and tungsten collimators are optimized for imaging not only Tc-99m but also photons with energies from Tl-201 to I-123. This higher energy resolution has also been shown to allow for simultaneous dual isotope imaging.

- Clinical trials have demonstrated that using these new ultrafast cameras and a conventional 1-day Tc-99m tetrofosmin rest/stress MPI protocol of 4- and 2-minute acquisitions, respectively, yielded studies that diagnostically agreed 90% of the time with 14- and 12-minute rest-stress conventional SPECT acquisitions.

- Some of these ultrafast camera systems allow for AC using a CT transmission scan. In addition, attenuation artifacts may be reduced because not all views are through the attenuator—some may view the heart from above or below, thus reducing breast attenuation artifacts.

BACKGROUND

Despite the clinical success of MPI, present clinical, scientific, and financial needs require further improvements in hardware and software to allow myocardial perfusion SPECT imaging to answer these challenges of modern health care. It is difficult to realize these improvements with the imaging hardware and software used in most nuclear cardiology laboratories today.

This chapter demonstrates, through patient examples, how MPI studies from conventional two-detector rotating SPECT systems compare to studies acquired with the new design cardiac-dedicated ultrafast SPECT cameras and with the new RRNR algorithms. These examples make evident that these advances are poised to meet present health care challenges by improving image quality while reducing study time, radiation dose to the patient, and ultimately reducing study cost.

ADVANCES IN IMAGE RECONSTRUCTION

Recent software improvements in iterative image reconstruction take into account the loss of resolution with distance inherent in parallel-hole collimators. Using this knowledge in conjunction with the imaging properties of the system allows for a mathematical correction of this resolution degradation known as resolution recovery. At the same time, noise is suppressed because additional counts are now correctly accounted for instead of being treated as noise. Moreover, noise regularization techniques have been implemented that go beyond simple smoothing by considering the expected noise for the regional count density. Because resolution recovery actually reduces noise while improving spatial resolution compared to FBP, resolution recovery can yield reconstructed images from studies acquired in less time with the same signal/noise as FBP images reconstructed from studies acquired over a longer time.

NEW ULTRAFAST CAMERA DESIGNS

Several manufacturers have begun to break away from the conventional SPECT imaging approach to create innovative designs for dedicated cardiac cameras. These cameras' designs have in common that all available detectors are constrained to imaging just the cardiac field of view. These new designs vary in the number and type of scanning or stationary detectors, and whether NaI, CSI, or CZT solid-state detectors are used. They all have in common the potential for a 5- to 10-fold increase in count sensitivity at no loss or even a gain in resolution, resulting in the potential for acquiring a stress myocardial perfusion scan in 2 minutes or less if injected with a standard dose. Some of this gain in sensitivity can be traded for a linear reduction in the injected dose to reduce the patient's exposure to radiation. Thus, in an ultrafast camera with a 10-fold increase in sensitivity using conventional radiopharmaceutical doses, the dose could be reduced by half and still maintain a 5-fold increase in sensitivity.

REDUCED DOSE VERSUS INCREASED EFFICIENCY

It is clear that these more efficient hardware/software imaging systems also allow for high-quality images obtained using a lower injected radiopharmaceutical dose and thus a decrease in the radiation dose absorbed by the patient and staff. This reduction in dose comes at an increase in acquisition time, even if the total time is less than what has been traditionally used in conventional systems. Since currently there are no financial incentives for using a lower radiopharmaceutical dose, a laboratory interested in just reducing costs would tend to opt for the most efficient protocol possible.

Recently, the American Society of Nuclear Cardiology published an information statement recommending that laboratories use imaging protocols that achieve, on average, a radiation exposure of 9 mSv or less in 50%

of studies by 2014. Although there are many different protocols that may be implemented to accomplish this exposure goal, use of the more efficient hardware/ software described herein would greatly facilitate this goal and allow for increases in efficiency over the imaging protocols used today.

| **Case 18-1** | **Half-Time Resolution Recovery Normal Study (Figure 18-1)** |

A 52-year-old, 5-foot 8-inch, 181-lb male smoker with hypertension, hypercholesterolemia, and family history of premature CAD underwent exercise and rest imaging on a standard dual-detector gamma camera for evaluation of an LAD stenosis that had been previously diagnosed with angiography in 2000. Twenty seconds per stop rest and gated stress acquisitions with 60 projections (10 minutes + rotation time) were reconstructed with OSEM. Ten seconds per stop rest and gated stress acquisitions with 60 projections (5 minutes + rotation time) were reconstructed with OSEM, incorporating correction for detector and collimator response.

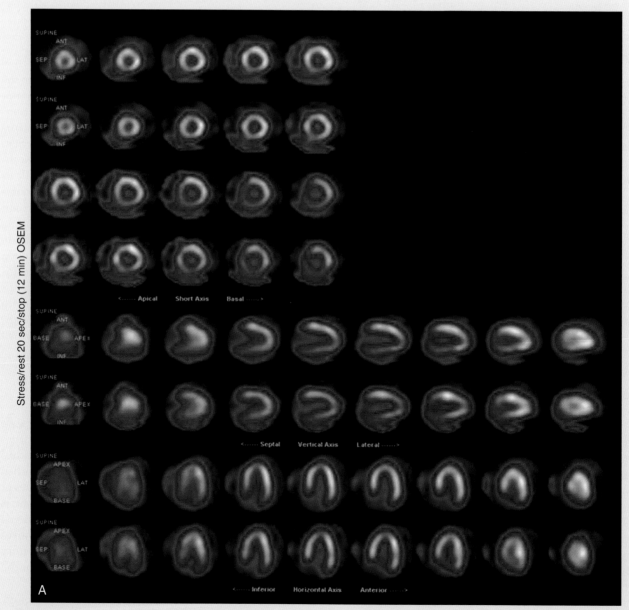

■ **Figure 18-1** Half-time resolution recovery normal study. **A,** Stress and rest slices (alternating rows) in short-axis, vertical long-axis, and horizontal-axis views. This image was acquired using standard imaging times (10-minute + rotation time), and reconstructed using OSEM without corrections. This is a normal distribution.

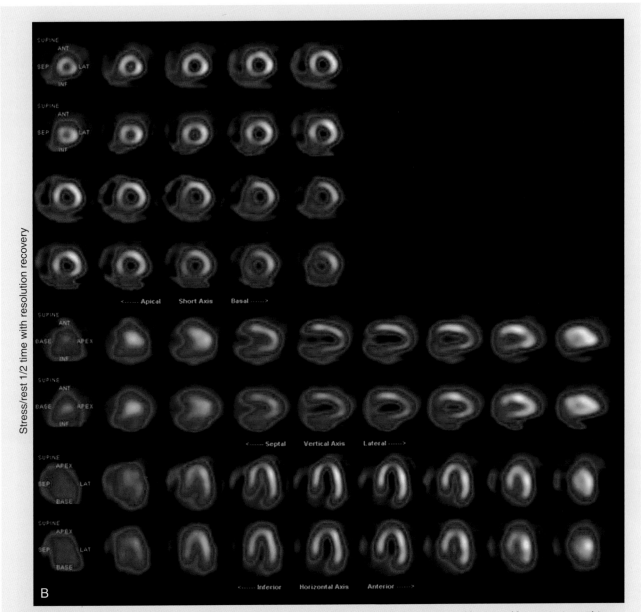

■**Figure 18-1—Cont'd B,** Stress and rest slices (alternating rows) in short-axis, vertical long-axis, and horizontal long-axis views. This image was acquired using a half-time protocol, and reconstructed iteratively using resolution recovery. Note the normal distribution of this patient and its similarity to that seen in the full-time images **(A)**, but with higher image contrast.

(Continued)

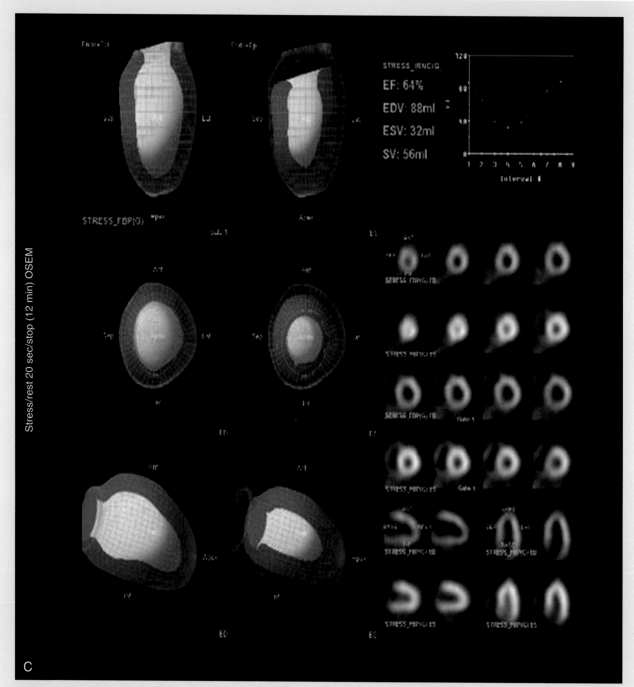

■**Figure 18-1—Cont'd C,** To the *left* are shown 3D views of the LV, with a green mesh epicardium and solid white endocardium. The *far left column* shows 3D end-diastolic frames in an anterior, apical, and septal view, from *top* to *bottom*. The next column shows the same views in the end-systolic frame. To the *right* is shown the LV volume curve on top, and then four rows of alternating end-diastolic and end-systolic short-axis slices. The *bottom two rows* show two vertical long-axis and two horizontal long-axis slices, with end-diastole on top and end-systole on bottom. This image corresponds to **A**; it is from a full-time acquisition reconstructed without resolution recovery.

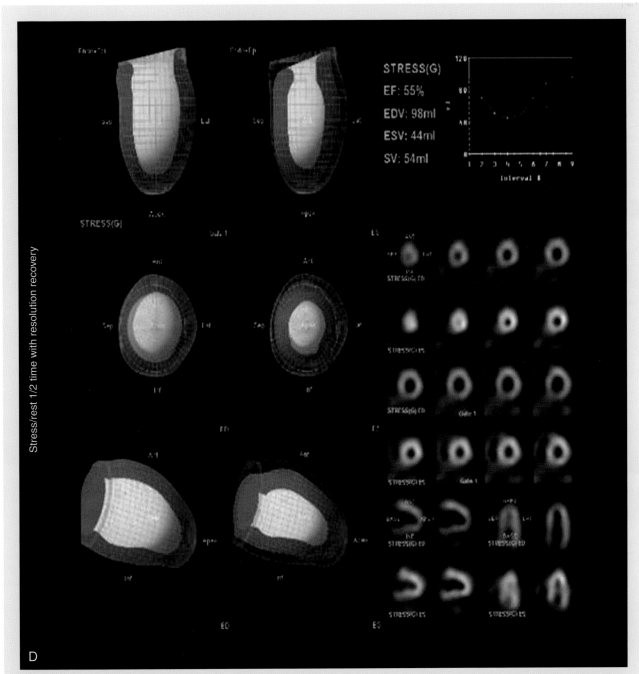

Stress/rest 1/2 time with resolution recovery

STRESS(G)
EF: 55%
EDV: 98ml
ESV: 44ml
SV: 54ml

■ **Figure 18-1—Cont'd D,** To the *left* are shown 3D views of the LV, with a green mesh epicardium and solid white endocardium. The *far left column* shows end-diastolic frames in an anterior, apical, and septal view, from *top* to *bottom*. The next column shows the same views in the end-systolic frame. To the right is shown the LV volume curve on top, and then four rows of alternating end-diastolic and end-systolic short-axis slices. The *bottom two* rows show two vertical long-axis and two horizontal long-axis slices, with end-diastole on top and end-systole on bottom. This image corresponds to **B**; it is from a half-time acquisition reconstructed with resolution recovery. Note the higher image resolution and higher contrast LV chamber compared to **C**.

COMMENTS

This is an example of a patient with normal myocardial perfusion in which half-time imaging reconstructed with resolution recovery algorithms is diagnostically equivalent to full-time imaging reconstructed without resolution recovery. Note the appearance of sharper myocardial boundaries and the higher myocardium/chamber contrast resulting from the increased resolution. Functional measurements are also similar for both studies; although the LVEF is somewhat reduced because of increased end-systolic volume, which is seen with some resolution recovery algorithms. Note that the decreased count rates resulting from the half-time imaging do not appear to adversely affect gated image quality; however, the increased resolution of the detector response corrected images may cause different volumetric measurements so that serial studies reconstructed differently may not be comparable.

Case 18-2	Half-Time Resolution Recovery With Improved Defect Contrast (Figure 18-2)

A 75-year-old, 6-foot 1-inch, 157-lb man with hypertension, hypercholesterolemia, and a history of CAD diagnosed with angiography 1 year previously underwent dipyridamole ECG gated stress imaging and static rest imaging using a standard dual-detector rotating gamma camera. Twenty seconds per stop rest and gated stress acquisitions with 60 projections (10 minutes +) were reconstructed with OSEM. Ten seconds per stop rest and gated stress acquisitions with 60 projections (5 minutes +) were reconstructed with OSEM, incorporating correction for detector and collimator response.

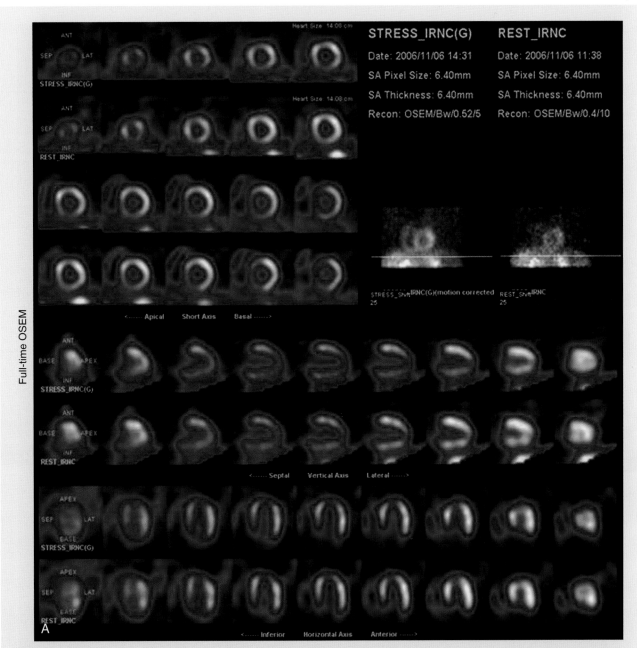

■ **Figure 18-2** Half-time resolution recovery with improved defect contrast. **A,** Stress and rest slices (alternating rows) in short-axis, vertical long-axis, and horizontal long-axis views. The *upper right* shows stress *(left)* and rest *(right)* planar projections. This image was acquired using standard imaging times and reconstructed using OSEM without corrections. This patient's LV has a small apical defect.

(Continued)

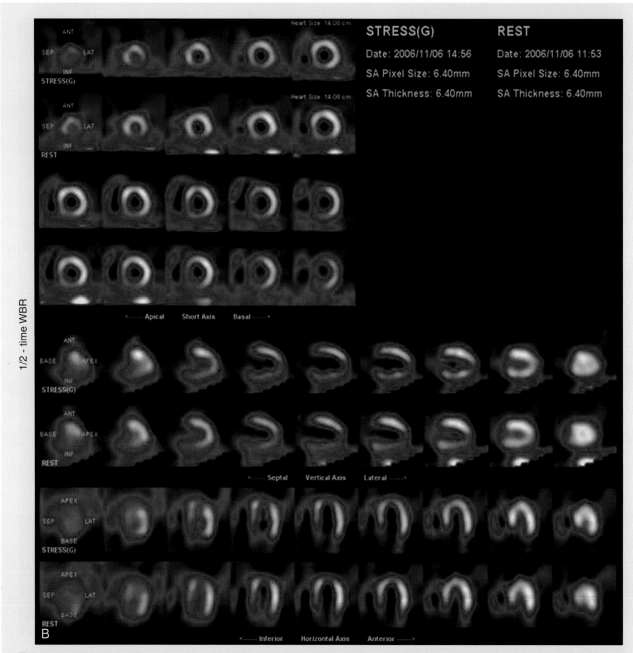

■ **Figure 18-2—Cont'd B,** Stress and rest slices (alternating rows) in short-axis, vertical long-axis, and horizontal long-axis views. This image was acquired using a half-time protocol, and reconstructed iteratively using resolution recovery. Note the improved visualization of the apical defect, attributable to the higher resolution of this image compared to **A.**

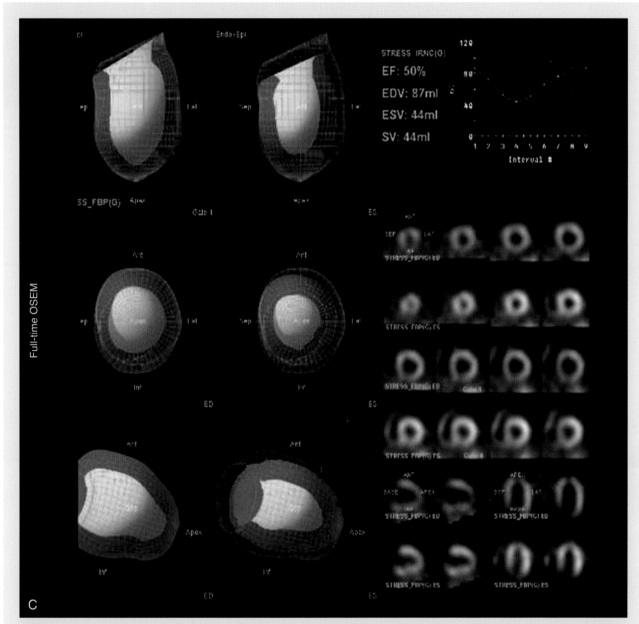

■ **Figure 18-2—Cont'd C,** To the *left* are shown 3D views of the LV, with a green mesh epicardium and solid white endocardium. The *far left* column shows end-diastolic frames in an anterior, apical, and septal view, from *top* to *bottom*. The next column shows the same views in the end-systolic frame. To the *right* is shown the LV volume curve on top, and then four rows of alternating end-diastolic and end-systolic short-axis slices. The *bottom two rows* show two vertical long-axis and two horizontal long-axis slices, with end-diastole on *top* and end-systole on *bottom*. This image corresponds to **A**; it is from a full-time acquisition reconstructed without resolution recovery.

(Continued)

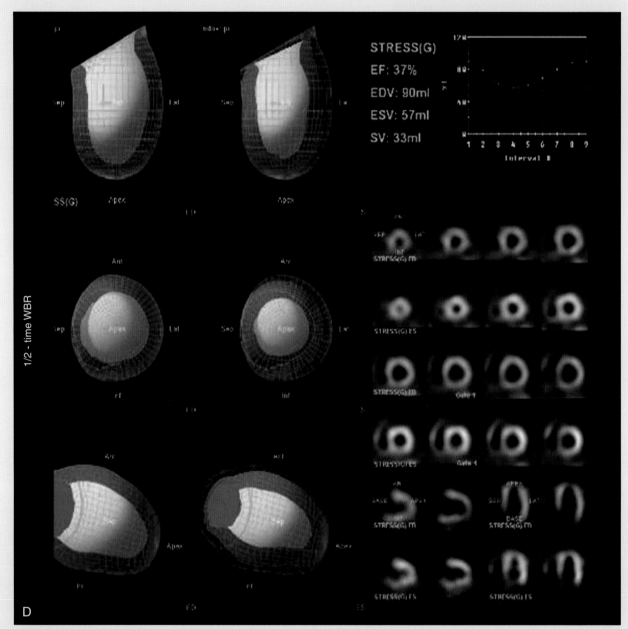

■ **Figure 18-2—Cont'd D,** To the *left* are shown 3D views of the LV, with a green mesh epicardium and solid white endocardium. The *far left* column shows end-diastolic frames in an anterior, apical, and septal view, from *top* to *bottom*. The next column shows the same views in the end-systolic frame. To the *right* is shown the LV volume curve on top, and then four rows of alternating end-diastolic and end-systolic short axis slices. The *bottom two rows* show two vertical long-axis and two horizontal long-axis slices, with end-diastole on top and end-systole on bottom. This image corresponds to **B**; it is from a 5-minute acquisition reconstructed with resolution recovery. Note the larger end-systolic volume, visualized best in the 3D images, in this dataset compared to **C**. This causes a reduced EF in this resolution recovered dataset. This is probably the more accurate measurement, given the known CAD status in this patient.

COMMENTS

This is an example of a patient with a small apical defect. This can be seen somewhat better in the image with resolution recovery. Otherwise, the images are diagnostically similar. The EF measurements in this patient are appreciably different, primarily due to the increased end-systolic volume measured with resolution recovery. This tends to be a result of the higher resolution and increased chamber volume contrast.

Case 18-3   **Normal Woman, Tc-99m Perfusion Study, Solid-State Ultrafast Camera (Figure 18-3)**

A 52-year-old, 5-foot 1-inch, 117-lb woman with nonanginal chest pain and no prior cardiac history underwent adenosine Tc-99m tetrofosmin myocardial perfusion SPECT using a 1-day rest (12 mCi)-stress (35 mCi) protocol. Acquisition times for the rest and stress studies were 4 and 2 minutes, respectively. The resting ECG was normal. The patient experienced no chest pain and there were no electrocardiographic changes during stress. SPECT images were acquired using a DNM (Discovery) 530c solid-state multipinhole 19-detector camera. Rest and poststress ECG gating was performed using eight frames per cardiac cycle.

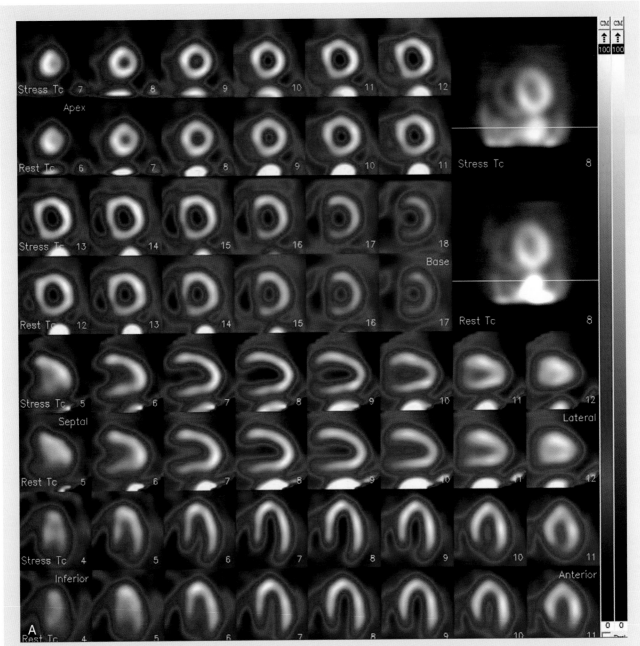

■ **Figure 18-3** Normal female, Tc-99m perfusion study, solid-state ultrafast camera. **A,** *Top right B/W panels* are the planar reprojection images demonstrating excellent image contrast. Color images are the corresponding tomographic slices display with the resting results interleaved between the stress slices. *Top four rows* display the LV short-axis from apex *(top left)* to base *(bottom right)*. Next two rows display the stress and rest vertical long-axis slices from the septum to the lateral wall and the last two rows show the stress and rest horizontal long-axis slices from the inferior to the anterior wall. Note the high image spatial and contrast resolution and homogeneous tracer uptake throughout the LV for studies acquired in 4 minutes (rest) and 2 minutes (stress).

Normal file: Female - 1 day R/S myoview NM530c   Distance-weighted polar maps

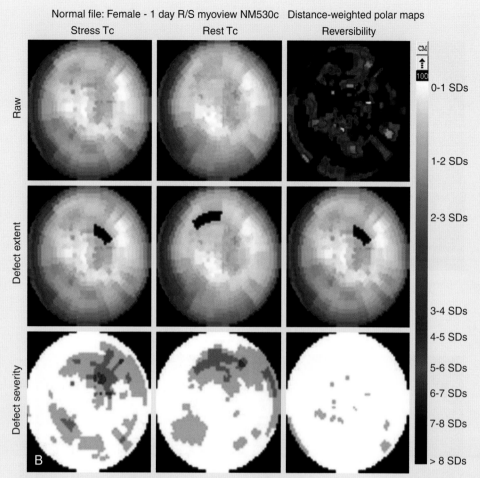

■ Figure 18-3—Cont'd B, Polar maps representation and quantification of this patient's LV tracer uptake. The *three panels in the top* row correspond to the stress, rest, and reversibility (normalized rest-stress) LV distributions. The brighter colors represent higher counts (perfusion) and the darker colors fewer counts as depicted by the translation table on the *rightmost column*. Note the relative homogeneity of the stress and rest polar maps. The *middle row* is the defect extent polar maps display, where areas that are abnormal in comparison to this protocol's normal database are highlighted in *black*. Note that there are two small, but insignificant blackout regions (one stress and one rest) indicating a totally normal study. The *bottom row* is the defect severity polar maps display where each pixel (voxel) is color coded to the number of standard deviations below the mean normal distribution with the scale shown next to the translation table.

(Continued)

Estimated scores

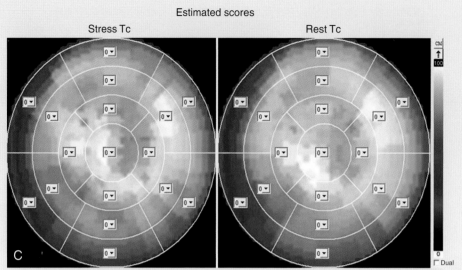

0: Normal   1: Equivocal   2: Moderate reduction   3: Severe reduction   4: Absent

Summed stress score (SSS) : 0   Summed rest score (SRS) : 0

Summed difference score: 0

Normal file: Female - 1 day R/S myoview NM530c

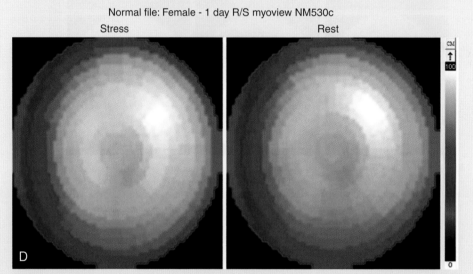

■**Figure 18-3—Cont'd C,** Stress and rest LV myocardial perfusion polar maps with superimposed 17-segment coordinate system using the 0-to-4 score for each segment. Note that for this patient, the sum of all 17-segment scores at stress *(SSS)* and at rest *(SRS)* is 0, indicating a normal perfusion study. **D,** Mean normal LV stress and rest Tc-99m myocardial perfusion distribution in females generated from a population of 30 female patients with < 5% probability of CAD. Note the general homogeneous perfusion distribution compared to the normal distributions in females imaged with conventional SPECT (see Figure 1-2D). Note that, compared to normal results from conventional SPECT, there is no count reduction in the anterior wall typically seen when using 180° acquisition corresponding to the anterior wall RV insertion location.

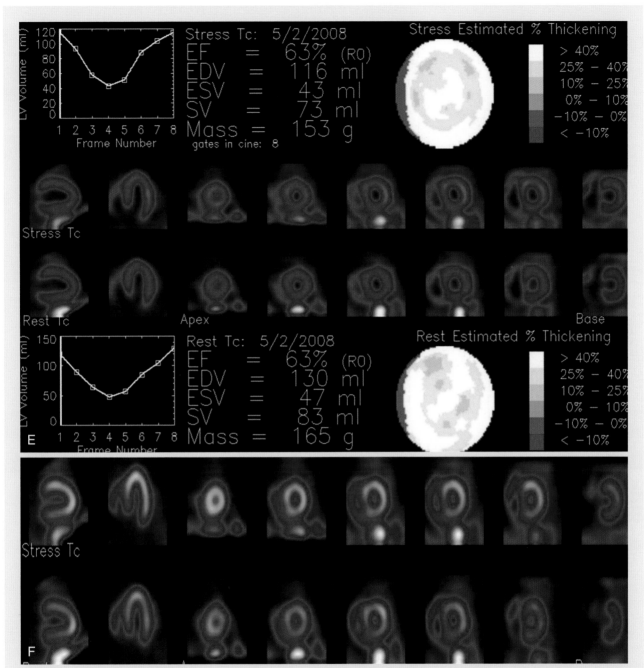

■ **Figure 18-3—Cont'd E and F,** The two rows of color images show end-diastolic **(E)** and end-systolic **(F)** poststress *(top)* and rest *(bottom)*, vertical, horizontal, and short-axis LV tomographic display of this patient's ECG-gated images. Note the uniform, regional significant inward LV and RV endocardial wall motion between diastole and systole typical of patient's normal cardiac function. Also note the uniform, regional significant change in myocardial color from diastole to systole due to the significant thickening seen in patients with normal LV thickening. The color polar maps in **E** represent the quantification of the poststress *(top)* and rest *(bottom)* regional thickening. Note the labeled thickening scale to the right of the maps. The *top left* (poststress) and *bottom left* (rest) panels show the patient's average volume-time curve per cycle, LVEF, EDV, ESV, SV, and LV mass. Note that both the rest and poststress LVEFs are above the 50% normal threshold for this quantitative program. These panels are accompanied by dynamic displays (Video 18-1).

(Continued)

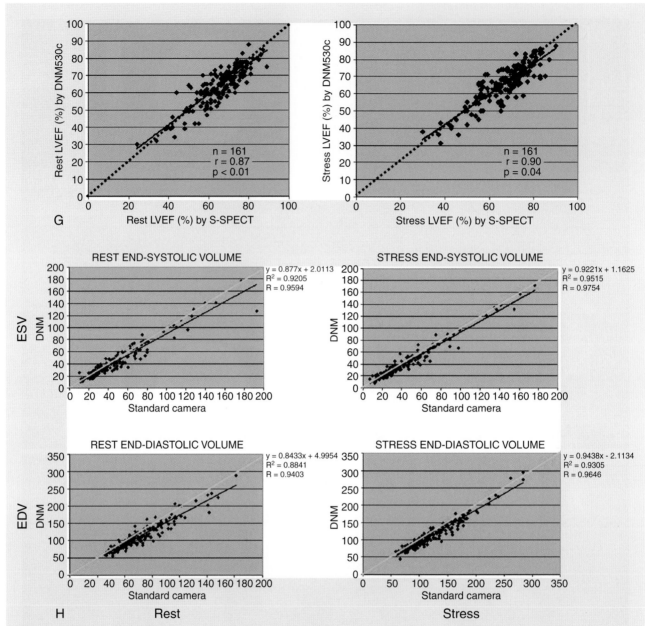

■ **Figure 18-3—Cont'd G,** Correlation of rest and stress LV EFs between eight-frame DNM and S-SPECT images. **H,** Correlations between rest and stress LV end-systolic volumes and end-diastolic volumes. The *dark line* represents the line of regression; the *dotted line* is the line of identity. *(G, H from* J Nucl Cardiol *16:927-934, 2009. Multicenter trial performed at Rambam Medical Center, Mayo Clinic and Emory University.)*

COMMENTS

This is an example of a woman with a normal perfusion study of excellent image quality performed with a new ultrafast camera. Compare these images to those from the same patient imaged with conventional SPECT and acquisitions times of 14 minutes for the rest and 12 minutes for the stress seen in Case 1-2. Note that, compared to conventional SPECT images (see Figure 1-2), both the stress and rest tomographic images from this solid-state camera exhibit higher spatial and contrast resolution, as depicted by the well-defined endocardial and epicardial myocardial borders and a well-defined LV chamber. Note the uniform count distribution throughout the LV myocardium consistent with homogeneous relative perfusion typical of patients with no significant coronary obstructions. Note also from regression lines how well the rest and stress LV EFs and volumes correlate between the new DNM 530c camera and standard SPECT (S-SPECT) cameras.

| Case 18-4 | **Normal Man, Rest Tl-201/ StressTc-99m Tetrofosmin Study, Solid-State Ultrafast Camera (Figure 18-4)** |

A 57-year-old, 5-foot 5-inch, 136-lb male patient suspected for CAD with a history of hypertension and end-stage renal disease. The patient underwent both standard dual-head rotating SPECT study and ultrafast solid-state MPI study, using the same injected dose. Rest Tl-201(3 mCi)–stress Tc-99m sestamibi (15 min) myocardial perfusion SPECT was performed using a 1-day dual isotope protocol. Rest and stress acquisitions times were 5 and 3 minutes for the DNM 530c system and 20 and 14 minutes for conventional SPECT. The patient underwent exercise testing using a modified Bruce protocol. The resting ECG was normal. The patient experienced no chest pain and there were no electrocardiographic changes during exercise. ECG gating of the poststress study was performed using eight frames per cardiac cycle.

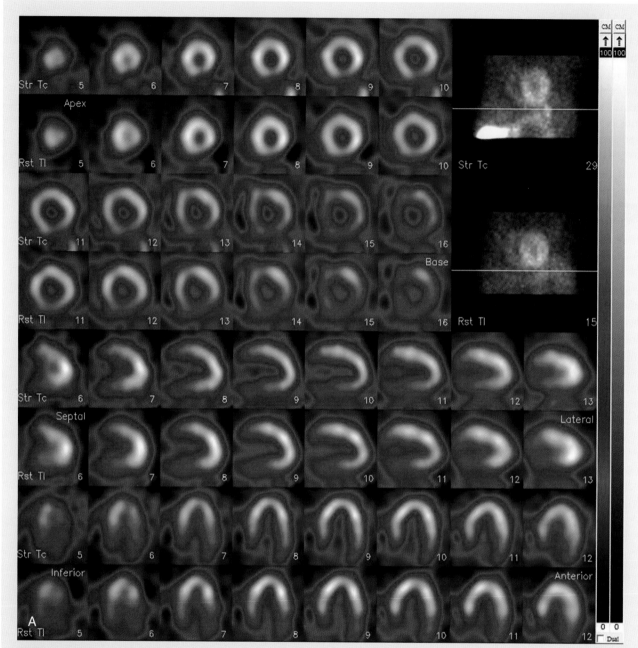

■**Figure 18-4** Normal male rest Tl-201/stress Tc-99m tetrofosmin study, solid-state ultrafast camera. **A,** Standard SPECT study. Color images are the tomographic slices display with the resting results interleaved between the stress slices. *Top four rows* display the LV short-axis from apex *(top left)* to base *(bottom right)*. Next two rows display the stress and rest vertical long-axis slices from the septum to the lateral wall, and the last two rows show the stress and rest horizontal long-axis slices from the inferior to the anterior wall. Note the image quality and homogenous tracer uptake throughout the LV.

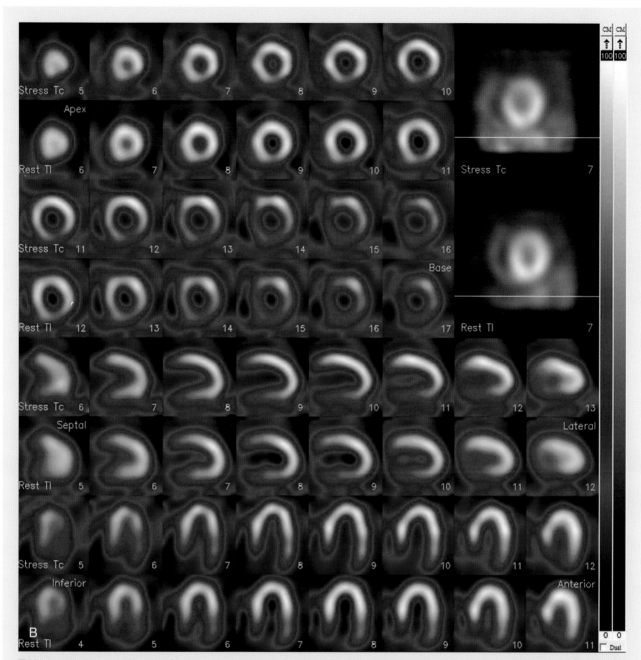

■ **Figure 18-4—Cont'd B,** Ultrafast CZT camera study. Color images are the tomographic slices corresponding to the orientations in **A.** Note the higher spatial and contrast resolution of these tomograms compared to those from **A,** even though they were acquired at a fraction of the time. Note, in particular, the high image quality of the Tl-201 images where the anterior papillary muscle is well-resolved.

(Continued)

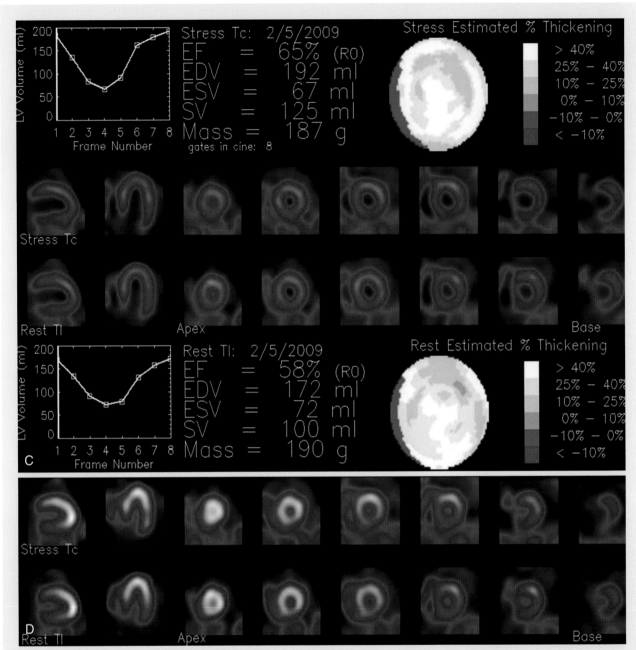

■ **Figure 18-4—Cont'd** The row of color images show end-diastolic **(C)** and end-systolic **(D)** poststress vertical long-axis, horizontal long-axis, and short-axis LV tomographic display of this patient's ECG-gated images acquired with the solid-state camera. Note the uniform, regional significant inward LV and RV endocardial wall motion between diastole and systole typical of patients with normal cardiac function. Also note the uniform, regional significant change in myocardial color from diastole to systole due to the significant thickening seen in patients with normal LV thickening. Note how the quality of the Tl-201 ED and ES images match those of the Tc-99m study, confirming the high energy resolution of the CZT detectors. The poststress and rest LVEFs are calculated to be well above the 50% normal threshold for this quantitative program. These panels are accompanied by dynamic displays (Video 18-2).

COMMENTS

This is an example of a male patient undergoing dual isotope imaging. Although the quality of the conventional SPECT images are satisfactory, the DNM 530c images, which were acquired in about 25% of the conventional time, demonstrate superior spatial and contrast resolution, particularly for the Tl-201 resting images.

| Case 18-5 | MPI Study of a Man With LCX Disease: Comparison Between Standard and Ultrafast SPECT Imaging (Figure 18-5) |

An 87-year-old, 5-foot 11-inch, 146-lb man with dyslipidemia, LV hypertrophy, and known history of CAD, including a previous MI, underwent rest/stress Tc-99m tetrofosmin myocardial perfusion imaging (using 10 mCi for rest and 30 mCi for stress). Standard dual-detector SPECT rest and stress acquisitions were 14 and 12 minutes, respectively. Ultrafast SPECT rest and stress acquisitions were 4 and 2 minutes, respectively. The patient was exercised using the Bruce protocol. ECG gating of the poststress study was performed using eight frames per cardiac cycle.

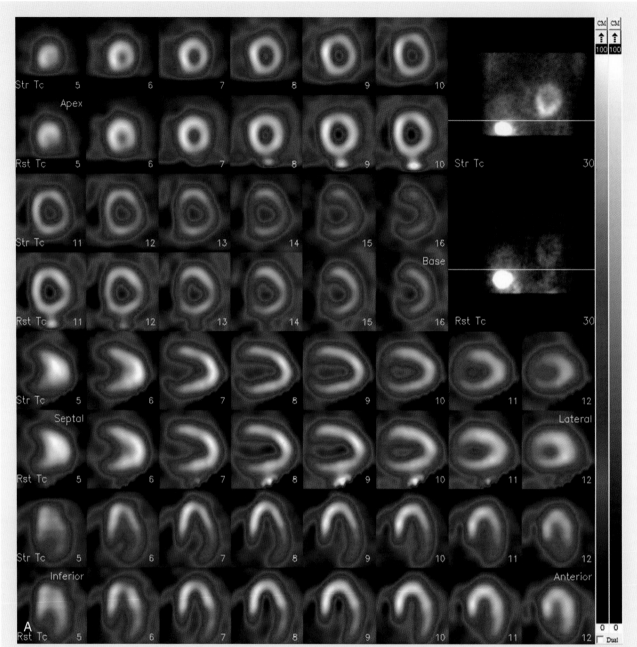

■ **Figure 18-5** MPI study of a man with LCX disease—comparison between standard and ultrafast SPECT imaging. **A,** Standard SPECT images. *Top right B/W panels* are the stress and rest planar reprojection images demonstrating excellent image quality. Color images are the corresponding tomographic slices display with the resting results interleaved between the stress slices. *Top four rows* display the LV short-axis from apex *(top left)* to base *(bottom right)*. Next two rows display the stress and rest vertical long-axis slices from the septum to the lateral wall and the last two rows show the stress and rest horizontal long-axis slices from the inferior to the anterior wall. Note the high image quality and the reversible perfusion defect in the LV lateral wall.

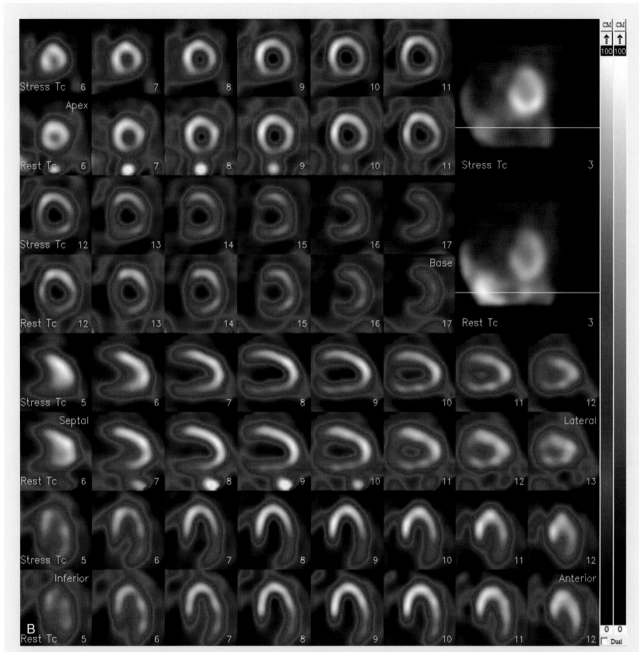

■**Figure 18-5—Cont'd B,** Ultrafast SPECT images. *Top right B/W panels* are the reprojection images demonstrating excellent image contrast. Color images are the corresponding tomographic slices display with the resting results interleaved between the stress slices. Format is the same as in **A.** Note the high image spatial and contrast resolution throughout the LV for studies acquired for 4 minutes (rest) and 2 minutes (stress). Note that the degree of reversibility of the lateral wall is even more marked in this study as compared to standard SPECT in A.

(Continued)

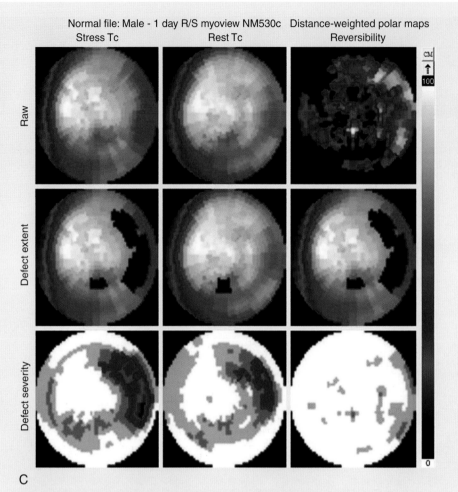

C

■ **Figure 18-5—Cont'd C,** Polar maps representation and quantification of this patient's LV tracer uptake using the ultrafast camera. The *three panels in the top row* correspond to the stress, rest, and reversibility (normalized rest/stress) LV distributions. The brighter colors represent higher counts (perfusion) and the darker colors represent fewer counts, as depicted by the translation table in the *rightmost column*. The *middle row* is the defect extent polar maps display where areas that are abnormal in comparison to this protocol's normal database are highlighted in *black*. Note that there is a large blacked-out area in the lateral wall region of the stress polar map identifying the extent of the hypoperfusion. The *bottom row* is the defect severity polar maps display, where each pixel (voxel) is color coded to the number of standard deviations below the mean normal distribution.

Estimated scores

Stress Tc

Rest Tc

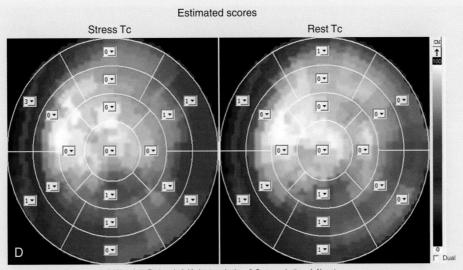

0: Normal   1: Equivocal   2: Moderate reduction   3: Severe reduction   4: Absent

Summed stress score (SSS) : 11   Summed rest score (SRS): 7

Summed difference score: 4

Normal file: Male - 1 day R/S myoview NM530c

Stress

Rest

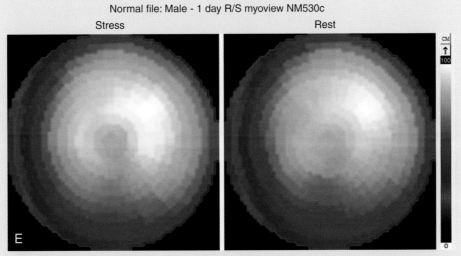

■ **Figure 18-5—Cont'd D,** Stress and rest LV myocardial perfusion polar maps with superimposed 17-segment coordinate system using the 0-to-4 score for each segment. Note that for this patient the automated *SSS* is 11 and the *SRS* is 7. Note that the lateral wall scores in the rest polar map have normalized to 0. **E,** Mean normal LV stress and rest Tc-99m myocardial perfusion distribution in males generated from a population of 30 male patients with less than 5% probability of CAD. Note the general homogeneous perfusion distribution. Compared to the normal distributions in females imaged with ultrafast SPECT (see Figure 18-3, *D*), the male normal distribution is quite similar.

(Continued)

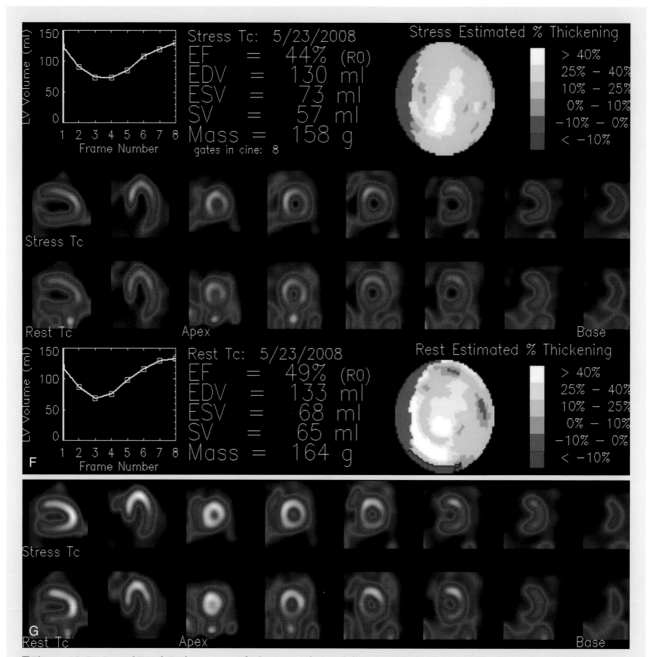

■ **Figure 18-5—Cont'd F and G,** The two rows of color images show end-diastolic (**F**) and end-systolic (**G**) poststress *(top)* and rest *(bottom)*, vertical-, horizontal-, and short-axis LV tomographic display of this patient's ECG-gated images. Note that the inward LV wall motion and the wall thickening (given by the change in color) between diastole and systole is somewhat reduced compared to the normal example in Figure 18-3. Note that the rest and poststress LVEFs are 49% and 44%, respectively, which are below the 50% normal threshold for this quantitative program. These panels are accompanied by dynamic displays (Video 18-3).

COMMENTS

This is an example of a male patient who underwent both standard and ultrafast solid-state SPECT during the same imaging session for purposes of comparison. Figure 18-5, *A*, shows that the conventional MPI tomograms are of high quality and that the LV lateral wall exhibits a stress perfusion defect that is reversible at rest, indicative of ischemia in the LCX vascular territory. Figure 18-5, *B*, shows that the tomograms from the solid-state DNM 530c camera are of even higher image quality with higher spatial and contrast resolution, even though they were acquired in one-sixth (stress) to one-fourth (rest) of the standard time. Note how the reversible lateral wall defect is even more pronounced in the ultrafast HLA images.

| Case 18-6 | Normal MPI Study of a Woman With Breast Attenuation Seen in the Standard SPECT Images but Absent in the Ultrafast Solid State DNM 530c SPECT Images (Figure 18-6) |

A 77-year-old, 5-foot 4-inch, 206-lb woman with a history of hypertension, diabetes, dyslipidemia, and known CAD with a previous stent in the LAD underwent rest/stress Tc-99m tetrofosmin myocardial perfusion imaging (using 10 mCi for rest and 30 mCi for stress). Standard dual-detector SPECT rest and stress acquisitions were 14 and 12 minutes, respectively. Ultrafast SPECT rest and stress acquisitions were 4 and 2 minutes, respectively. The patient was exercised using the Bruce protocol. ECG gating of the poststress and rest studies were performed using eight frames per cardiac cycle.

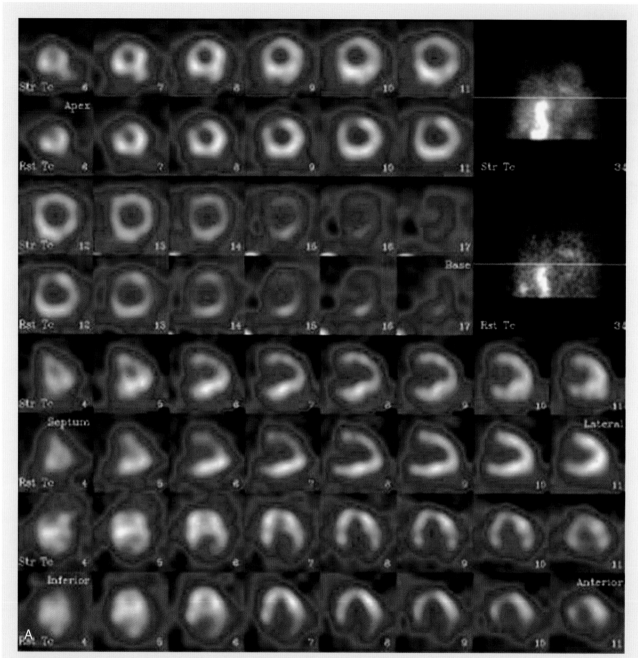

■ **Figure 18-6** Normal MPI study of a woman with breast attenuation seen in the standard SPECT images but absent in the ultrafast SPECT images. **A,** Standard SPECT images. *Top right B/W panels* are the stress and rest planar reprojection images demonstrating an anterior and anterolateral reduction in counts due to breast attenuation. *Color images* are the corresponding tomographic slices display with the resting results interleaved between the stress slices. Note from the short- and vertical long-axis slices there is a similar fixed reduction in counts in the anterior and anterolateral walls due to breast attenuation.

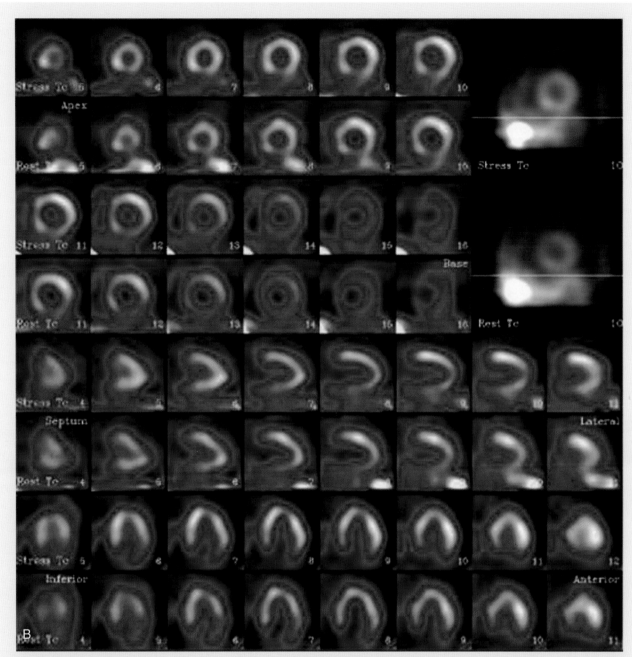

■ **Figure 18-6—Cont'd B,** Ultrafast Solid State SPECT images. *Top right B/W panels* are the planar reprojection images demonstrating the lack of breast attenuation artifact. *Color images* are the corresponding tomographic slices display with the resting results interleaved between the stress slices. Format is the same as in **A.** Note the high image spatial and contrast resolution and the absence of breast attenuation of the anterior and anterolateral LV walls. Note that now there is a mild fixed inferior wall count reduction that is commonly seen in diaphragmatic attenuation.

(Continued)

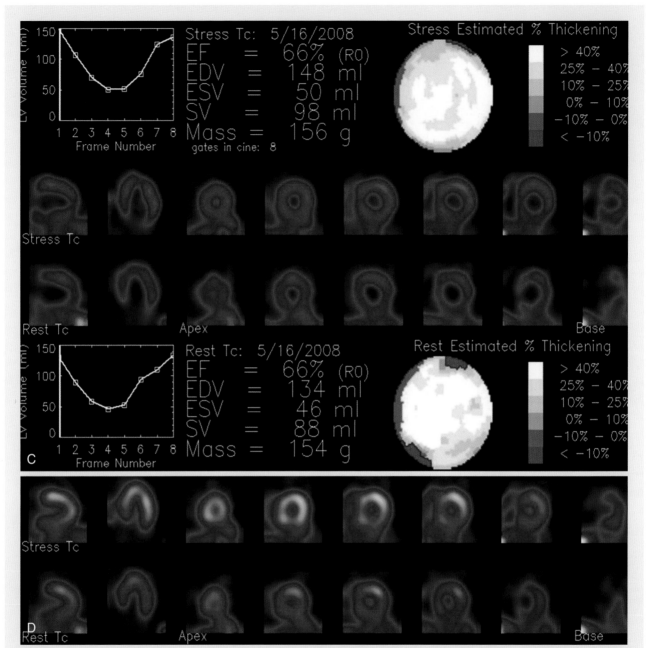

■ **Figure 18-6—Cont'd C and D,** The two rows of color images show end-diastolic **(E)** and end-systolic **(F)** poststress *(top)* and rest *(bottom)*, vertical-axis, horizontal-axis, and short-axis LV tomographic display of this patient's ECG-gated images acquired with the solid-state camera. Note the uniform, regional significant inward LV and RV endocardial wall motion between diastole and systole typical of patient's with normal cardiac function. Also note the uniform, regional significant change in myocardial color from diastole to systole due to the significant thickening seen in patients with normal LV thickening. The color polar maps in **E** represent the quantification of the poststress *(top)* and rest *(bottom)* regional thickening. Note the labeled thickening scale to the *right* of the maps. Note also that both the rest and poststress LVEFs are above the 50% normal threshold for this quantitative program. The normal global and regional function is consistent with the absence of a previous MI. These panels are accompanied by dynamic displays (Video 18-4).

COMMENTS

This is an example of a female patient who underwent both standard and ultrafast solid-state SPECT during the same imaging session for purposes of comparison. Figure 18-6, *A,* shows that the conventional MPI tomograms are of acceptable quality and that the LV anterior and anterolateral walls exhibit a fixed perfusion abnormality consistent with breast attenuation in both the tomograms and B/W projections. Figure 18-6, *B,* shows that the tomograms from the solid-state DNM 530c camera are of high image quality with higher spatial and contrast resolution even though they were acquired in one-sixth (stress) to one-fourth (rest) of the standard time. Note that both the B/W planar projections and the tomograms from the DNM 530c system do not show anterior and anterolateral wall attenuation artifacts due to the 3D geometry of the detectors' distribution in this solid-state system. A mild inferior wall attenuation pattern is now seen. Note in Figure 18-6, *C* and *D,* how both the global and regional LV function is normal consistent with the absence of an anterior wall MI.

SELECTED READINGS

DePuey EG, Gadraju R, Clark J, et al: Ordered subset expectation maximization and wide beam reconstruction "half-time" gated myocardial perfusion SPECT functional imaging: a comparison to "full-time" filtered back projection, *J Nucl Cardiol* 15:547–563, 2008.

Garcia EV, Faber TL: New trends in camera and software technology in nuclear cardiology, *Cardiol Clin* 27:227–236, 2009.

Garcia EV, Faber TL: Advances in nuclear cardiology instrumentation, clinical potential of SPECT and PET, *Curr Cardiovasc Imaging Rep* 2(3):230–237, 2009.

Garcia EV, Faber TL, Esteves FP: Cardiac dedicated ultrafast SPECT cameras: new designs and clinical implications, *J Nucl Med,* 2011; 52:210-217.

Sharir T, Slomka PJ, Berman DS: Solid-state SPECT technology: fast and furious, *J Nucl Cardiol* 17(5):890–896, 2010.

Chapter 19

Myocardial Perfusion SPECT/CT: The Added Value of CT Imaging

Fabio P. Esteves, Cesar A. Santana, Paolo Raggi, and Ernest V. Garcia

KEY POINTS

- Artifactual perfusion defects may develop in the AC image if the CT image is not correctly registered with the SPECT image prior to reconstruction. Therefore, the CT image should be quality controlled prior to SPECT image interpretation.

- The radiation exposure from CT attenuation is small.

- AC eliminates the dependence of body habitus on the normal count distribution of myocardial perfusion images. As a result, the specificity and the normalcy rate of AC images are superior to non-AC images.

- Line sources for simultaneous transmission and emission imaging are the second most common alternative method for attenuation correction.

- Noncontrast CT images may be used to assess the presence and extent of coronary artery calcium. Because coronary calcium is pathognomonic of CAD, it could change the risk stratification of patients without known CAD who have a normal SPECT MPI.

- The absence of coronary artery calcium is associated with a very low (<5%) probability of inducible myocardial ischemia on SPECT imaging. This information should be used in conjunction with the patient's pretest probability of CAD to increase the diagnostic confidence of the physician in excluding obstructive CAD.

- The radiation exposure from coronary calcium scoring is small.

- SPECT MPI may underestimate the ischemic burden in patients with multivessel obstructive CAD because of the relative nature of perfusion distribution. In such cases, CT coronary angiography may help determine the true extent of myocardium at jeopardy.

- It may be difficult to determine the culprit artery in patients with multivessel CAD and inducible ischemia (such as in the anterolateral [LAD or LCX territory] or inferolateral [RCA or LCX territory]) walls. Software fusion of SPECT and CT angiography images may prove useful in isolating the culprit vessel.

- The radiation exposure from combined SPECT perfusion and CT angiography is of concern and might be a reason against its routine use.

BACKGROUND

Hybrid SPECT/CT cameras are becoming more available in the nuclear cardiology community. These two imaging modalities, whether or not performed in the same setting, can pave the way to a more comprehensive assessment of CAD. While CT imaging allows detection and localization of anatomic CAD, SPECT imaging reflects the functional consequences of the disease process. Non-contrast CT images can be used for SPECT AC and coronary artery calcium scoring and contrast-enhanced images are used for CT coronary angiography. The clinical and economic effects of this technology have not yet been established. Optimal clinical use of hybrid imaging requires the appropriate selection of patients and an understanding of SPECT/CT quality control issues.

The attenuation image used for SPECT AC is obtained either with gadolinium line sources or with a CT scanner. While the gadolinium attenuation image is obtained simultaneously with the emission image, the CT attenuation image is acquired either before or after the emission image, increasing the likelihood of misregistration between the emission and transmission images. Artifactual perfusion defects may develop in the AC image if the CT image is not correctly registered with the SPECT image prior to reconstruction.

Case 19-1

SPECT/CT Registration Artifact: LV–Lung Mismatch (Figure 19-1)

A 60-year-old woman reported an episode of a heavy feeling in her chest lasting 5 to 10 minutes 2 weeks prior to an outpatient clinic visit. Chest pain was not associated with exertion and resolved spontaneously. Her only risk factor for CAD was hypercholesterolemia. Her physical examination was unremarkable. She exercised for 5 minutes on the treadmill, achieving 92% of maximum predicted heart rate. The ECG was unremarkable at baseline. Stress ECG showed no ischemic changes. The rest/stress (5/20 mCi) sestamibi SPECT images were obtained using a solid-state-detector camera equipped with multiple pinholes. A single CT attenuation image was obtained prior to rest SPECT imaging using a stand-alone 64-row CT scanner. The CT image was used for attenuation correction of the rest and stress SPECT images.

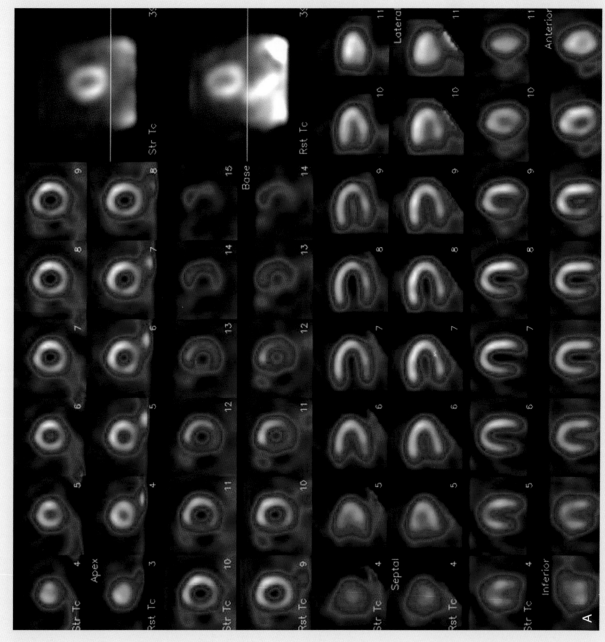

Figure 19-1 SPECT/CT registration artifact: LV–lung mismatch. **A,** The non-AC tomographic SPECT images are normal by visual analysis. A mild fixed count reduction in the inferior wall is consistent with diaphragm attenuation. There is also a small area of mild count reduction in the anterior wall on the stress image (*top row*).

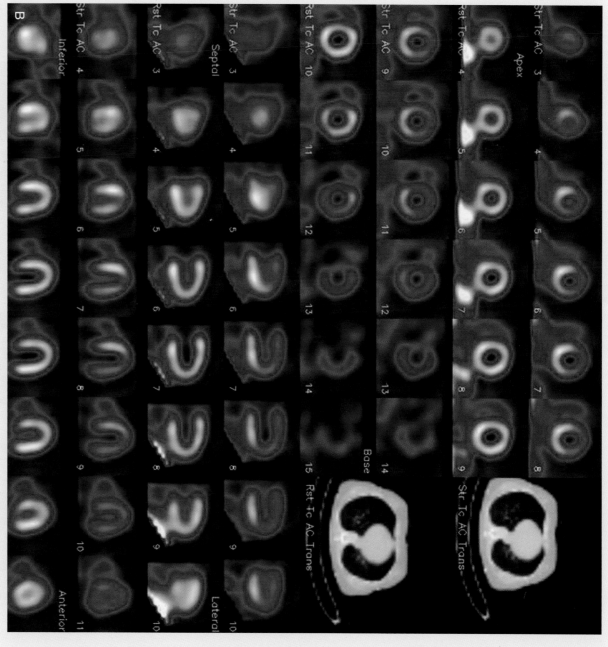

Figure 19-1—Cont'd. B, The AC tomographic SPECT images are abnormal. There is a large and severe reversible defect involving the apical, anterior, and lateral walls.

(Continued)

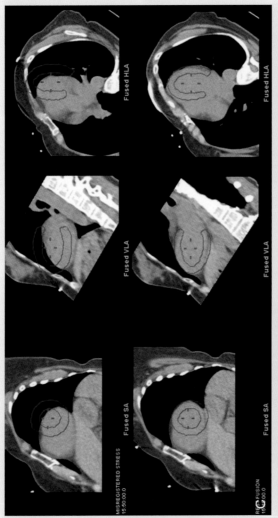

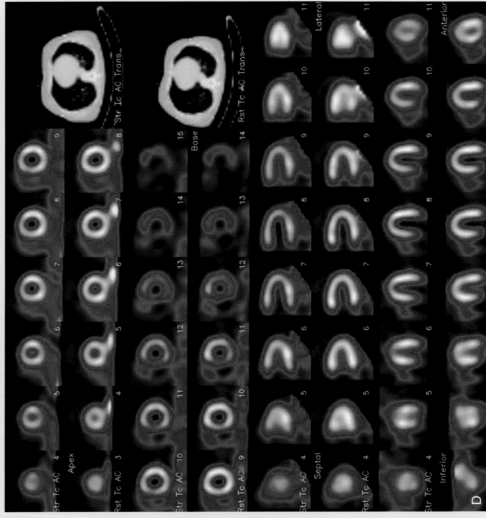

■ **Figure 19-1—Cont'd.** C, Fused stress (*top row*) and rest (*bottom row*) images. The *red* contours were extracted from the emission data and represent the endocardial and epicardial borders of the LV. Note that there is gross misregistration of the stress emission and the CT images. The apical, anterior, and lateral walls on the stress emission image overlay lung tissue on the CT image. The rest emission and the CT image are well registered. Manual rigid registration of the stress images was subsequently performed using manufacturer-provided software. Following registration and reconstruction of the stress SPECT images, the AC SPECT images no longer demonstrate perfusion defects (**D**).

COMMENTS

Emission-transmission misregistration of the stress images, but not the rest images, resulted in a large artifactual reversible perfusion defect in the AC SPECT images. Significant count losses in the myocardium are usually seen when the LV wall on the SPECT image overlays lung tissue on the CT image. The quality of the CT image can have a substantial impact on the quality of the AC SPECT image. For example, CT images with streaking artifacts and dark bands, which are commonly seen in

patients with implantable metal devices (such as defibrillator leads), may result in artificially increased myocardial uptake in the corresponding AC SPECT image because of incorrect scaling of the Hounsfield units into the attenuation map. Also, hypoinflated or hyperinflated lungs on CT can be a source of artifacts in the AC SPECT images (see Figure 20-2). The CT and fused images should always be available at the time of SPECT image interpretation to ensure CT image quality and proper alignment of the emission and transmission images.

Case 19-2

SPECT/CT: Improving Image Quality With Attenuation Correction (Figure 19-2)

A 45-year-old man presented to the outpatient clinic with a history of daily atypical chest pain in the past month. He had no accompanying shortness of breath, nausea, or vomiting. His risk factors for CAD included a 10-pack-year history of smoking and a family history of CAD. The physical examination was unremarkable (215 lb, BMI 28 kg/m²). He underwent vasodilator stress testing with 0.4 mg IV regadenoson. The baseline ECG showed normal sinus rhythm and first-degree AV block. Stress ECG showed no ischemic changes. The rest/stress (5/20 mCi) sestamibi SPECT images were obtained using a solid-state–detector camera equipped with multiple pinholes. A single CT attenuation image was obtained prior to rest SPECT imaging using a stand-alone 64-row CT scanner. The CT image was used for AC of the rest and stress SPECT images. Emission and transmission images were well-registered prior to AC SPECT image reconstruction.

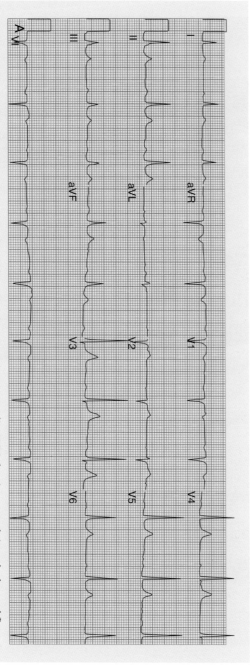

■ **Figure 19-2** SPECT/CT: improving image quality with attenuation correction. **A,** Baseline ECG showing normal sinus rhythm and first-degree AV block.

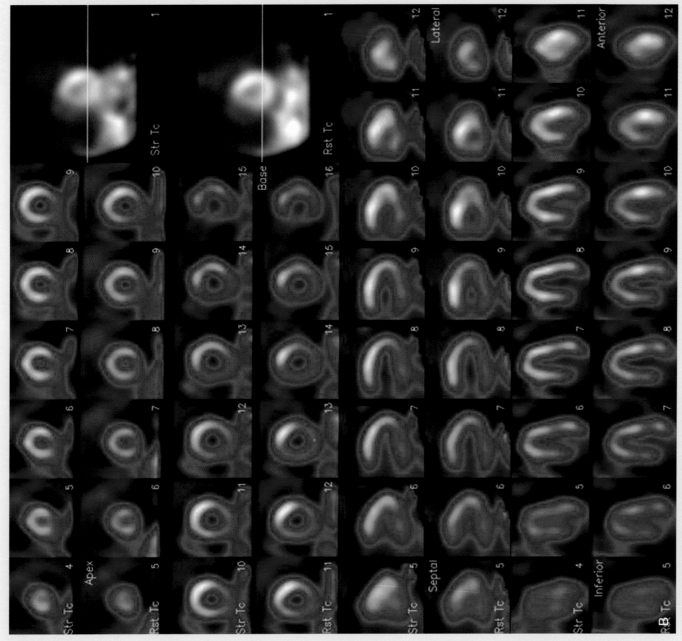

■ **Figure 19-2—Cont'd B**, The non-AC tomographic SPECT images show a fixed mild to moderate count reduction in the inferior wall, extending into the inferoseptal and inferolateral walls.

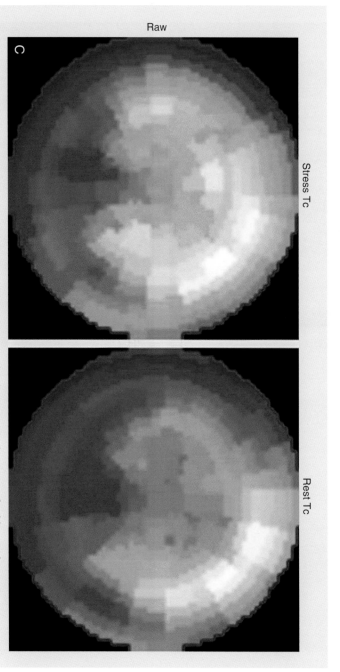

Raw

Stress Tc

Rest Tc

■ **Figure 19-2—Cont'd C,** The raw stress (*left*) and rest (*right*) polar maps also demonstrate a large area of mild to moderate count reduction in the inferior wall with normal perfusion in the remaining LV walls.

(Continued)

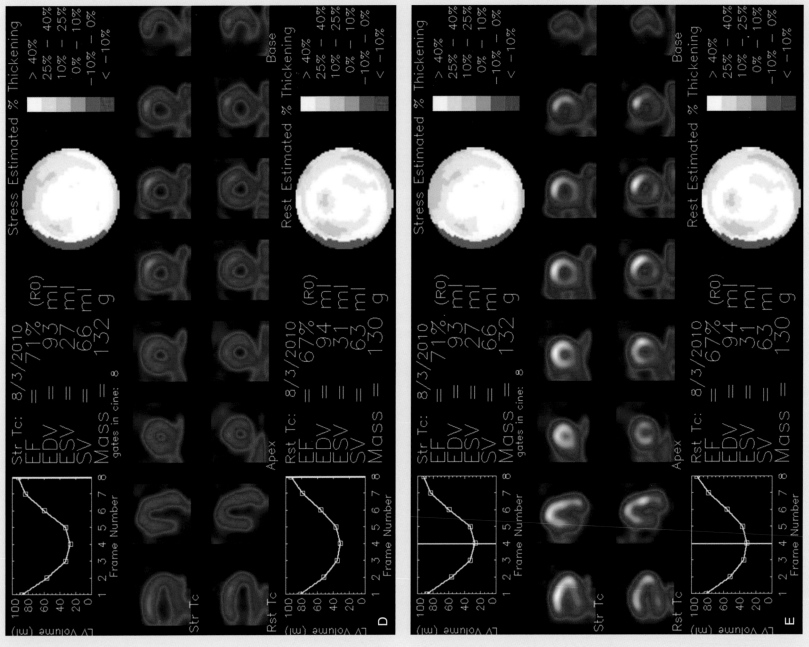

Figure 19-2—Cont'd End-diastolic (**D**) and end-systolic (**E**) poststress (*top*) and rest (*bottom*), VLA, HLA, and SA LV tomographic display of the ECG-gated images. The rest and poststress gated images reveal normal LV wall motion, volumes, and LVEF (67% at rest and 71% poststress).

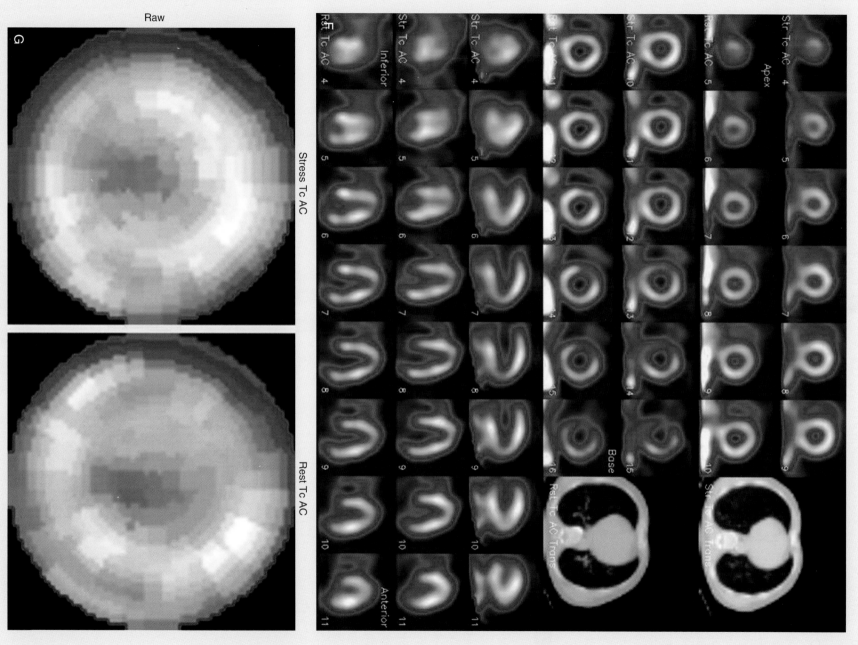

■ **Figure 19-2—Cont'd F,** The AC tomographic SPECT images are normal. The fixed count reduction in the inferior wall seen on non-AC images resolved. **G,** AC raw stress (*left*) and rest (*right*) polar maps show improved count homogeneity and no apparent defects.

COMMENTS

Myocardial perfusion SPECT images are susceptible to soft tissue attenuation artifacts. These artifacts can be misinterpreted as perfusion defects and increase the false-positive rate of SPECT imaging. AC images have higher LV count homogeneity in normal patients than non-AC images because AC eliminates the dependence of body habitus on the normal count distribution. AC algorithms will include not only correction for photon absorption, but also correction for scatter and for the degradation of resolution with depth. The correction for these phenomena improves image quality and increases the interpretive certainty of the physician.

Compensation for soft tissue attenuation and scatter resulted in a more homogeneous count distribution in the LV and is not consistent with hemodynamically significant CAD. The fixed count reduction in the inferior wall was attributed to diaphragmatic attenuation because, in addition to resolution of the defect on AC images, there was normal inferior wall motion on gated images and there were no Q-waves on the ECG.

There is increasing evidence that the specificity and the normalcy rate of AC images are superior to non-AC images. However, one should not expect that AC will yield perfect results every time. AC SPECT image quality may be compromised because of CT artifacts, truncation, misregistration, etc., which should all be quality controlled prior to AC SPECT interpretation. Today, the American Society of Nuclear Cardiology recommends AC as an adjunct to myocardial perfusion SPECT studies, whenever available.

Case 19-3   SPECT/CT: Improving Risk Stratification With Coronary Artery Calcium Scoring (Figure 19-3)

A 56-year-old man without known CAD presented to the outpatient clinic having suffered 2 episodes of atypical chest pain over the past week. The chest discomfort was not associated with exertion and resolved spontaneously. There were no associated symptoms. His risk factors for CAD included a 40-pack-year history of smoking and a strong family history of CAD (father had fatal MI at age 45). The physical examination was unremarkable. He was exercised using the standard Bruce protocol. The baseline ECG was normal. He exercised for 11 minutes, reached target heart rate, and stopped because of fatigue. Stress ECG showed no ischemic changes. The rest/stress (10/30 mCi) sestamibi SPECT images were obtained using a standard dual-detector SPECT camera covering a 180-degree imaging arc from the 45-degree RAO projection to the 45-degree LPO projection. A non-contrast breath-hold ECG-gated chest CT was obtained prior to rest SPECT imaging, using a stand-alone 64-row CT scanner.

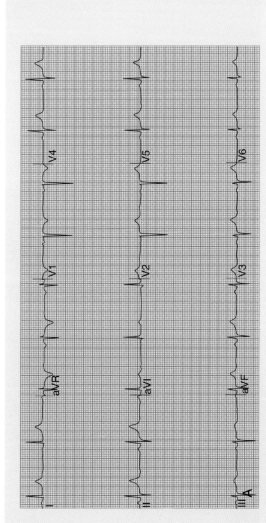

■ **Figure 19-3** SPECT/CT: improving risk stratification with coronary artery calcium scoring. A, Baseline ECG shows normal sinus rhythm and no ST-T changes.

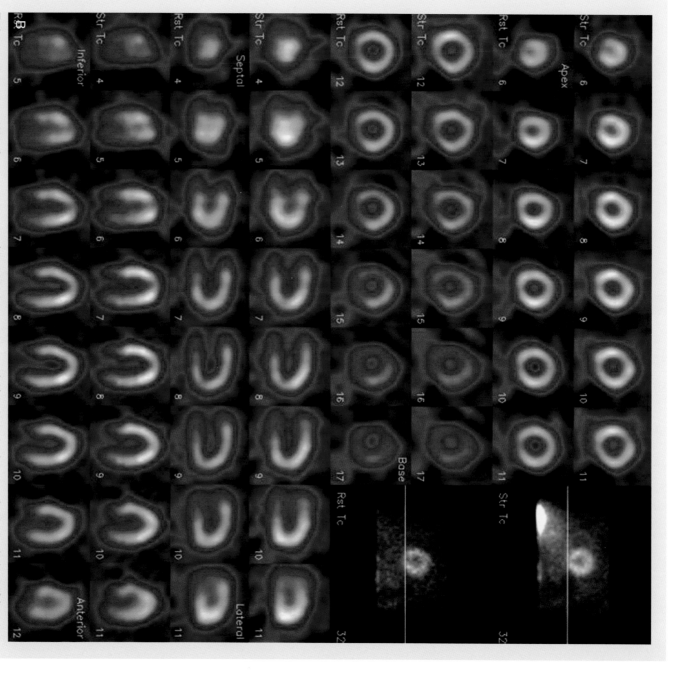

■ **Figure 19-3—Cont'd B,** The non-AC tomographic SPECT images are normal. There is minimal count reduction in the base of the inferior wall that is due to diaphragmatic attenuation.

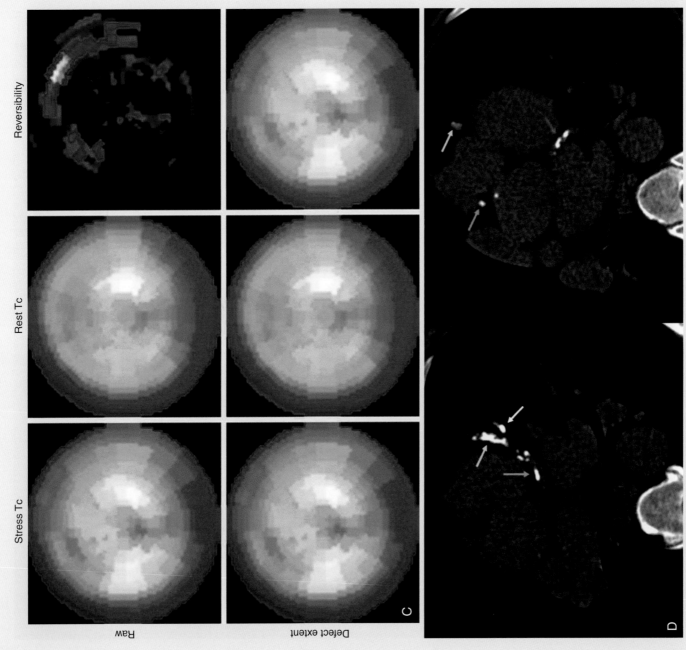

Figure 19-3—Cont'd C, The extent polar maps are also normal. There are no blackout regions in the defect extent polar maps (*bottom row*) indicating a normal study by quantitative analysis. The gated images show normal segmental and global LV wall motion and normal LV ejection fraction. The calcium scoring CT revealed dense calcifications in the coronary arteries. **D,** Transaxial CT images demonstrate calcifications in the distal LM (*orange arrow*), mid and proximal LAD (*yellow arrows*), second diagonal (*white arrow*), LCX (*red arrow*), and RCA (*green arrow*). Total calcium scoring was 563, distributed as follows: LM 24, LAD 231, LCX 130, RCA 178.

COMMENTS

A normal myocardial perfusion SPECT study markedly reduces the possibility of hemodynamically significant CAD, but it does not exclude nonobstructive CAD. The CT image can be used to detect the presence and extent of coronary artery calcifications (as well as to diagnose other incidental thoracic pathologies). Because coronary artery calcium is pathognomonic of CAD, it provides additional diagnostic information in patients without known CAD who have normal myocardial perfusion SPECT imaging. In addition, calcium scoring quantifies the burden of calcified coronary atherosclerosis and provides prognostic information beyond that of traditional cardiovascular risk factors. Therefore, coronary calcium scoring can be used to reclassify the risk of patients with low to intermediate likelihood of CAD and normal myocardial perfusion SPECT imaging, thereby indicating whether initiation of medical therapies should be considered.

This case illustrates how coronary calcium scoring can improve risk stratification in patients without known CAD and with a normal SPECT study. This patient had intermediate likelihood of CAD based on Diamond and Forrester criteria, but a low (<10%) 10-year risk of hard cardiovascular events based on the Framingham risk score. The presence of extensive coronary artery calcium reclassified the patient's cardiovascular risk and he was started on aspirin and statin therapy soon thereafter.

Coronary calcium scoring is not expected to have additional diagnostic value in patients with known CAD or in patients with inducible myocardial ischemia because patient management is unlikely to be altered. Similarly, patients with normal myocardial perfusion SPECT imaging and a high (>20%) 10-year risk of hard cardiovascular events based on the Framingham risk score are also less likely to benefit from calcium scoring CT because their clinical risk already warrants the initiation of medical therapies and lifestyle changes.

Case 19-4

SPECT/CT: Improving Diagnostic Confidence With Coronary Artery Calcium Scoring (Figure 19-4)

A 54-year-old man presented with shortness of breath on exertion. There were no associated symptoms. He quit smoking 20 years ago. His risk factors for CAD included hypercholesterolemia and family history of CAD. Exercise treadmill testing was attempted but baseline ECG showed LBBB. The patient was referred for stress echo, which revealed a mildly compromised LV function with an EF of 50% and mild hypokinesis of the anterior and anteroseptal walls during stress. To establish whether the patient's LV functional abnormalities were due to the LBBB rather than obstructive CAD, he was subsequently scheduled for myocardial perfusion SPECT imaging. He underwent pharmacologic stress testing with an infusion of adenosine over 4 minutes. The rest/stress (4/30mCi) dual-isotope (rest thallium, stress Tc-99m tetrofosmin) SPECT images were obtained using a standard dual-detector SPECT camera covering a 180-degree imaging arc from the 45-degree RAO projection to the 45-degree LPO projection. A non-contrast breath-hold ECG-gated chest CT was obtained prior to rest SPECT imaging using a stand-alone 64-row CT scanner.

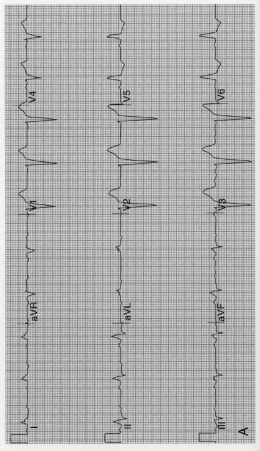

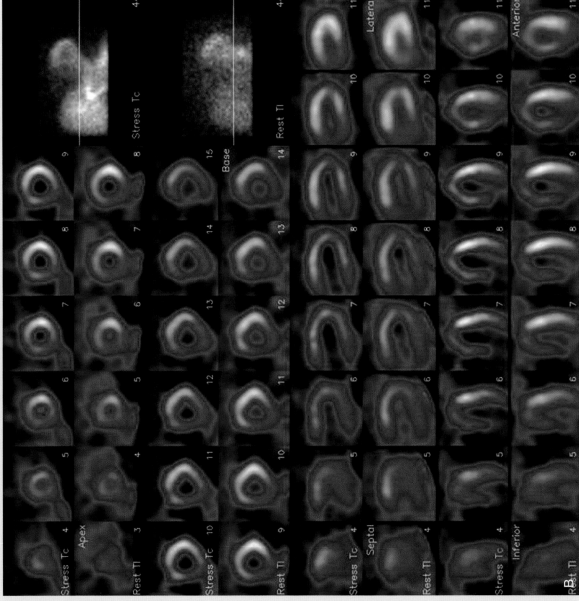

■ **Figure 19-4** SPECT/CT: improving diagnostic confidence with coronary artery calcium scoring. **A,** Baseline ECG shows normal sinus rhythm and LBBB. **B,** The non-AC tomographic SPECT images are abnormal. There is a large area of mild to moderate count reduction in the apical, septal, anteroseptal, and inferoseptal walls in the rest and stress images.

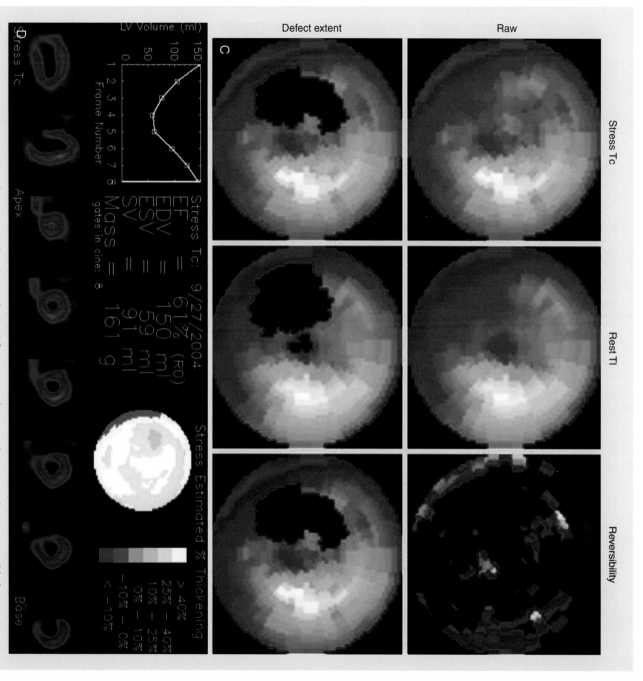

Figure 19-4—Cont'd C, The polar maps are also abnormal. The defect extent polar maps (*bottom row*) demonstrate a blackout region indicating that the regional count reduction is significant when compared to the corresponding rest and stress normal databases. The absence of whiteout areas (*bottom right*) suggests no inducible ischemia by the quantitative analysis. End-diastolic **(D)** and end-systolic **(E)** poststress VLA, HLA, and SA LV tomographic display of the ECG-gated images. The gated images show paradoxical motion of the septal wall and normal LV volumes and ejection fraction (EDV 150 ml, ESV 59 ml, LVEF 61%). The coronary artery calcium score was zero.

(Continued)

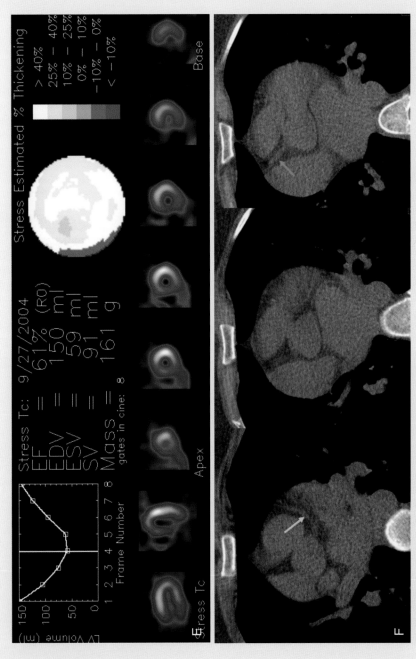

■ **Figure 19-4—Cont'd. E,** see previous page for legend. **F,** Transaxial CT images demonstrates absent calcifications in the proximal LAD (*yellow arrow*), proximal LCX (*red arrow*), and proximal RCA (*green arrow*).

COMMENTS

Coronary artery calcium scoring has been increasingly used as an adjunct to SPECT image interpretation with the advent of hybrid cameras. CAC scoring is not a good diagnostic tool in symptomatic patients with suspected CAD because the association between calcium score and obstructive disease is only modest. However, the absence of coronary calcium is associated with a very low (<5%) probability of inducible myocardial ischemia on SPECT imaging. This information can be extremely valuable for physicians interpreting challenging SPECT studies where perfusion defects may develop in the absence of hemodynamically significant coronary stenosis. Classic examples include patients with LVH, pacemakers, and LBBB.

The non-invasive detection of myocardial ischemia in patients with LBBB remains a challenge. Exercise-induced ST-segment changes on ECG are nondiagnostic and myocardial perfusion SPECT images often show septal/anteroseptal defects that are not associated with significant LAD stenosis on coronary angiography (see Chapter 7).

This case illustrates how absent coronary calcium, used in conjunction with the patient's pretest probability of CAD, can increase the diagnostic confidence of the physician in excluding obstructive CAD because coronary calcifications usually precede obstructive disease by many years. In fact, calcium scoring studies of over 9000 symptomatic patients using coronary angiography as the gold standard suggest that a score of zero can exclude obstructive CAD with a negative predictive value nearing 97%. Therefore, the SPECT perfusion defects seen on this patient are unlikely a result of significant CAD. Moreover, only in the presence of very high CAC may one rightfully suspect obstructive CAD because calcium is associated with almost all stages of intermediate to advanced atherosclerosis.

Case 19-5   SPECT/CT: Helpful Extracoronary Findings on CT (Figure 19-5)

A 79-year-old woman with history of systemic hypertension, hyperlipidemia, and hypothyroidism presented to the ED after a prolonged episode of atypical chest discomfort accompanied by dyspnea. She also reported increasing fatigue and shortness of breath for a few weeks prior to admission. An echocardiogram performed at an outside institution 3 weeks earlier revealed normal chambers size, normal LV systolic function (with an EF of 65%), but decreased compliance. There was also minimal sclerosis of the mitral valve with trace insufficiency. She was referred for pharmacologic stress testing with infusion of adenosine over 4 minutes at 140 mcg/kg/min. The rest/stress (10/30 mCi Tc-99m sestamibi) SPECT images were obtained using a standard dual-detector SPECT camera covering a 180-degree imaging arc from 45-degree RAO projection to the 45-degree LPO projection. A non-contrast chest CT was obtained prior to rest SPECT imaging using a stand-alone 64-row CT scanner.

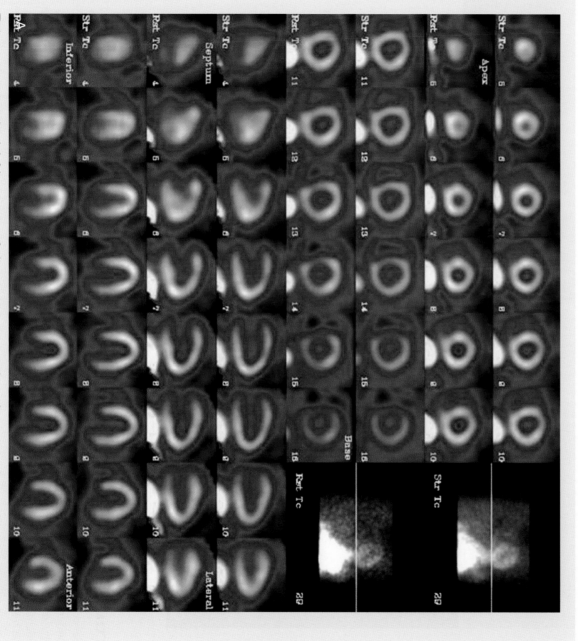

■ **Figure 19-5** SPECT/CT: helpful extracoronary findings on CT. **A,** Tomographic perfusion images showing a homogeneous uptake of the tracer in all segments of the left ventricle.

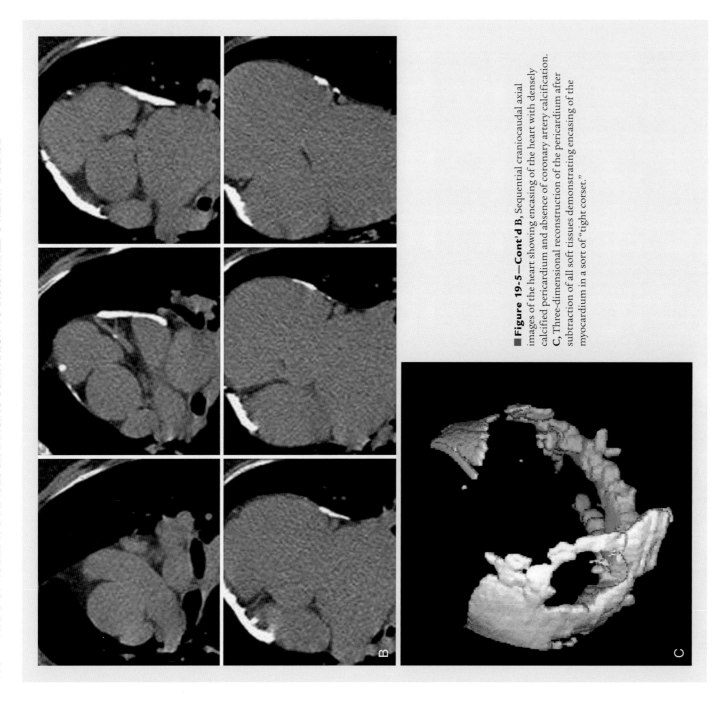

Figure 19-5—Cont'd *B*, Sequential craniocaudal axial images of the heart showing encasing of the heart with densely calcified pericardium and absence of coronary artery calcification. *C*, Three-dimensional reconstruction of the pericardium after subtraction of all soft tissues demonstrating encasing of the myocardium in a sort of "tight corset."

COMMENTS

Several unexpected findings on the chest CT of patients undergoing hybrid imaging may be useful to elucidate the source of the symptoms. Noncoronary findings are encountered with a reported frequency of about 20% on chest CT studies performed to quantify coronary artery calcium screening. This underscores the need for adequate training in the interpretation of chest CT studies, beyond the implementation of CT imaging for attenuation correction, to avoid overlooking findings that may have a significant impact on the care of the patient.

This patient suffered from unsuspected constrictive pericarditis; the myocardial perfusion images showed homogeneous uptake of the tracer and the CT images showed the presence of minimal coronary calcium, thus enhancing the probability of normal coronary arteries. On the other hand, the pericardium was heavily calcified, which provided an explanation for her progressive shortness of breath and fatigue.

SPECT/CT: Improving Quantification of Ischemic Burden With CT Coronary Angiography (Figure 19-6)

A 62-year-old man with hypertension, paroxysmal atrial fibrillation, and CAD with PCI of the LAD and second diagonal branch 6 years ago reported new exercise-induced chest pain and was referred for myocardial perfusion SPECT and CT coronary angiography. He was exercised using the standard Bruce protocol. The baseline ECG was remarkable for LVH. He exercised for 7 minutes, reached target heart rate, developed chest pain, and 2-mm ST-segment depression in the inferolateral leads at peak stress. The rest/stress (10/30mCi) sestamibi SPECT images were obtained using a standard dual-detector SPECT camera covering a 180-degree imaging arc from the 45-degree RAO projection to the 45-degree LPO projection. CT angiography was performed using a stand-alone 64-row CT scanner.

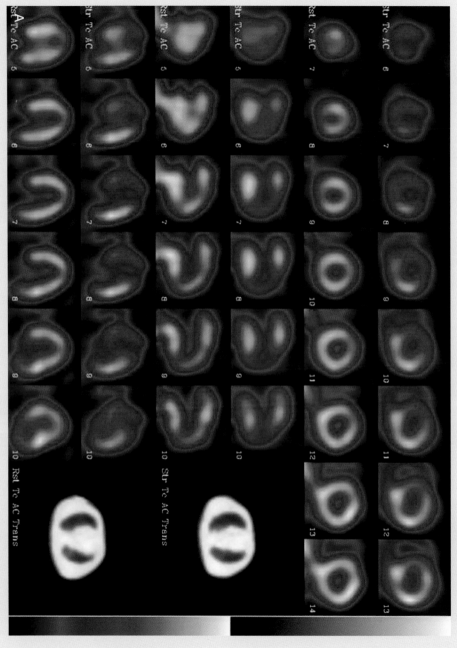

■ **Figure 19-6** SPECT/CT: improving quantification of ischemic burden with CT coronary angiography. **A,** AC SPECT tomographic images demonstrate a large and severe reversible perfusion defect in the apical, anteroapical, inferoapical, mid-anterior, and septal walls. Also note a small and mild reversible defect in the inferobasal wall.

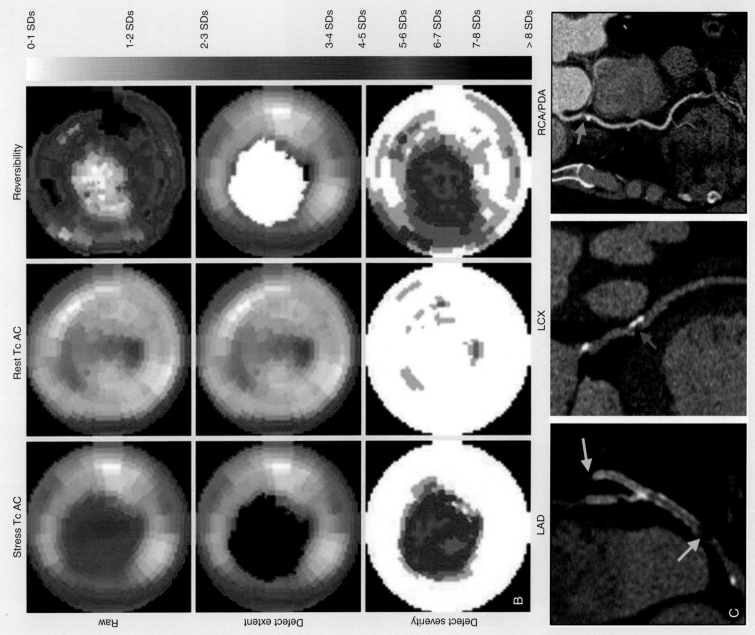

■ **Figure 19-6—Cont'd B,** Polar maps representation and quantification of the LV tracer uptake. The blackout region in the defect extent stress polar map (*middle row*) indicates that the stress images are abnormal by quantitative analysis. The whiteout region suggests complete reversibility in the LAD distribution. **C,** Multiplanar reconstructions of the coronary arteries on CT angiography show calcifications within the three major coronary arteries. There is obstructive disease in the LAD (before and after the stent, *yellow arrows*), LCX (*red arrow*), and RCA (*green arrow*).

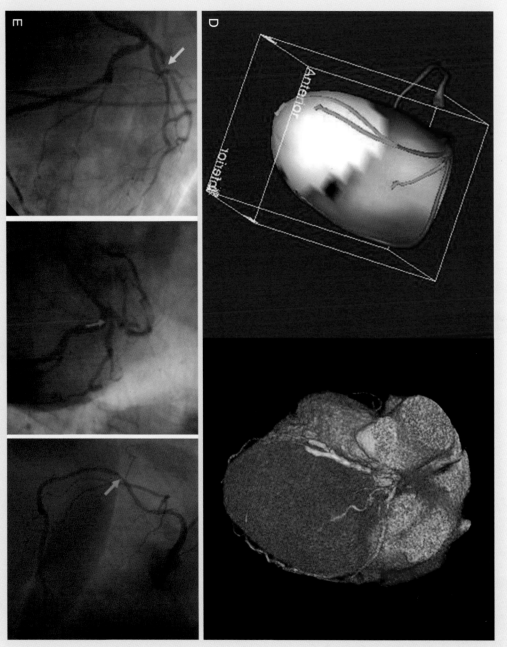

Figure 19-6—Cont'd D, Three-dimensional rendered images of the coronary arteries on CT angiography *(right)* show the course of the LAD and LCX in the LV epicardial surface. Fused display of the SPECT and CT angiography images *(left)* shows a large whiteout area in the LAD distribution, suggesting inducible ischemia. The *green* segments of the coronary arteries are segments distal to the stenosis detected by CT angiography. **E,** Multiplanar views of the coronary arteries on invasive angiography show obstructive stenosis within the LAD *(yellow arrow),* LCX *(red arrow),* and RCA *(green arrow).*

COMMENTS

Myocardial perfusion SPECT imaging is limited by the relative nature of LV perfusion distribution. In other words, the myocardial region with highest count density is normalized to 100% and the perfusion distribution in the remainder of the LV is scaled to that region. As a result, there may be underestimation of the ischemic burden in patients with multivessel CAD because perfusion defects may develop only in segments supplied by the artery with the highest degree of intraluminal obstruction. Furthermore, in patients who have a similar degree of obstruction in all three major coronary arteries, there may be a uniform count reduction in LV tracer uptake and, as a result, the SPECT images will occasionally appear completely normal.

This case illustrates how myocardial perfusion SPECT can underestimate ischemic burden in patients with multivessel CAD. The large reversible defect in the apical, anterior, and septal walls correlated well with obstructive disease in the proximal LAD. However, SPECT images failed to demonstrate significant perfusion abnormalities in the LCX and RCA territories. While SPECT imaging suggested flow-limiting stenosis in only one vessel, CT angiography showed three-vessel disease. Because invasive coronary angiography also revealed three-vessel obstructive stenosis, the patient underwent CABG. It should be noted that physiologic assessment of coronary stenosis using fractional flow reserve showed that only a minority of patients with three-vessel disease by invasive angiography have, in fact, physiologically significant stenoses in all three vessels.

Case 19-7

SPECT/CT: Improving Assessment of the Culprit Lesion With Fusion of SPECT and CT Coronary Angiography (Figure 19-7)

A 55-year-old man with multivessel CAD and previous MI presented with recurrent angina. Invasive coronary angiography demonstrated a short LM, 70% stenosis in the mid LAD, 70% stenosis in the proximal LCX and 95% stenosis before the second marginal, a dominant RCA with 70% stenosis in the distal segment, and 60% stenosis in the PDA. Rest/stress (10/30 mCi) tetrofosmin SPECT images were then obtained using a standard dual-detector SPECT camera covering a 180-degree imaging arc from the 45-degree RAO projection to the 45-degree LPO projection. Subsequently, the patient underwent CT coronary angiography using a stand-alone 16-row CT scanner. This case is from a European hospital where this work-up is used to identify the culprit lesion for selective target vessel PTCA/stenting.

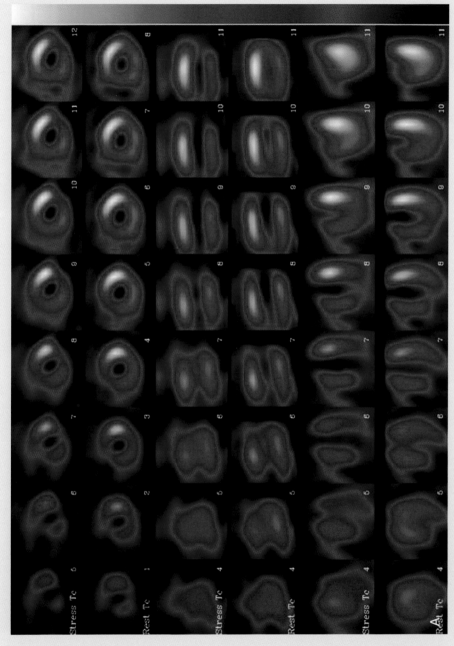

■ **Figure 19-7** SPECT/CT: improving identification of the culprit artery with CT coronary angiography and image fusion. **A**, Non-AC SPECT tomographic images demonstrate a large and severe fixed perfusion defect in the apical, anteroapical, inferoapical, and septal walls, as well as a partially reversible defect of moderate size in the inferolateral wall.

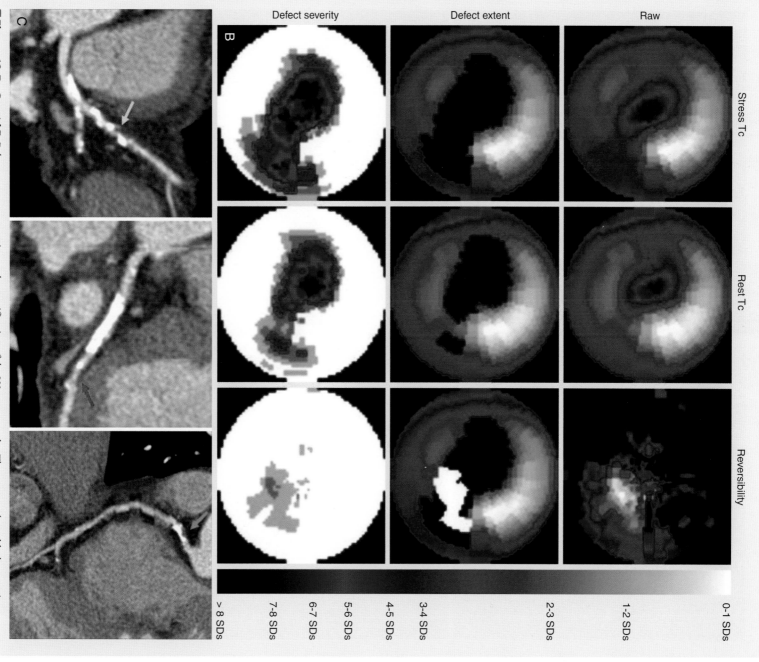

Defect severity   Defect extent   Raw

Stress Tc

Rest Tc

Reversibility

> 8 SDs
7-8 SDs
6-7 SDs
5-6 SDs
4-5 SDs
3-4 SDs
2-3 SDs
1-2 SDs
0-1 SDs

Figure 19-7—Cont'd B, Polar maps representation and quantification of the LV tracer uptake. The stress and rest blackout regions in the defect extent polar maps (*middle row*) indicate that the images are abnormal by quantitative analysis. The whiteout region suggests reversibility in the inferolateral wall. **C,** Multiplanar reconstructions of the coronary arteries on CT angiography show extensive calcifications throughout the three major coronary arteries. There are multiple borderline obstructive stenosis, including 70% stenosis within the LAD (*yellow arrow*), 70% stenosis in the LCX (*red arrow*), and 70% stenosis in the RCA (*green arrow*).

(*Continued*)

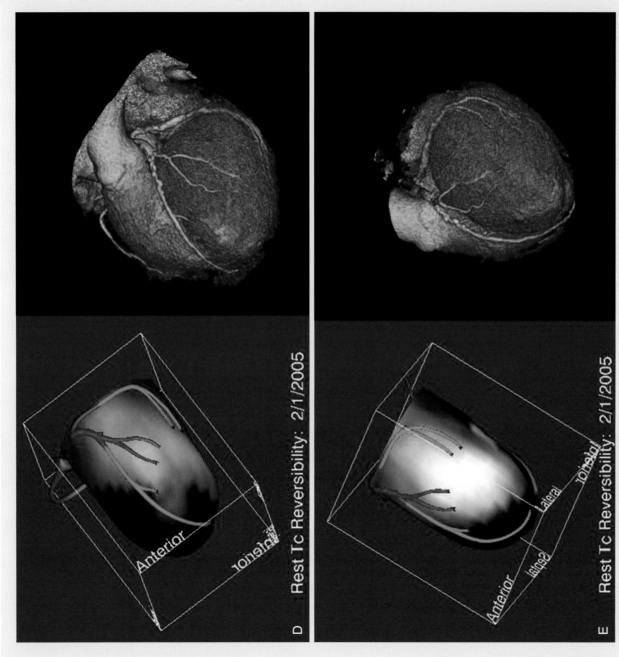

D   Rest Tc Reversibility: 2/1/2005

E   Rest Tc Reversibility: 2/1/2005

■ **Figure 19-7—Cont'd D,** Three-dimensional rendered images of the coronary arteries on CT angiography (*right*) show the course of the LAD and LCX (and their major branches) in the LV epicardial surface. Fused display of the SPECT and CT angiography images (*left*) shows a blackout area in the LAD distribution, suggesting scar tissue but no inducible ischemia. The *green* segments of the coronary arteries are segments distal to the stenosis detected by CT angiography. **E,** Three-dimensional rendered images of the coronary arteries on CT angiography (*right*) show the course of the LAD and LCX (and their major branches) in the LV epicardial surface. Fused display of the SPECT and CT angiography images (*left*) shows no significant perfusion abnormalities in the LCX distribution, suggesting no flow-limiting stenosis. The *green* segments of the coronary arteries are segments distal to the stenosis detected by CT angiography.

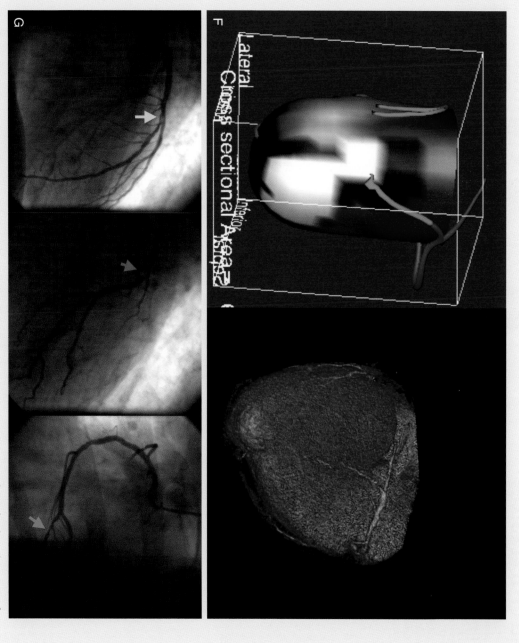

Figure 19-7—Cont'd F, Three-dimensional rendered images of the coronary arteries on CT angiography (*right*) show the course of the RCA in the LV epicardial surface. Fused display of the SPECT and CT angiography images (*left*) shows a whiteout area in the RCA distribution, suggesting inducible ischemia. The green segments of the coronary arteries are segments distal to the stenosis detected by CT angiography. **G,** Multiplanar views of the coronary arteries on invasive angiography show borderline obstructive stenosis within the LAD (*yellow arrow*), LCX (*red arrow*), and RCA/PDA (*green arrow*).

COMMENTS

In current clinical practice, the cardiologist subjectively performs the integration of anatomic and physiologic information from angiograms or CT coronary angiography with SPECT. However, in patients with inducible ischemia and multivessel CAD, it may be difficult to determine the culprit artery, especially if the degree of stenosis is between 50% and 70%. Such stenoses may or may not be associated with inducible myocardial ischemia.

The image fusion on this patient with multivessel CAD helped in the identification of the culprit artery. The SPECT images demonstrated a large and fixed perfusion defect suggestive of scar tissue in the LAD distribution. However, a partially reversible inferolateral wall perfusion defect could be the result of obstructive disease in the LCX or RCA. SPECT or CT coronary angiography images alone were unable to isolate the culprit lesion. However, fusion of the SPECT and CT angiography images proved successful in identifying the artery associated with inducible ischemia. The inferolateral wall ischemia was secondary to obstructive disease in the RCA and not the LCX. Subsequently, the patient underwent successful PTCA/stenting of the RCA, which resulted in resolution of his angina.

SELECTED READINGS

Faber TL, Galt JR: SPECT/CT and PET/CT hybrid imaging and image fusion. In Iskandrian AE, Garcia EV, editors: *Nuclear Cardiac Imaging*, ed 4, New York, 2008, Oxford University Press, pp 202–217.

Iskandrian AE, Garcia EV: Practical issues: ask the experts. In Iskandrian AE, Garcia EV, editors: *Nuclear Cardiac Imaging*, ed 4, New York, 2008, Oxford University Press, pp 703–718.

Kaufmann PA, Gaemperli O: Hybrid cardiac imaging. In Zaret BL, Beller GA, editors: *Clinical Nuclear Cardiology: State of the Art and Future Directions*, ed 4, Philadelphia, 2010, Mosby Elsevier, pp 121–131.

Raggi P: Cardiac computed tomography for the nuclear cardiology specialist. In Iskandrian AE, Garcia EV, editors: *Nuclear Cardiac Imaging*, ed 4, New York, 2008, Oxford University Press, pp 688–702.

Venuraju S, Yerramasu AK, Goodman DA, et al: Coronary artery calcification: pathogenesis, imaging, and risk stratification. In Zaret BL, Beller GA, editors: *Clinical Nuclear Cardiology: State of the Art and Future Directions*, ed 4, Philadelphia, 2010, Mosby Elsevier, pp 332–355.

Chapter 20

Cardiac PET and PET/CT: Artifacts and Tracers

Fabio P. Esteves and Ernest V. Garcia

KEY POINTS

- PET imaging is ideal for the quantitative assessment of myocardial blood flow, metabolism, viability, and innervation.

- PET imaging can be done with or without on-site cyclotrons, but the tracers are different.

- The radiation exposure from PET studies is generally less than that of SPECT studies.

- Attenuation correction is routinely used for PET imaging, unlike SPECT imaging, where it is optional and not widely used.

- Misregistration artifacts have become more prevalent with the advent of hybrid cameras because of the difference in temporal resolution between the PET and the CT image. Artifactual count losses may develop if lung tissue on the CT image overlays LV wall activity on the PET image and there is not proper alignment of the images prior to reconstruction.

- Overcorrection of the inferior wall is another artifact that results from the difference in scanning times between PET and CT images. This artifact is typically seen in patients with hypoinflated lungs on CT imaging.

- Thirteen percent of rubidium decays are associated with a prompt-gamma that correlates in time with the annihilation photons. Prompt-gammas may represent a significant problem when imaging in the 3D mode. Artifactual defects may develop in the PET image if there is no adequate correction for these unwanted events in the reconstruction algorithm.

- N-13-ammonia has favorable physical characteristics over rubidium. However, it has not entered the mainstream of nuclear cardiology because it requires an on-site cyclotron for production.

● F-18 flurpiridaz is a new tracer developed in an attempt to allow exercise stress testing in myocardial perfusion PET and to facilitate the quantification of myocardial blood flow. The diagnostic performance of F-18 flurpiridaz myocardial perfusion PET has not yet been determined.

● The image quality is improved with glucose-loading protocols relative to fasting protocols in FDG myocardial viability imaging. Glucose-loading protocols stimulate the release of endogenous insulin, decreasing plasma levels of free fatty acids and optimizing the myocardial transport and utilization of FDG. As a result, it decreases the blood pool activity and improves image contrast.

BACKGROUND

There has been an exponential growth in cardiac PET imaging in the past decade. The growing interest in this technology is a result of the increased availability of PET cameras, changes in reimbursement, and the scientific evidence documenting its clinical efficacy in the evaluation of patients with CAD. In this chapter, we will illustrate common artifacts in cardiac PET imaging, briefly review the physical characteristics and kinetics of myocardial perfusion PET tracers, and discuss the differences between fasting and glucose-loading protocols in FDG viability imaging.

Case 20-1   PET/CT Artifact: LV–Lung Mismatch (Figure 20-1)

A 53-year-old woman presented to the ED with new-onset atypical angina. Her risk factors included hyperlipidemia, hypertension, and family history of CAD. She was first ruled out for MI by ECG and serial troponin I. Subsequently she was referred for rubidium myocardial perfusion PET. The physical findings were remarkable for obesity (weight 230 lb, BMI 35 kg/m^2) and hypertension. She underwent vasodilator stress testing with regadenoson. The ECG showed sinus rhythm at baseline. Stress ECG showed an isolated PVC and no ischemic changes. The images were obtained using a PET/CT camera operating in the 3D mode.

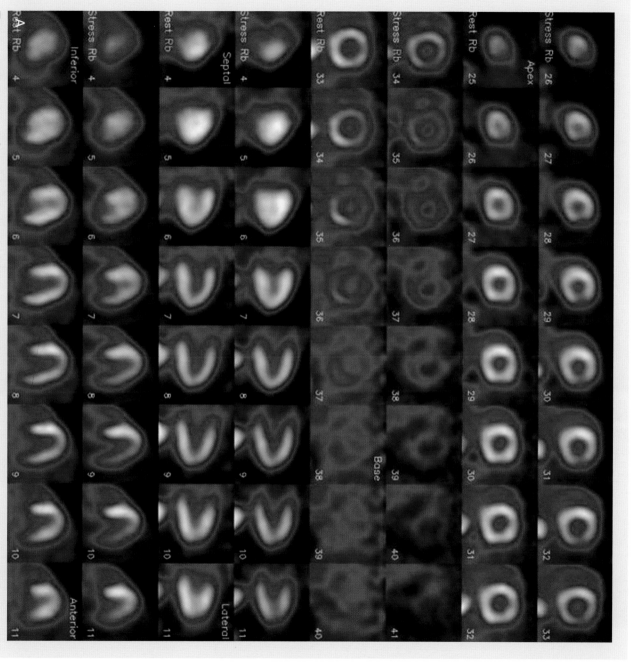

■ **Figure 20-1** PET/CT artifact: LV-lung mismatch. **A.** Tomographic slices display with the resting results interleaved between the stress slices. *Top four rows* display the LV SA from apex (*top left*) to base (*bottom right*). *Next two rows* display the stress and rest VLA slices from the septum to the lateral wall and the *last two rows* show the stress and rest HLA slices from the inferior to the anterior wall. Note there is a large reversible defect of moderate severity in the anterolateral wall.

(Continued)

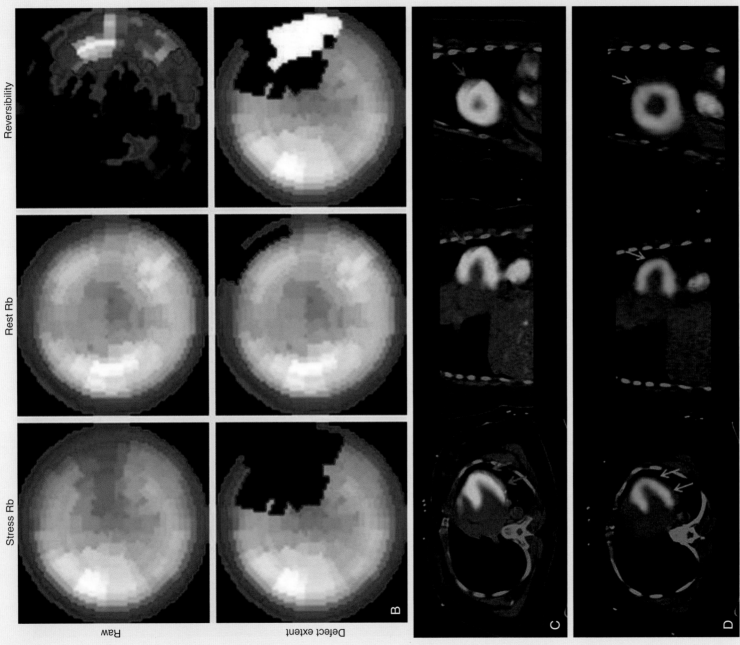

Figure 20-1—Cont'd B, Polar maps representation of perfusion distribution. The *three panels in the top row* correspond to the stress, rest, and reversibility (normalized rest/stress) LV distributions. The *bottom row* is the defect extent polar maps display where areas that are abnormal in comparison to the normal database are highlighted in *black*. Note there is a blackout region in the anterolateral wall at stress indicating an abnormal study by quantitative analysis. The defect extent reversibility polar map *(bottom right)* shows a whiteout area in the anterolateral wall suggesting ischemic changes. **C,** Fused transaxial, coronal, and sagittal stress images. There is misregistration of the stress emission *(color images)* and the CT image *(B/W images)*. The apical, anterior, and lateral walls on the stress emission image overlay lung tissue on the CT image *(red arrows)*. The rest emission and the CT image are well-registered (images not shown). **D,** Fused transaxial, coronal, and sagittal stress images following emission-driven registration. The software artificially replaced lung tissue with soft tissue attenuation in the misregistered voxels *(blue arrows)*.

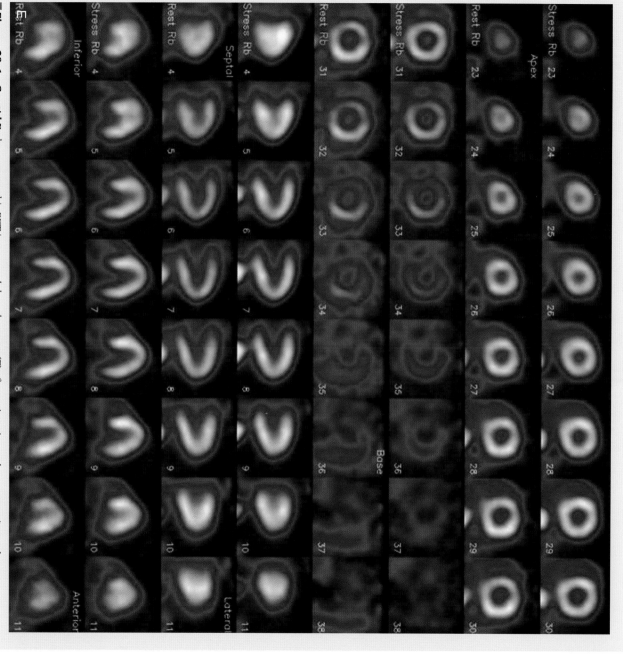

Figure 20-1—Cont'd **E,** the tomographic PET images and the polar maps **(F)** after registration and reconstruction no longer demonstrate perfusion defects.

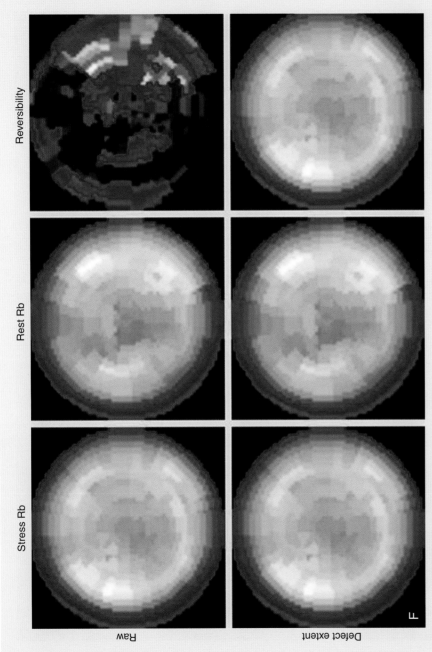

Stress Rb   Rest Rb   Reversibility

Raw

Defect extent

F

■ **Figure 20-1—Cont'd F**, see previous page for legend.

COMMENTS

Hybrid PET/CT cameras are rapidly replacing stand-alone PET cameras in cardiac imaging. While on stand-alone cameras, rotating sources (germanium or cesium) are used to obtain the attenuation image, on hybrid cameras, the CT image is used for PET attenuation correction. This reduces the attenuation scan time from minutes (3 to 10 minutes) to seconds (5 to 20 seconds). The PET image is averaged over a few minutes (about 5 minutes for rubidium). Because the CT scan time is short, sometimes the image does not match the LV–lung interface of the PET image. This increases the emission-transmission misalignment rate in cardiac PET. If the images are not properly aligned prior to reconstruction, perfusion defects may develop. The artificially low attenuation value of the LV wall on the CT image (lung tissue instead of soft tissue) decreases the expected photon attenuation and scatter from that region. When the images are reconstructed, the count density of the misregistered LV wall is artifactually decreased.

The original reconstructed PET images show a large reversible defect of moderate severity in the anterolateral wall. The stress perfusion defect is secondary to misalignment of the PET and CT images in the LV–lung

interface. There is lung tissue on CT images overlaying LV activity in the anterolateral wall on PET images. Registration of the stress images was subsequently performed using an emission-driven method. This method is proprietary and not commercially available. It modifies the heart outline of the CT image based on the PET data. The program expects to find soft tissue attenuation on the CT image if the corresponding voxel on the PET image contains LV wall activity. If there is an inconsistency and lung tissue on the CT image overlays LV wall activity on the PET image, the attenuation value of the voxel is modified to match that of soft tissue. Following registration and reconstruction of the images, the PET images are normal.

Different CT protocols have been proposed in an attempt to minimize the emission-transmission misregistration rate on PET/CT imaging. At our institution, the "solution" to this problem has been to coach the patients to shallow breathe during the acquisition and to average the CT data over a longer time by slowing the rotational speed of the gantry and increasing the pitch. Despite these efforts, the CT attenuation scan time on multislice CT scanners is still typically under 20 seconds. We have tested other CT protocols including ECG-gated (with breath-hold), ungated (with and without breath-hold), "slow," "fast," and cine CT. The misregistration rate was highest with ECG-gated breath-hold CT (about 60%) and lowest with cine CT and "slow" ungated CT (about 20% each). Regardless of the CT protocol used for attenuation correction, it is important that the reader remembers to review the quality control images. The fused images should be available at the time of interpretation to ensure proper registration was performed prior to image reconstruction.

Case 20-2   PET/CT Artifact: LV–Diaphragm Mismatch (Figure 20-2)

A 42-year-old man was referred for rubidium myocardial perfusion PET because of worsening shortness of breath on exertion. He had type 2 diabetes and hyperlipidemia. Calcium scoring CT performed 1 year prior showed a total Agatston score of 102. He underwent vasodilator stress testing with regadenoson. There were no ST changes on ECG. The images were obtained using a PET/CT camera operating in 3D mode.

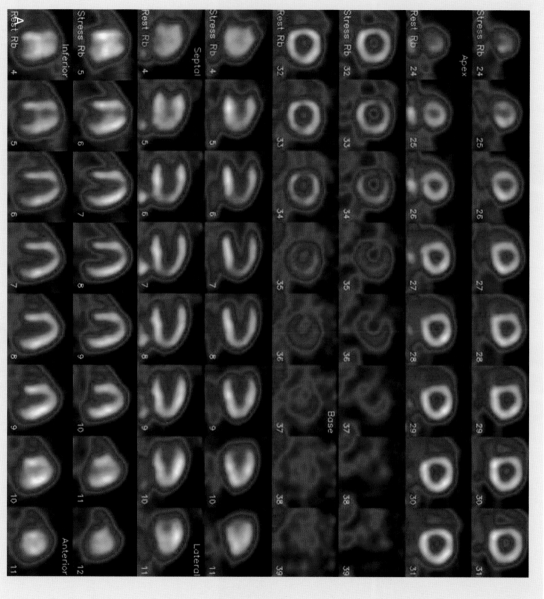

■ **Figure 20-2** PET/CT artifact: LV–diaphragm mismatch. **A,** Tomographic slices display with the resting results interleaved between the stress slices. *Top four rows* display the LV SA from apex (*top left*) to base (*bottom right*). *Next two rows* display the stress and rest VLA slices from the septum to the lateral wall and the *last two rows* show the stress and rest HLA slices from the inferior to the anterior wall. Note that there is relatively increased uptake in the inferior wall, which is slightly more pronounced on the stress images.

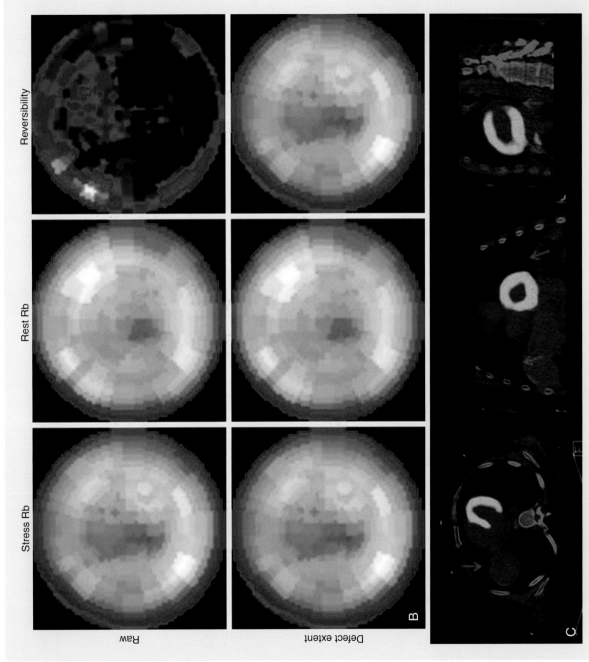

■ **Figure 20-2—Cont'd B,** Polar maps representation of perfusion distribution. Note the absence of blackout regions in the defect extent polar maps, indicating a normal study by quantitative analysis. **C,** Fused transaxial, coronal, and sagittal stress images. There is no LV–lung mismatch between the stress emission (*color images*) and the CT image (*B/W images*). However, the CT images show hypoinflated lungs, the diaphragm is elevated (*red arrows*).

COMMENTS

The PET images in this patient show relatively increased uptake in the inferior wall, which is slightly more pronounced on the stress images. Fused stress PET/CT attenuation images reveal no LV–lung mismatch. However, there is LV-diaphragm mismatch. The lungs on the CT image are hypoinflated relative to the averaged lung volumes of the PET image. The elevation of the diaphragm on the CT image increases the expected photon attenuation from tissues in the same axial plane of the inferior LV wall because lung attenuation is replaced by soft tissue attenuation from the subdiaphragmatic organs. As a result, the reconstructed PET images show an artifactually increased count density in the inferior LV wall.

The LV–diaphragm mismatch is less prevalent than the LV–lung mismatch; it occurs in about 5% of cases at our institution. When severe, the "hot spot" in the inferior wall can produce downscaling in the remainder of the LV and artifactual perfusion defects may develop in the LAD and LCX distributions. These artifactual defects are sometimes "reversible," particularly when the patient hyperventilates during the stress PET acquisition.

Can we prevent "reversible" artifacts by performing a CT scan post-stress for stress PET attenuation correction? At our institution, we use the same rest CT image for rest and stress PET attenuation correction. We have not been able to demonstrate an improvement in registration rate of the stress images by adding a CT attenuation scan post-stress. This is because we use regadenoson

for pharmacologic stress testing. By the time the stress PET acquisition is finished and a second CT attenuation scan is obtained, hyperventilation and tachycardia have usually subsided (the same applies for adenosine). As a result, the CT image poststress is essentially another rest CT attenuation scan that does not improve the stress PET image quality.

Case 20-3   Rubidium 3D PET Artifact: Prompt-Gammas (Figure 20-3)

A 63-year-old woman was referred for rubidium myocardial perfusion PET because of one episode of unexplained syncope. Her risk factors for CAD were hypertension and hyperlipidemia. She underwent vasodilator stress testing with adenosine. Baseline ECG showed sinus rhythm, no Q waves, and no ST-T abnormalities. Stress ECG was unremarkable. The images were obtained using a PET/CT camera operating in 3D mode.

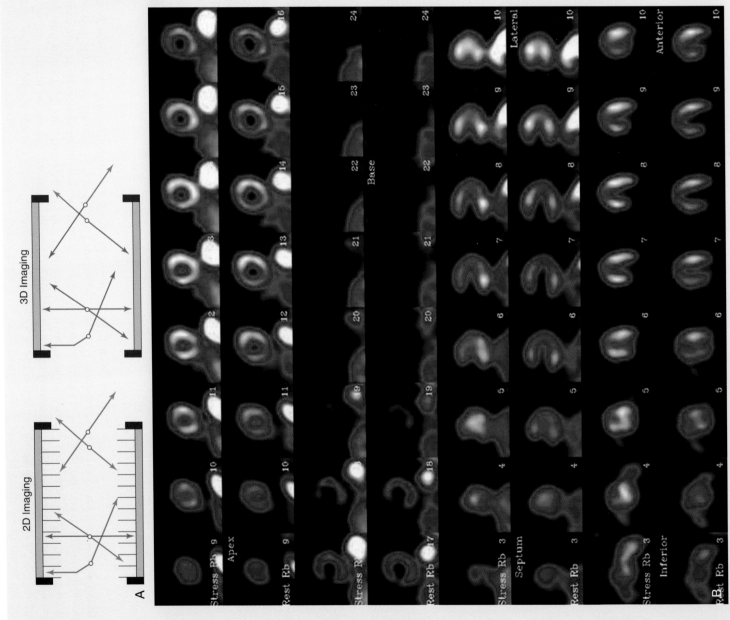

■ **Figure 20-3** Rubidium 3D PET artifact: prompt-gammas. **A,** Schematic representation of 2D and 3D PET imaging. Note the presence of septa in the 2D mode. The lack of septa in the 3D mode increases the count sensitivity to coincident, random, and scattered events. The *blue arrows* represent recorded coincident events. The *red arrows* represent unrecorded photons. **B,** The tomographic PET images show a large, moderate to severe, predominately-fixed defect involving the apical, septal, and anterior walls. In the apical wall, the perfusion defect is more severe at rest. Note the background activity is nearing zero.

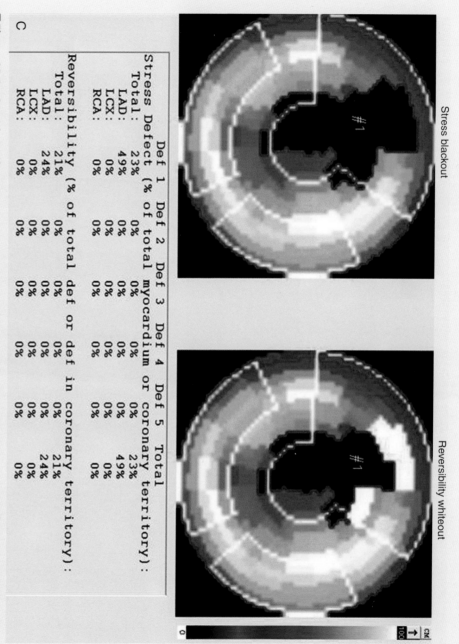

Stress blackout

Reversibility whiteout

Stress Defect (% of total myocardium or coronary territory):	Def 1	Def 2	Def 3	Def 4	Def 5	Total
Total:	23%	0%	0%	0%	0%	23%
LAD:	49%	0%	0%	0%	0%	49%
LCX:	0%	0%	0%	0%	0%	0%
RCA:	0%	0%	0%	0%	0%	0%
Reversibility (% of total def or def in coronary territory):						
Total:	21%	0%	0%	0%	0%	21%
LAD:	24%	0%	0%	0%	0%	24%
LCX:	0%	0%	0%	0%	0%	0%
RCA:	0%	0%	0%	0%	0%	0%

C

■ **Figure 20-3—Cont'd. C,** Polar maps representation and quantification of perfusion defects. The perfusion defect in the LAD territory involves 23% of the LV, of which 21% is reversible by quantitative analysis (in the mid and basal anterior wall).

(Continued)

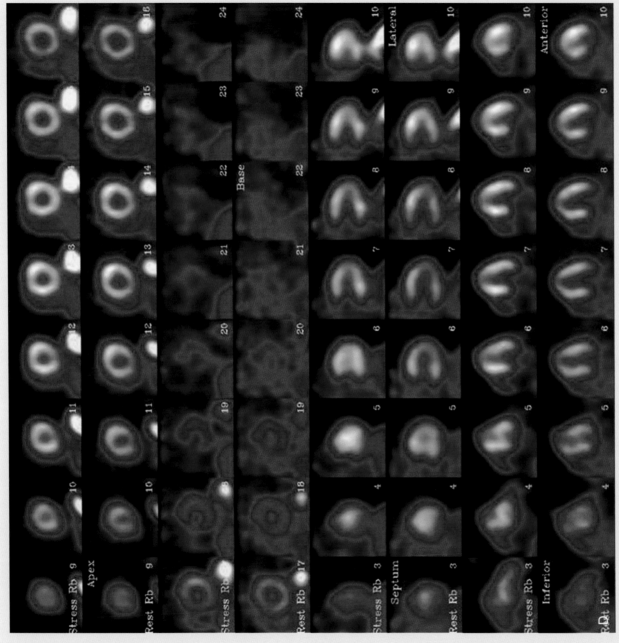

Figure 20-3—Cont'd. D, Upon reconstruction of the images applying prompt-gamma correction, there is resolution of the defects, both visually in the tomographic display.

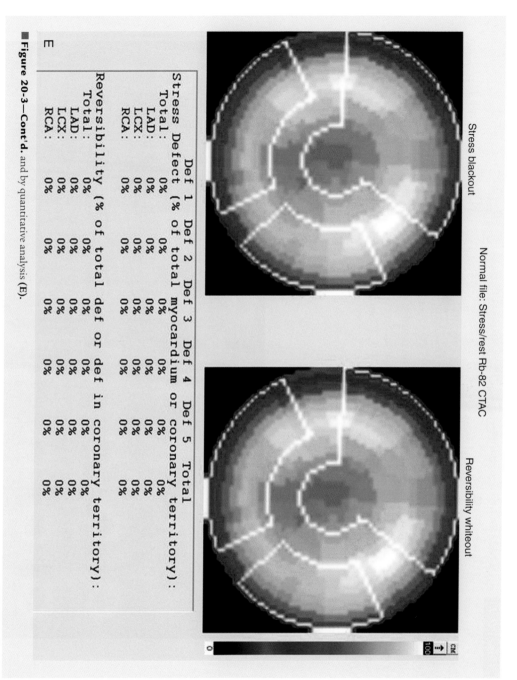

Stress blackout   Normal file: Stress/rest Rb-82 CTAC   Reversibility whiteout

	Def 1	Def 2	Def 3	Def 4	Def 5	Total
Stress Defect (% of total myocardium or coronary territory):						
Total:	0%	0%	0%	0%	0%	0%
LAD:	0%	0%	0%	0%	0%	0%
LCX:	0%	0%	0%	0%	0%	0%
RCA:	0%	0%	0%	0%	0%	0%
Reversibility (% of total def or def in coronary territory):						
Total:	0%	0%	0%	0%	0%	0%
LAD:	0%	0%	0%	0%	0%	0%
LCX:	0%	0%	0%	0%	0%	0%
RCA:	0%	0%	0%	0%	0%	0%

E

■ **Figure 20-3—Cont'd.** and by quantitative analysis (E).

COMMENTS

The perfusion defects seen on the images without prompt-gamma correction are artifactual. While the defects are mostly fixed, the patient did not have a history of MI, there were no Q waves on the ECG, and the gated images showed no segmental wall motion abnormality. In addition, the background activity in the rest and stress images is nearly absent, which is not expected on rubidium images.

PET images are obtained either in 2D or 3D mode. While in the 2D mode, there are thin septa of lead or tungsten separating each crystal ring; in the 3D mode, the septa are absent. The lack of septa increases the count sensitivity of the camera because it widens the axial acceptance angle to incident photons. It is desirable to increase the sensitivity of the PET cameras to true coincidence events as it results in better image contrast and allows faster imaging times. However, 3D imaging increases not only the sensitivity to true coincidence events but also the sensitivity to random and scattered events. Therefore, the 3D PET reconstruction must correct for these unwanted events in order to optimize image quality. Thirteen percent of rubidium decays are associated with a 776-keV prompt-gamma emission in addition to the positron. Because the prompt-gammas correlates

in time with the annihilation photons, coincidences between either one or both of the annihilation photons can be produced if the prompt-gamma down scatters into the PET energy window. The sensitivity to prompt-gamma coincidences is significantly increased in 3D imaging. If there is no adequate correction for these unwanted events, artifactual perfusion defects may develop in the PET image. Conventional image reconstruction (in 2D or 3D) assumes that events detected outside the body are either random or scattered events. As a result, after random events correction, scatter correction fails to account for prompt-gamma coincidence events. It fails to account for prompt-gamma coincidence events remain but also prompt-gamma coincidence events remain, producing a scatter distribution that is overscaled. When scatter correction is applied, too many counts are subtracted from the image and photopenic areas develop. In the LV, these artifactual defects are usually seen in the septal and anterior walls where the scatter distribution peaks in the image.

Rubidium is the only PET radionuclide used in clinical practice that emits prompt-gammas. N-13 and F-18 are not prompt-gamma emitters. Further studies are needed to better understand the impact of prompt-gammas on each 3D PET camera.

Case 20-4   Rubidium Myocardial Perfusion PET: Normal Patient (Figure 20-4)

A 45-year-old woman presented to the ED complaining of atypical chest pain. She was ruled out for MI by ECG and serial troponin I. Her risk factors for CAD were hypertension and tobacco use. The patient was obese (195 lb, 5 feet 8 inches, BMI 30 kg/m²). She underwent regadenoson stress rubidium myocardial perfusion PET to exclude unstable angina. Baseline ECG was unremarkable. Stress ECG showed no ischemic changes. The images were obtained using a PET/CT camera operating in 3D mode.

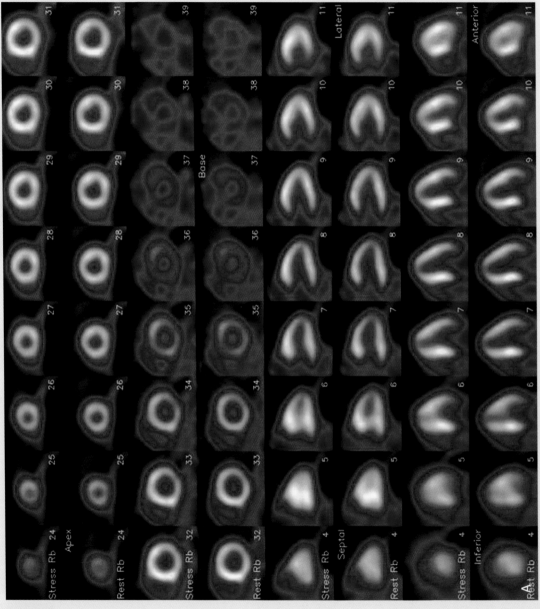

■ **Figure 20-4** Rubidium myocardial perfusion PET: normal patient. **A,** Tomographic slices display with the resting results interleaved between the stress slices. Top four rows display the LV SA from apex (*top left*) to base (*bottom right*). *Next two rows* display the stress and rest VLA slices from the septum to the lateral wall and the *last two rows* show the stress and rest HLA slices from the inferior to the anterior wall. Note the high-contrast resolution and homogeneous tracer uptake throughout the LV.

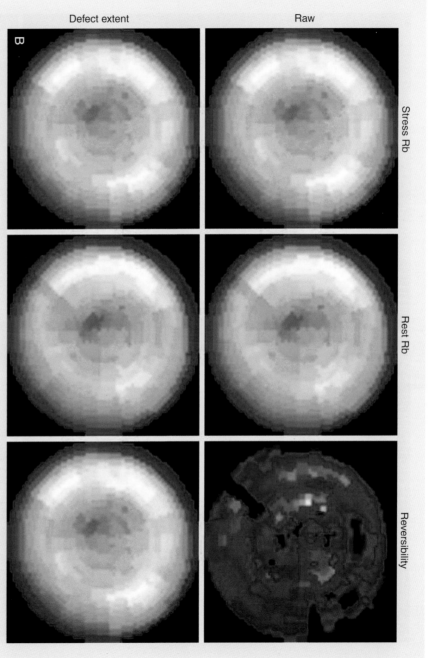

Figure 20-4—Cont'd B, Polar maps representation and quantification of this patient's LV tracer uptake. The *three panels in the top row* correspond to the stress, rest, and reversibility (normalized rest/stress) LV distributions. The brighter colors represent higher counts (perfusion) and the darker colors represent fewer counts. Note the relative homogeneity of the stress and rest polar maps. The *bottom row* is the defect extent polar maps display where areas that are abnormal in comparison to this protocol's normal database are highlighted in *black*. Note the absence of blackout regions at stress and rest indicating a totally normal study.

(Continued)

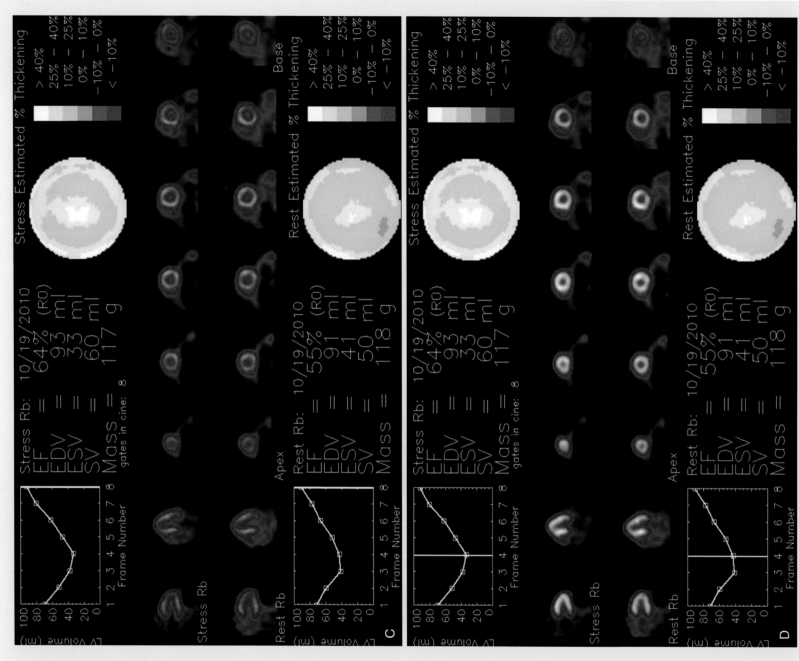

■ **Figure 20-4—Cont'd C and D,** The *two rows of color images* show end-diastolic (**C**) and end-systolic (**D**) stress (*top*) and rest (*bottom*), vertical-axis, horizontal-axis, and short-axis LV tomographic display of this patient's ECG-gated images. Note the uniform LV wall change in myocardial color from diastole to systole, consistent with normal LV thickening. The color polar maps in **C** represent the quantification of the stress (*top*) and rest (*bottom*) regional thickening. Note the labeled thickening scale to the right of the maps. The *top left* (stress) and *bottom left* (rest) show the patient's average volume-time curve per cycle, LVEF, EDV, ESV, SV, and LV mass.

COMMENTS

The PET images are normal by visual and quantitative analysis. The images show high contrast resolution. The end-diastolic and end-systolic images demonstrate normal LV wall thickening at rest and stress. Note that the

LVEF increased from 55% at rest to 64% at stress, which is normal. Different from gated SPECT, the LVEF in rubidium stress PET is not a post-stress EF. It does reflect hemodynamic changes at stress because the images are acquired during pharmacologic stress testing.

Case 20-5

Rubidium Myocardial Perfusion PET: Ischemic Patient (Figure 20-5)

A 75-year-old man had worsening typical angina. He had DM and chronic renal insufficiency. The baseline ECG showed normal sinus rhythm and right bundle branch block. The patient underwent vasodilator stress testing with regadenoson and developed 1- to 2-mm horizontal ST depressions in the lateral leads. The images were obtained using a PET/CT camera operating in 3D mode.

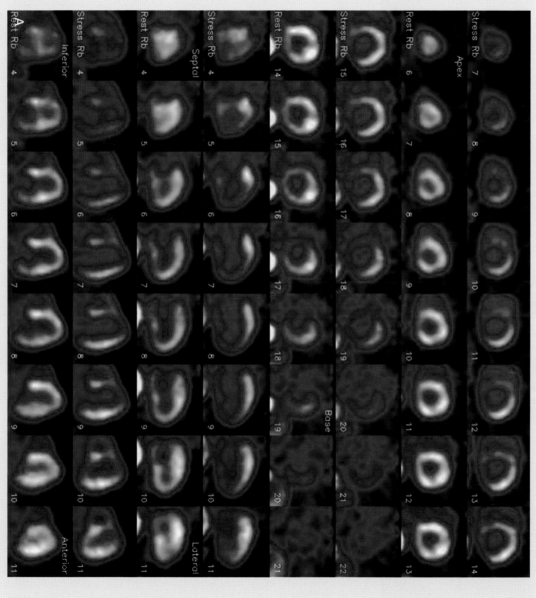

■ **Figure 20-5.** Rubidium myocardial perfusion PET: ischemic patient. **A.** Tomographic slices display with the resting results interleaved between the stress slices. *Top four rows* display the LV SA from apex (*top left*) to base (*bottom right*). *Next two rows* display the stress and rest VLA slices from the septum to the lateral wall and the *last two rows* show the stress and rest HLA slices from the inferior to the anterior wall. There is inducible ischemia in the apical, septal, anterior, and inferior walls. The TID index is abnormal at 1.58, suggesting multivessel CAD.

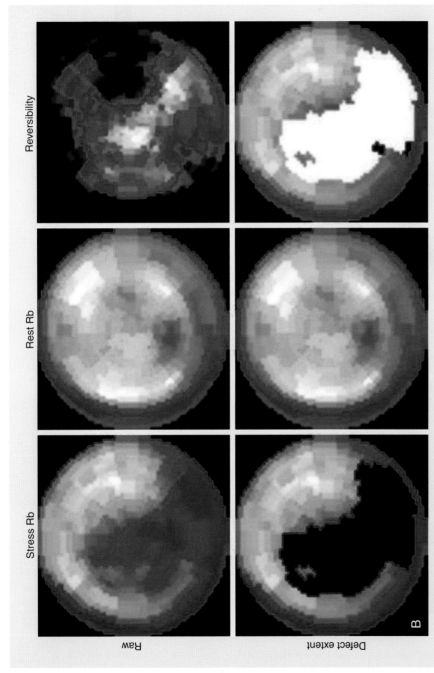

Figure 20-5—Cont'd B, Polar maps representation and quantification of this patient's LV tracer uptake. The *three panels in the top row* correspond to the stress, rest, and reversibility (normalized rest/stress) LV distributions. The *brighter colors* represent higher counts (perfusion) and the *darker colors* represent counts. Note the large and severe perfusion defects in the LAD and RCA territories at stress and a mild count reduction in the inferior wall at rest. The *bottom row* is the defect extent polar maps display where areas that are abnormal in comparison to this protocol's normal database are highlighted in black. The defect extent reversibility polar map (*bottom right*) shows a large whiteout area, suggesting near-complete reversibility of the stress defects.

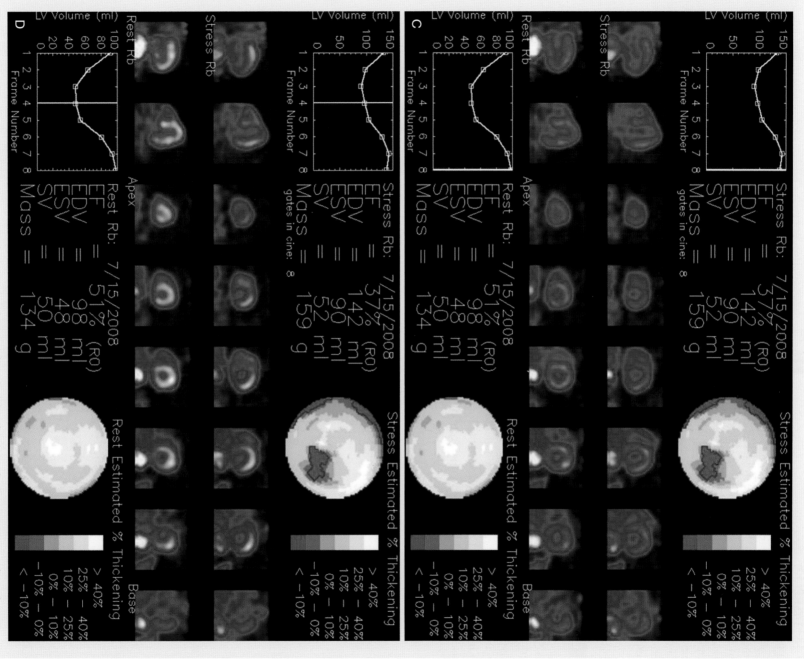

■ Figure 20-5—Cont'd C and D, The two rows of color images show end-diastolic (**C**) and end-systolic (**D**) stress (*top*) and rest (*bottom*), vertical-axis, horizontal-axis, and short-axis LV tomographic display of this patient's ECG-gated images. The color polar maps in C represent the quantification of the stress (*top*) and rest (*bottom*) regional thickening. Note the labeled thickening scale to the right of the maps. There is paradoxical thickening of the septal-basal and mid-inferolateral walls. The *top left* (stress) and *bottom left* (rest) show the patient's average volume-time curve per cycle, LVEF, EDV, ESV, SV, and LV mass.

COMMENTS

The PET images are markedly abnormal. There are large and severe reversible perfusion defects in the LAD and RCA territories. Subendocardial ischemia is present in the lateral wall as well. The TID index is 1.58 (upper limit of normal is 1.15). The images are also abnormal by quantitative analysis. The extent polar maps show reversibility in 42% of the LV. The end-diastolic and end-systolic images demonstrate normal LV wall thickening at rest, but paradoxical motion of the septal-basal and mid-inferolateral walls at stress. Note that the LVEF decreased from 51% at rest to 37% at stress, which is an independent predictor of future adverse events.

Following PET imaging, the patient underwent invasive coronary angiography that revealed 75% stenosis in the distal LM, 75% proximal and 90% mid LAD, 80% ostial first diagonal branch, normal LCX, and an occluded proximal RCA. These angiographic findings suggest that there was an underestimation of ischemic burden by quantitative analysis, which is often seen in patients with multivessel obstructive CAD (see Case 19-6). The patient underwent CABG 2 weeks later.

Case 20-6   N-13-Ammonia Myocardial Perfusion PET: Normal Patient (Figure 20-6)

A 52-year-old woman was referred for N-13-ammonia myocardial perfusion PET because of worsening shortness of breath. Her risk factors for CAD were hypertension and diet-controlled diabetes. The patient was obese (215 lb, 5 feet 6 inches, BMI 35 kg/m²). She was scheduled for vasodilator stress testing with adenosine. Baseline ECG was remarkable for LBBB. The images were obtained using a stand-alone PET camera operating in 2D mode.

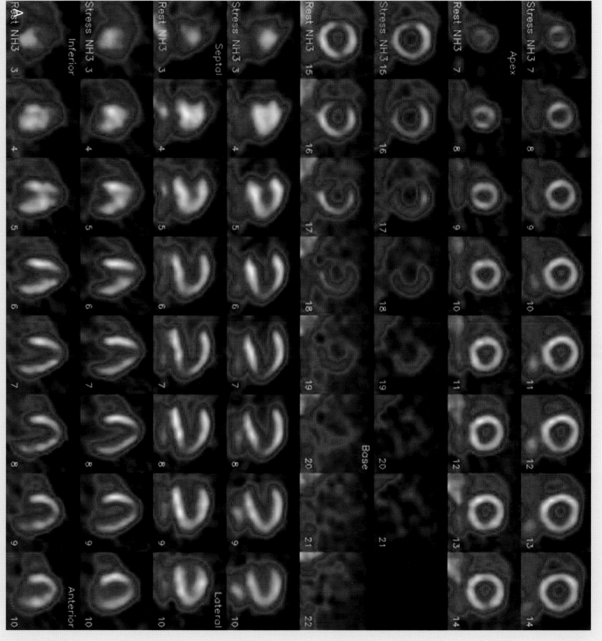

■ **Figure 20-6** N-13-ammonia PET: normal patient. **A,** The tomographic PET images demonstrate a mild fixed count reduction in the apical wall that represents apical thinning. There is also a mild fixed count reduction in the lateral wall. The emission and transmission images are well registered; that is, there is no LV–lung mismatch (images not shown).

(Continued)

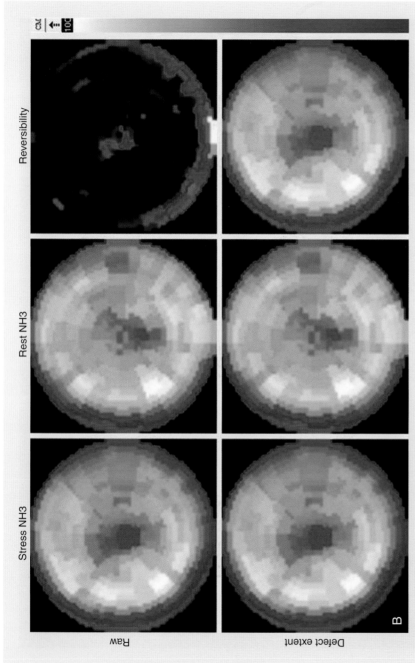

■ **Figure 20-6—Cont'd B,** Polar maps representation of perfusion distribution. The *three panels in the top row* correspond to the stress, rest, and reversibility (normalized rest/stress) LV distributions. The *bottom row* is the defect extent polar maps display where areas that are abnormal in comparison to the normal database are highlighted in *black*. Note the absence of blackout regions, indicating a normal study by quantitative analysis.

COMMENTS

The PET images are normal. The images show high spatial and contrast resolution with well-defined endocardial and epicardial borders. A mild fixed count reduction in the apical wall represents apical thinning. Note that there is also a mild fixed count reduction in the lateral wall. The emission and transmission images are well registered; that is, there is no LV–lung mismatch (images not shown). The normal database quantification accounts for this relative count reduction in the lateral wall and does not highlight this area as abnormal in the extent polar maps.

N-13 has favorable physical characteristics over rubidium. The longer half-life (10 minutes *vs* 1.3 minutes) allows longer imaging times, increasing the count density of the PET images. Image quality is further improved by

the lower energy of the positron (1.2 *vs* 3.3 MeV), which results in better spatial resolution. This is because the higher the energy, the longer is the distance traveled by the positron (on average) before annihilation occurs. In other words, the annihilation event that originates from a high energy positron is more likely to be a few millimeters distant from the decay event and "blur" the image.

N-13-ammonia has a higher retention fraction than rubidium at rest (85% *vs* 65%). Higher retention fractions of N-13-ammonia are preserved for blood flows up to 2.5 ml/min/g, which is an advantage if measurement of myocardial blood flow is desired. The quantification of myocardial blood flow with N-13-ammonia PET is an attractive tool to prevent underestimation of ischemic burden in patients with multivessel CAD.

A 64-year-old man was referred for N-13-ammonia myocardial perfusion PET after a 3-week history of atypical chest pain. The risk factors included hypertension and hypercholesterolemia. Physical examination was positive for obesity (230 lb, 6 feet 0 inches, BMI 31 kg/m²). The resting ECG was normal. The patient underwent vasodilator stress testing with adenosine. There were no ECG changes during adenosine infusion. The images were obtained using a stand-alone PET camera operating in 2D mode.

Case 20-7

N-13-Ammonia Myocardial Perfusion PET: Ischemic Patient (Figure 20-7)

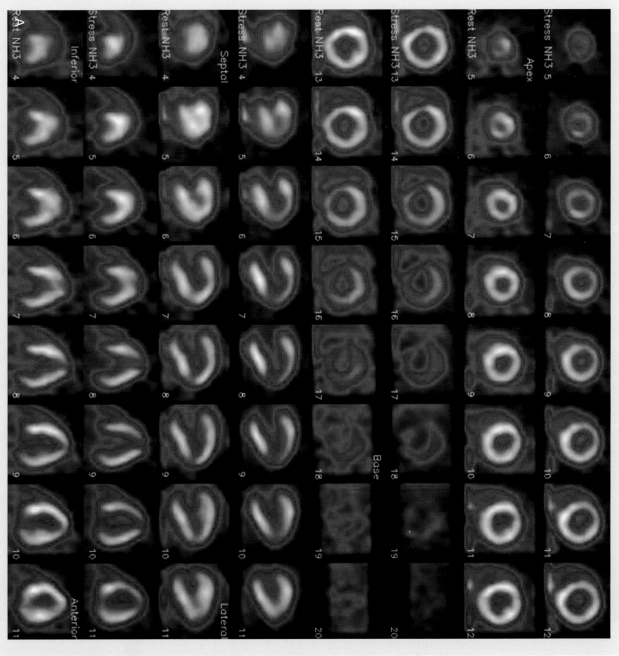

■ **Figure 20-7** N-13-ammonia PET: ischemic patient. **A,** The tomographic PET images are abnormal. There is a moderate-sized reversible defect of moderate severity in the LAD distribution involving the apical, mid-to-distal anterior, and septal walls.

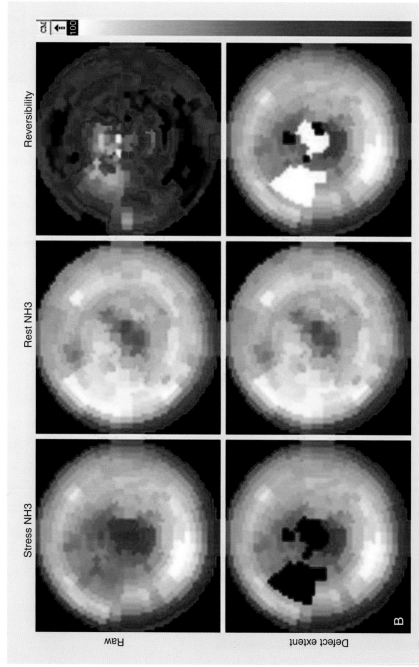

■ **Figure 20-7—Cont'd B,** Polar maps representation of perfusion distribution. The three panels in the *top row* correspond to the stress, rest, and reversibility (normalized rest/stress) LV distributions. The *bottom row* is the defect extent polar maps display, where areas that are abnormal in comparison to the normal database are highlighted in *black.* Note there is a blackout region in the anteroseptal and apical walls at stress, indicating an abnormal study by quantitative analysis. The defect extent reversibility polar map *(bottom right)* shows a whiteout area in the same area, suggesting ischemic changes.

COMMENTS

The PET images are abnormal. There is a moderate-sized reversible defect of moderate severity in the LAD distribution involving the apical, mid-to-distal anterior, and septal walls. The stress images are also abnormal by quantitative analysis and the extent polar maps show reversibility in the LAD distribution.

N-13-ammonia has not entered the mainstream of nuclear cardiology because it requires an on-site cyclotron for production. Rubidium PET is just logistically easier to perform because the radiotracer is always available and the patient throughput is higher.

Case 20-8   **F-18 Flurpiridaz Myocardial Perfusion PET: Normal Patient (Figure 20-8)**

A patient with low pretest probability of CAD underwent 1-day rest and exercise stress F-18 flurpiridaz imaging using 2.4mCi at rest and 8.4mCi at stress. Rest and stress imaging times were 15 minutes each. The images were obtained using a PET/CT camera operating in 3D mode.

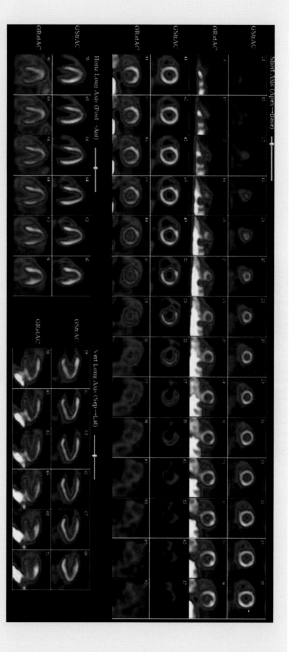

■ **Figure 20-8** F-18 flurpiridaz PET: normal patient. Tomographic slices display with the resting results interleaved between the stress slices. *Top four rows* display the LV SA from apex (*top left*) to base (*bottom right*). The *last two rows* display the stress and rest HLA slices from the inferior to the anterior wall (*bottom left*) and the stress and rest VLA slices from the septum to the lateral wall (*bottom right*). There are no perfusion defects to suggest obstructive CAD.

COMMENTS

The tomographic PET images are normal. Subdiaphragmatic activity is present in the rest, but not in the stress images. Note that there is high spatial and contrast resolution evidenced by well-defined myocardial borders and a well-defined LV chamber. The RV walls are faintly visualized.

There are two essential limitations to rubidium PET imaging. First, because of the very short half-life of the isotope (1.3 minutes), imaging has to start shortly after tracer infusion. Therefore, stress testing is always pharmacologic. Second, there is a nonlinear relationship between tracer extraction and myocardial blood flow; that is, tracer extraction decreases as the blood flow increases. This phenomenon complicates the mathematical model for the quantitative analysis and can cause a significant underestimation of myocardial blood flow reserve.

In an attempt to overcome these limitations, a new myocardial perfusion PET tracer has been developed. F-18 flurpiridaz has a high first-pass extraction at rest (about 90%), which is maintained over a wide range of myocardial blood flows. In addition, it does not show delayed redistribution like thallium.

Case 20-9

F-18 Flurpiridaz Myocardial Perfusion PET: Ischemic Patient (Figure 20-9)

A 76-year-old man status post-CABG had typical exertional angina. He underwent 1-day rest and adenosine stress F-18 flurpiridaz imaging using 2.0 mCi at rest and 6.1 mCi at stress. Rest and stress imaging times were 10 minutes each.

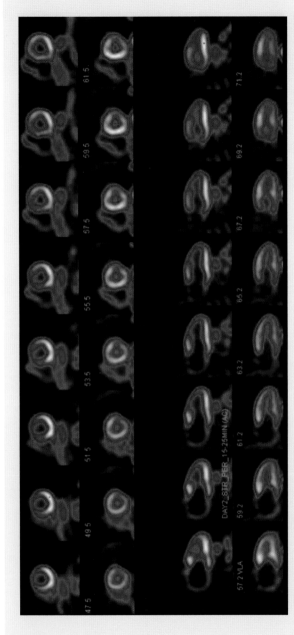

■ **Figure 20-9** F-18 flurpiridaz PET: ischemic patient. Tomographic slices display with the resting results interleaved between the stress slices. *Top two rows* display the LV SA slices from apex (*left*) to base (*right*). The *bottom two rows* display the stress and rest VLA slices from the septum (*left*) to the lateral wall (*right*). There is a large and severe reversible defect in the mid-to-distal anteroseptal and apical walls suggesting inducible ischemia in the LAD territory. (*Courtesy of Dr. Jamish Maddahi, Dr. Daniel Berman, and Lantheus Medical Imaging.*)

COMMENTS

The tomographic PET images are abnormal. There is a large and severe reversible defect in the mid-to-distal anteroseptal and apical walls. The patient underwent invasive coronary angiography, which showed 99% LAD disease past a small first diagonal, severe, and diffuse distal LAD disease and a patent LIMA. Based on the angiographic findings, stress-induced ischemia was expected in the anteroseptal and apical regions due to severe and diffuse LAD disease past the LIMA insertion point.

F-18 flurpiridaz may represent an alternative to rubidium because the half-life of the isotope (110 minutes) will allow distribution of the radiotracer from a central cyclotron facility to many nuclear cardiology laboratories as is currently done with F-18 FDG. Ordering unit doses of F-18 flurpiridaz will likely become more cost-effective to imaging centers with low volume of myocardial perfusion PET studies. This is because rubidium generators are replaced every 28 days at a fixed cost of about $30,000 per month.

The diagnostic performance of F-18 flurpiridaz myocardial perfusion PET has not yet been determined. A Phase 2 multicenter clinical trial for the development of 1-day rest/stress imaging protocols is now closed. Enrollment of patients into Phase 3 is expected to start in the first quarter of 2011.

Case 20-10   **F-18 FDG Myocardial Viability PET: Fasting Protocol (Figure 20-10)**

An 83-year-old man with a history of hypertension, anemia of chronic disease, and chronic renal insufficiency was admitted to the hospital with an acute coronary syndrome in acute heart failure. Cardiac catheterization revealed severe three-vessel obstructive CAD. Transthoracic echocardiogram revealed an LVEF of 20% to 25% with moderate mitral regurgitation. Baseline ECG showed RBBB and Q waves in V_1–V_4. Myocardial viability PET imaging was performed using rest rubidium and fasting FDG protocol (no glucose or insulin administered). Patient's glucose level was 118mg/dl. FDG PET images were obtained 60 minutes after tracer injection. The images were obtained using a PET/CT camera operating in 3D mode.

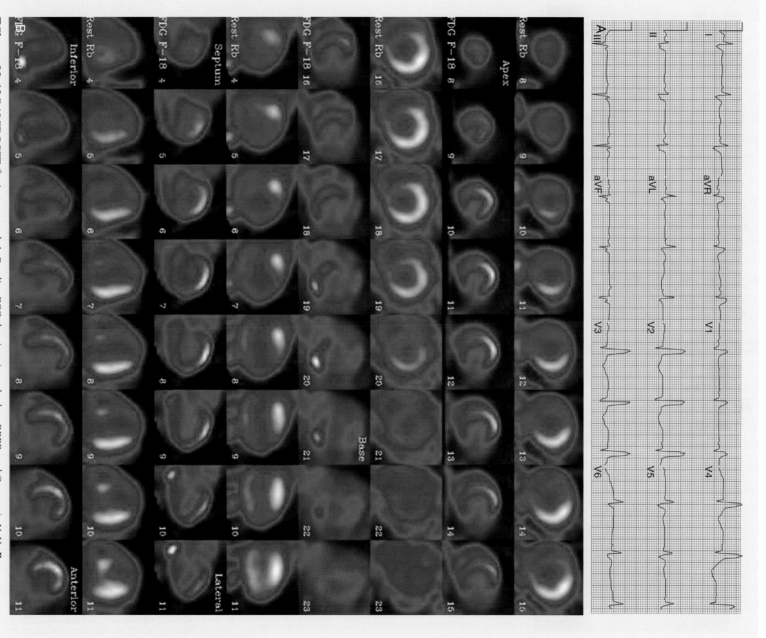

Figure 20-10 F-18 FDG PET: fasting protocol. **A,** Baseline ECG showing sinus rhythm, RBBB, and Q waves in V_1-V_4. **B,** Tomographic slices display with the resting rubidium results interleaved between the FDG slices. *Top four rows* display the LV SA from apex (*top left*) to base (*bottom right*). *Next two rows* display the VLA slices from the septum to the lateral wall, and the *last two rows* show the HLA slices from the inferior to the anterior wall. The tomographic rest rubidium and FDG PET images are abnormal. There is a large and severe perfusion defect involving the apical, anterior, septal, inferior, and inferoseptal walls. The FDG images show increased FDG uptake in the apical, anterior, and septal walls; only mild uptake in the inferior and inferoseptal walls; and absent uptake in the lateral wall.

(Continued)

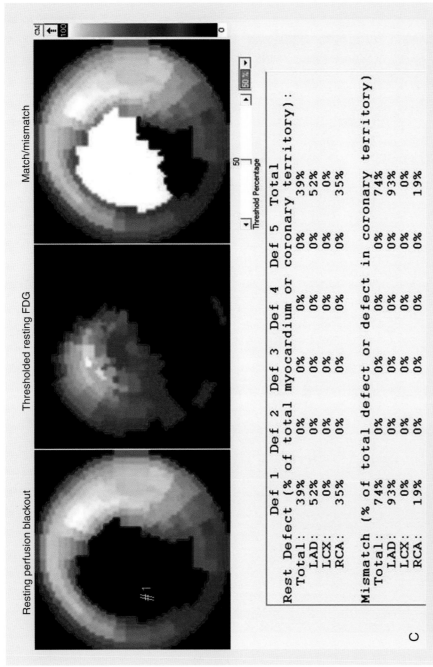

Resting perfusion blackout	Thresholded resting FDG	Match/mismatch

	Def 1	Def 2	Def 3	Def 4	Def 5	Total
Rest Defect (% of total myocardium or coronary territory):						
Total:	39%	0%	0%	0%	0%	39%
LAD:	52%	0%	0%	0%	0%	52%
LCX:	0%	0%	0%	0%	0%	0%
RCA:	35%	0%	0%	0%	0%	35%
Mismatch (% of total defect or defect in coronary territory)						
Total:	74%	0%	0%	0%	0%	74%
LAD:	93%	0%	0%	0%	0%	93%
LCX:	0%	0%	0%	0%	0%	0%
RCA:	19%	0%	0%	0%	0%	19%

C

■ **Figure 20-10—Cont'd** C, Polar maps representation and quantification of rest perfusion distribution (*center*), and matched/mismatched defects (*right*). The *left* is the rest rubidium defect extent polar map display where areas that are abnormal in comparison to the normal database are highlighted in *black*. The resting perfusion blackout map (*left*) reveals a 39% perfusion defect size. The *right* is the matched/mismatched defect extent polar map where areas that are matched are highlighted in *black* and areas that are mismatched are highlighted in *white*. The matched/mismatched polar map (*right*) was generated using a 50% threshold from the maximum. It demonstrates that 74% of the rest perfusion defect is mismatched (apical, septal, and anterior walls) while 26% (inferior and inferoseptal walls) is matched.

COMMENTS

The tomographic rest rubidium and FDG PET images are abnormal. There is a large and severe perfusion defect involving the apical, anterior, septal, inferior, and inferoseptal walls (LAD and RCA distributions). The metabolic images show increased FDG uptake in the apical, anterior, and septal walls, only mild uptake in the inferior and inferoseptal walls, and absent uptake in the lateral wall. The resting perfusion blackout map reveals a 39% perfusion defect size. The match/mismatch polar map was generated using a 50% threshold; that is, myocardium with a count density equal or greater than 50% from the maximum was considered viable. It demonstrates that 74% of the perfusion defect is mismatched. In other words, 74% of the resting perfusion defect shows increased FDG uptake, while 26% (inferior and inferoseptal walls) does not. The gated images (not shown) demonstrate severe global hypokinesis with LVEF of 15% (EDV 65 ml, ESV 55 ml). Because the mismatched defect size is large (>20%) and because there is no significant LV

dilatation, the patient is likely to recover LV function if revascularization is performed.

FDG is more sensitive than myocardial perfusion radiotracers in the assessment of myocardial viability. Different from the perfusion radiotracers, the myocardial uptake of FDG is not driven by blood flow. Instead it reflects whether or not glucose is being used as a metabolic substrate during the uptake phase (up to 30 to 45 minutes postinjection). Under fasting conditions, ischemic myocardium demonstrates glucose avidity, whereas myocardium with normal perfusion and scar tissue do not. Under glucose-loaded conditions, not only ischemic myocardium, but also myocardium with normal perfusion, demonstrates glucose avidity. The use of glucose as opposed to free fatty acids by the ischemic myocardium represents a metabolic adaptation to anaerobic conditions. On the other hand, the use of glucose by the normal myocardium is induced by increased serum levels of insulin (endogenous or exogenous).

Case 20-11   F-18 FDG Myocardial Viability PET: Glucose-Loading
Protocol (Figure 20-11)

A 49-year-old man with ischemic cardiomyopathy, hypertension, hyperlipidemia, and
insulin-dependent diabetes presented to the outpatient clinic with 6-week history of
worsening shortness of breath on exertion. He had undergone three-vessel CABG
and cardiac defibrillator implantation 5 years prior. Transthoracic echocardiogram
revealed an EF of 30% to 35% with mild mitral regurgitation. Baseline ECG showed
an electronic atrial pacemaker and nonspecific ST changes in the anterolateral
leads (Figure 20-11, *A*). The patient fasted overnight and withheld the a.m. insulin
dose. Patient's glucose level was 180 mg/dl. Myocardial viability PET imaging was
performed using rest rubidium and oral glucose–loaded FDG protocol (25 g glucose).
A total of 15 units of regular insulin was injected intravenously prior to FDG
injection. FDG PET images were obtained 90 minutes after injection. The images
were obtained using a PET/CT camera operating in 3D mode.

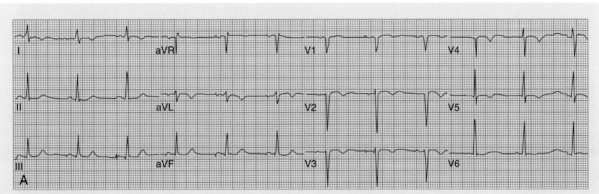

■Figure 20-11 F-18 FDG PET: glucose-loading protocol. **A,** Baseline ECG showing showing an electronic atrial pacemaker and
nonspecific ST changes in the anterolateral leads.

(Continued)

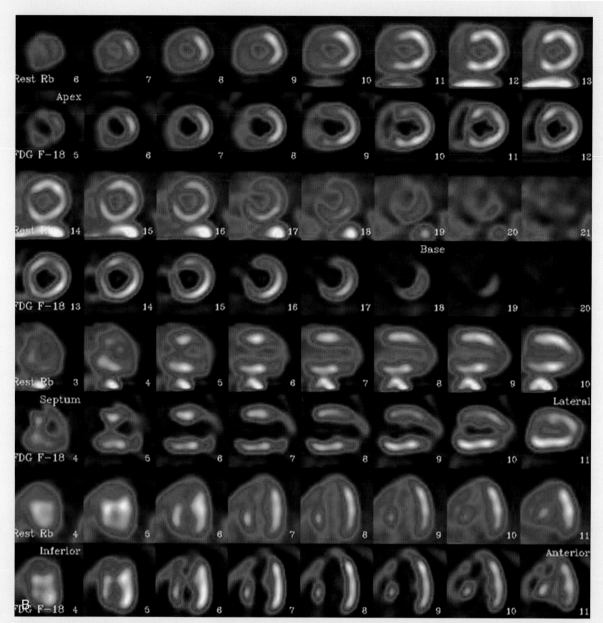

■**Figure 20-11—Cont'd B,** Tomographic slices display with the resting rubidium results interleaved between the FDG slices. *Top four rows* display the LV SA from apex *(top left)* to base *(bottom right). Next two rows* display the VLA slices from the septum to the lateral wall and the *last two rows* show the HLA slices from the inferior to the anterior wall. The tomographic rest rubidium and FDG PET images are abnormal. There is a large and severe perfusion defect involving the apical, distal anterior, septal, and inferoapical walls. The FDG images show no significant uptake in these regions.

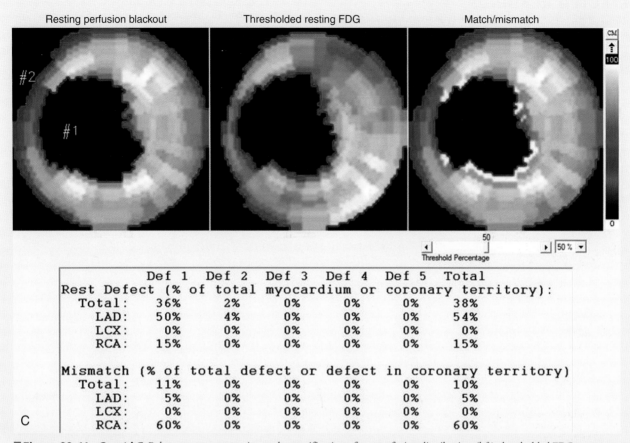

| | Resting perfusion blackout | Thresholded resting FDG | Match/mismatch |

	Def 1	Def 2	Def 3	Def 4	Def 5	Total
Rest Defect (% of total myocardium or coronary territory):						
Total:	36%	2%	0%	0%	0%	38%
LAD:	50%	4%	0%	0%	0%	54%
LCX:	0%	0%	0%	0%	0%	0%
RCA:	15%	0%	0%	0%	0%	15%
Mismatch (% of total defect or defect in coronary territory)						
Total:	11%	0%	0%	0%	0%	10%
LAD:	5%	0%	0%	0%	0%	5%
LCX:	0%	0%	0%	0%	0%	0%
RCA:	60%	0%	0%	0%	0%	60%

■ **Figure 20-11—Cont'd C,** Polar maps representation and quantification of rest perfusion distribution *(left)*, thresholded FDG distribution *(center)*, and matched/mismatched defects *(right)*. The *left* is the rest rubidium defect extent polar map display where areas that are abnormal in comparison to the normal database are highlighted in *black*. The resting perfusion blackout map *(left)* reveals a 38% perfusion defect size. The *right* is the match/mismatch defect extent polar map, where areas that are matched are highlighted in *black* and areas that are mismatched are highlighted in *white*. The match/mismatch polar map *(right)* was generated using a 50% threshold from the maximum. It demonstrates that only 10% of the rest perfusion defect is mismatched, while 90% is matched.

COMMENTS

The tomographic rest rubidium and FDG PET images are abnormal. There is a large and severe perfusion defect involving the LAD distribution (apical, anterior, septal, and inferoapical walls). The metabolic images show increased FDG uptake in the RCA and LCX territories but near absent uptake in the LAD territory. The resting perfusion blackout map reveals a 38% perfusion defect size. The match/mismatch polar map demonstrates that only 10% of the perfusion defect is mismatched, while 90% is matched and consistent with scar tissue. The gated images (not shown) demonstrate akinesis in the apical, septal, mid-to-distal anterior, and inferoapical walls. The LVEF is 37% (EDV 151 ml, ESV 95 ml). Because the mismatched defect size is small (<10%), the patient is unlikely to recover LV function if revascularization is performed.

Glucose-loading protocols (oral or intravenously) are used to stimulate the release of endogenous insulin in order to decrease plasma levels of free fatty acids and to optimize the myocardial transport and utilization of FDG. The image quality is improved with glucose loading protocols relative to fasting protocols because it decreases the blood pool activity, which improves image contrast. Also, FDG uptake in the normal myocardium facilitates the quantification of viable tissue because it often serves as a reference to scale the image for display and to define the threshold for viability.

SELECTED READINGS

Dilsizian V, Bacharach SL, Beanlands RS, et al: PET myocardial perfusion and metabolism clinical imaging. http://wwwasncorg/imageuploads/ImagingGuidelinesPETJuly2009pdf; 2008.

Esteves FP, Nye JA, Khan A, et al: Prompt gamma compensation in adenosine stress rubidium-82 myocardial perfusion 3-dimensional PET/CT, *J Nucl Cardiol* 17:247–253, 2010.

Faber TL, Galt JR: SPECT/CT and PET/CT hybrid imaging and image fusion. In Iskandrian AE, Garcia EV, editors: *Nuclear Cardiac Imaging*, ed 4, New York, 2008, Oxford University Press, pp 202–217.

Gould KL, Pan T, Loghin C, et al: Frequent diagnostic errors in cardiac PET/CT due to misregistration of CT attenuation and emission PET images: a definitive analysis of causes, consequences, and corrections, *J Nucl Med* 48:1112–1121, 2007.

Index

Note: Page numbers followed by *f* indicate figures and *t* indicate tables.